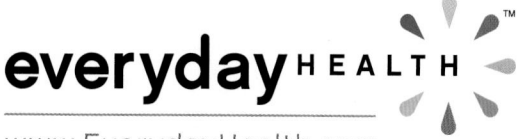

everyday HEALTH

www.EverydayHealth.com

MY calorie COUNTER

Complete nutritional information on more than 8,000 food items from popular brands, restaurant chains, and common groceries

The Editors of Everyday Health and Maureen Namkoong, MS, RD

ID1012796

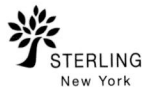

STERLING
New York

An Imprint of Sterling Publishing
1166 Avenue of the Americas
New York, NY 10036

Previous edition published in 2011 by Sterling Publishing Co., Inc., as
*Everyday Health™ My Calorie Counter: Complete Nutritional Information on More Than 8,000
Popular Brands, Fast-Food Chains, and Restaurant Menus* ISBN 978—1-4027-8619-8.

ISBN 978-1-4549-0665-0

Distributed in Canada by Sterling Publishing
c/o Canadian Manda Group, 664 Annette Street
Toronto, Ontario, Canada M6S 2C8

For information about custom editions, special sales, and premium and corporate purchases,
please contact Sterling Special Sales at 800-805-5489 or specialsales@sterlingpublishing.com.

Manufactured in China

4 6 8 10 9 7 5 3

www.sterlingpublishing.com

Nutritional data for Common Foods was obtained from the USDA Nutrient Data Laboratory

Contents

The Secret to Losing Weight?

We all wish there were a magic formula for losing weight and keeping it off for good. But the "secret" to shedding unwanted pounds the healthy way isn't banishing carbs or eating gallons of cabbage soup. Doctors and nutritionists

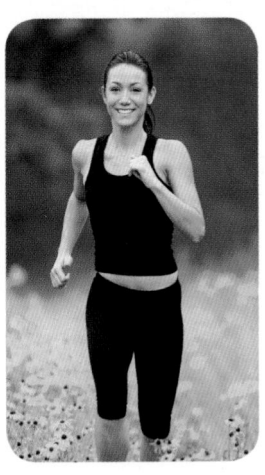

agree that sustained, healthy weight loss comes down to a pretty basic equation: fewer calories plus more exercise. By eating delicious, nutritious meals and snacks, and keeping track of how many calories you consume and burn every day, you can slim down, gain energy, and stave off a whole host of health problems.

Maintaining a healthy diet, however, isn't always easy. We're surrounded by super-size portions of tasty, high-calorie food that has little to no nutritional value—it's quick, it's cheap, and it tastes good. This is where *Everyday Health* can help. We provide the tools and the support you need to stick with your plan.

ONLINE   Look for this icon to learn about weight-loss tools on EverydayHealth.com.

HERE'S HOW IT ALL WORKS:

Use this book to look up the calories, portion sizes, and nutritional content (fat, sodium, carbohydrates, fiber, and protein) for thousands of foods and restaurant dishes.

It contains the most detailed, up-to-date information available, organized in three sections:

- Common Foods, such as vegetables, fruits, meats, grains, oils
- Store Brands, covering hundreds of common supermarket brands
- Restaurant and Fast Food menus, including appetizers, entrées, sides, drinks, and desserts

To get the most from *Everyday Health: My Calorie Counter*, start with this introductory section. You'll learn how to set realistic goals and find out why eating certain nutrients is key to successful weight loss.

Keep a daily calorie journal to stay on track. You can keep a notebook or visit EverydayHealth.com and use the free *Food and Fitness Journal*. Enter a food you've eaten, and the tool will tell you how many calories you consumed, as well as the number you have left for the day to stay within your target. It even factors in calories burned from exercise.

Share your progress (and pitfalls). Studies have shown that having a weight-loss buddy to encourage you when you falter, celebrate your weight-loss milestones, or just listen to a list of what you ate that day can help you stick to your goals. Visit the groups on EverydayHealth.com to find a weight-loss buddy, get advice, or just vent.

ONLINE Try the free *Food and Fitness Journal* and find support in the groups on EverydayHealth.com.

❝ I knew I was going to need some help to lose weight—and I found all the help I could ever want at EverydayHealth.com. I've made friends and met people who understand the everyday struggle of losing weight, sticking to an eating plan, and finding time to work out with a busy schedule. I've lost 54 lbs, four sizes, and 30 inches. ❞

HEATHER F.

Your Goal: A Healthy Weight

Don't be daunted by the number on the scale. Health professionals have found that if you're overweight, losing just five percent of your body weight can boost energy levels, relieve aching knees and hip joints, and improve serious health problems such as high blood pressure and Type 2 diabetes. Just as important is what losing weight can *prevent*, including:

- **Type 2 diabetes.** If you've been diagnosed with pre-diabetes, shedding pounds can keep you from developing the disease. And if you already have diabetes, you'll see improvements in blood sugar control and lower your risk of complications as you lose weight.

- **High blood pressure.** Losing weight can lower high blood pressure—the culprit behind many strokes and heart attacks—and you may undo some damage to your heart and blood vessels while you're at it.

- **Cancer.** That's right—slim down and your chance of getting many kinds of cancer drops. About half of all new cancer cases in women can be linked to being overweight or obese. For advanced breast cancer alone, overweight women are 10 percent more at risk than women who are a healthy weight; if you're obese that number jumps to 56 percent.

- **Osteoarthritis**. Overweight women are four times more likely to develop "wear and tear" arthritis than women in the healthy weight range. For men, the risk is five times greater. A recent study of overweight women showed that dropping just 11 pounds reduced their chances of developing knee arthritis by half.

If you're already at a healthy weight, calorie counting can help you stay there—for life. By tracking your calories using this book and the tools at EverydayHealth.com, you can immediately detect and avoid the empty calories that might creep into your daily diet, and continue to make healthy choices. When you're aware of calorie counts and portion sizes, it's much easier to keep your weight under control.

Getting Started

How do you know what a healthy weight is for you? It will only take a few minutes to assemble your stats. You'll need a measuring tape and a calculator. Or, use the calculators and tools on EverydayHealth.com.

FIRST, FIGURE OUT YOUR BMI.

The body mass index (BMI) is a quick and easy way to see if your weight is within the normal range for your height—and, if it's not, to determine how many pounds you should lose to get it there.

Check the BMI chart opposite for your height and weight. Or, use this formula:

1. Multiply your weight by 703.
2. Divide that number by your height in inches.
3. Divide that number again by your height in inches.
   - If your BMI is between 18.5 and 24.9, you're normal weight.
   - If your BMI is between 25 and 29.9, you're overweight.
   - If your BMI is between 30 and 39.9, you're obese—very overweight.
   - If your BMI is 40 or over, you're dangerously obese (sometimes called morbidly obese).

Height														
	5'0"	5'1"	5'2"	5'3"	5'4"	5'5"	5'6"	5'7"	5'8"	5'9"	5'10"	5'11"	6'0"	6'2"
100	20	19	18	18	17	17	16	16	15	15	14	14	14	13
110	22	21	20	20	19	18	18	17	17	16	16	15	15	14
120	23	23	22	21	21	20	19	19	18	18	17	17	16	15
130	25	25	24	23	22	22	21	20	20	19	19	18	18	17
140	27	27	26	25	24	23	23	22	21	21	20	20	19	18
150	29	28	27	27	26	25	24	24	23	22	22	21	20	19
160	31	30	29	28	28	27	26	25	24	24	23	22	22	21
170	33	32	31	30	29	28	27	27	26	25	24	24	23	22
180	35	34	33	32	31	30	29	28	27	27	26	25	24	23
190	37	36	35	34	33	32	31	30	29	28	27	27	26	24
200	39	38	37	36	34	33	32	31	30	30	29	28	27	26
210	41	40	38	37	36	35	34	33	32	31	30	29	29	27
220	43	42	40	39	38	37	36	35	34	33	32	31	30	28
230	45	44	42	41	40	38	37	36	35	34	33	32	31	30

(Weight)

Underweight	Healthy Weight	Overweight	Obese	Morbidly Obese

To see how many pounds you need to lose to enter a healthy weight range:

Place a finger on the square that corresponds to your height and weight on the BMI chart. Now slide your finger up until you hit the first weight in the healthy range. Subtract that weight from your current weight.

ONLINE Find your Body Mass Index using the BMI Calculator at EverydayHealth.com.

You may want to lose even more pounds to reach the middle or lower end of that healthy range, but this is a good starting point.

NEXT, WORK OUT YOUR BODY FAT PERCENTAGE.

Your body needs a certain amount of fat to function well. Fat stores energy for times when you may not be able to eat (if you have had a bad stomach bug, for instance), it helps keep you warm, and it protects you from bruising and cushions your body's organs. But you can have too much of a good thing. This is why your body fat percentage is another indicator of whether you need to lose weight.

The calculation for figuring this one out is complex, so use the body fat calculator at EverydayHealth.com.

Enter your gender, height, and weight. Then, using your measuring tape, enter the circumference, in inches, of your neck (measure in the middle of your throat), waist (at its smallest, just above your bellybutton), and hips (at their widest, around the buttocks).

For optimal health, your body fat percentage should be in the range of 21 to 36 percent for a woman, 8 to 25 percent for a man.

FINALLY, CONSIDER YOUR WAIST-TO-HIP RATIO.

Are you shaped like an apple or a pear? When it comes to health problems such as heart disease and Type 2 diabetes, where your body carries weight counts. If you're heavier around the abdomen—an apple—then you will need to be more vigilant about keeping your weight down. In general, women with a waist circumference of 35 inches or more are likely to develop weight-related health problems; for men, the number is 40 inches.

Pears aren't off the health-hook, of course. But their risk of developing heart disease is somewhat lower. Here's how to assess your waist-to-hip ratio (WHR):

Step 1: Measure your hips at their widest, around your buttocks.

Step 2: Measure your waist at its smallest, just above your bellybutton.

Step 3: Divide your waist measurement by your hip measurement. Then use the chart on the next page to check your health risk level.

ONLINE   To determine your Body Fat Percentage, use the Body Fat Calculator at EverydayHealth.com.

Waist-to-Hip Ratio Health Risk

Women	Men	Risk Based on WHR
0.80 or below	0.95 or below	low risk
0.81 to 0.85	0.96 to 1.0	moderate risk
0.85 or higher	1.0 or higher	high risk

How Many Calories Do You Need?

The answer depends on the body you're in and how active you are. About two-thirds of the calories you consume each day are used just to keep your systems functioning—your heart beating, your muscles moving, and so on. The rest of your calorie intake fuels your regular activities like walking around, exercising, typing an e-mail, doing a crossword. Anything left over is stored as fat. To work out how many calories you would need to maintain your current weight, let's do another quick calculation to find your basal metabolic rate, or BMR.

Step 1: Women, multiply your weight by 10. Men, multiply by 11. This is your BMR.

Step 2: Now, add to that:

- 20 percent of your BMR if you have a sedentary lifestyle (you don't move around much).
- 30 percent if you are somewhat active.

- 40 percent if you are moderately active.
- 50 percent if you are very active.

ONLINE To figure out your Basal Metabolic Rate, use the BMR Calculator at EverydayHealth.com.

So, let's say you're a somewhat active 145-pound woman. Your BMR is 1,450 calories a day, and your lifestyle quotient is 30 percent of that, or an additional 435 calories (1,450 x .30 = 435). Add them together, and you come up with a daily calorie total of 1,885 (1,450 + 435 = 1,885).

Now remember, this gives you the number of calories you need to consume each day to *stay at the weight you are now*. To lose weight, you'll need to cut calories, use some up by exercising, or both.

Take It One Pound at a Time

Whatever your final goal, you should aim to lose about one to two pounds each week. Most doctors caution against cutting your calories drastically. If you go below 1,200 calories a day for a woman or 1,500 calories a day for a man, it's difficult to get the nutrition you need, plus you'll feel hungry, tired, and grouchy. You'll also be at risk for some serious health problems, including gallstones and heart rhythm disruptions from the lack of minerals in your diet.

The good news: To lose one pound a week you only have to cut 500 calories from your diet each day. Why 500?

One pound of weight is the equivalent of approximately 3,500 calories that your body has stored but not used. If you cut 500 calories every day for seven days (500 x 7 = 3,500) your body will use up that pound.

The even *better* news: small changes make a big difference. Substitute diet drinks or water for regular sodas and you'll save about 150 calories per 12-ounce can. Swap your afternoon junk-food fix for a low-calorie snack, and you're well on your way to your goal—there are 250 calories in just two ounces of potato chips or one regular-size candy bar. Follow these tips for success:

KEEP YOUR CALORIES IN CHECK.

- Start today. If you wait for a good time to begin, it may never come.
- Look up the number of calories for every food you eat and write it down. You could also use the *Food and Fitness Journal* on EverydayHealth.com or download the *Calorie Counter* mobile app.
- Track your calories as soon after eating as you can. If you wait, you may forget a part of a meal or a snack.
- Be aware of portion size and track it accurately.
- Plan your meals using the calorie charts in this book and on EverydayHealth.com.
- Don't forget your exercise bonus! Add in half an hour of moderate walking each day and you can knock off about 100 calories from your daily total—as well as improve your blood sugar, blood pressure, and overall

WHAT'S A CALORIE ANYWAY?

A calorie is simply a unit used to measure how much energy is contained in a particular food. The more calories a food has, the more energy it contains.

When you eat something, your body converts that food into energy to keep you alive and moving. If you consume more calories than you need to keep your body going, you'll gain weight. Why? Because the body stores all that excess energy as fat. If you take in fewer calories than you use, you'll lose weight as your body burns those fat stores to make up for the missing energy.

fitness. Did you move even more? The *Food and Fitness Journal* at EverydayHealth.com will calculate your calorie rebate based on the exercise type, speed, and time.

- Track your exercise soon after you do it. As with food, you may forget the details if you wait.
- Share your ups and downs. There's nothing like a diet buddy to give you an extra boost to keep going. Check in regularly with the groups on EverydayHealth.com.

66 *On the* Food and Fitness Journal *you can see whether you really did blow it on a particular day. Sometimes, when I thought I had eaten really badly, I was pleasantly surprised to see I hadn't consumed that much at all. I used to give up if I'd had one really bad day! I've now lost a total of 70 lbs.* 99

JULIE G.

The Skinny on Carbs, Protein, Fat, and More...

To get the most out of calorie counting, it helps to have a basic understanding of what's in the food you eat. Once you know that, you can make good decisions about what types of calories to cut.

Carbohydrates

Carbs have gotten a bad rap lately. But they give you quick energy and they're an essential—and satisfying—part of any diet. The trick is to stick to the good ones—such 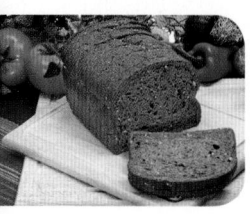 as whole grains, beans, vegetables, and fruit. These are what nutritionists call complex carbs: they take more time for the body to break down, so they keep you feeling full longer and give you a steady flow of energy. Refined carbs are the kind to avoid. They get absorbed quickly and give you a brief spike in energy, but that can be followed by an energy crash. You'll find the bad carbs in highly processed grains and sugars—which are the main ingredients in so many high-calorie, low-nutrition convenience foods and snacks—and in other white, starchy foods such as french fries.

One gram of any carbohydrate food contains 4 calories. That doesn't sound like much, but carb calories can add up fast. For instance, there are about 285 calories in a large bagel. Cutting back on carbs, especially highly processed carbs that have little nutrition, can have a big impact on your daily calorie count. Aim to get about half your daily calorie intake from high-quality carbs.

Protein

Protein comes from animal-based foods (meat, poultry, fish, eggs, and dairy products) and some plant-based foods (beans, soy, peas, nuts, and whole grains). Your body uses proteins to help build, maintain, and repair cells. Your body also uses proteins to help it produce hormones, enzymes, and many other chemical substances you need to function. With all the talk about high-protein diets, you may be 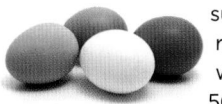 surprised by how little you really need: the recommended daily intake for an adult woman is just 46 grams; for an adult man, 56 grams. To put that in perspective, two roasted chicken drumsticks contain about 25 grams of protein, a slice of American cheese about 5 grams, an egg around 6 grams. One gram of fat contains four calories.

Fat

If you've ever been on any sort of diet, you've been told to cut back on fat. One gram of fat contains 9 calories, so eating less of it means consuming fewer calories. The problem: you're also cutting back on flavor and nutrition. Fat is what makes food taste good and satisfies your hunger. Cut back too much and you may end up consuming more calories than you save just to feel full. Plus, you could deplete your body's supplies of vitamin A, vitamin E, folic acid, calcium, iron, and zinc. So, how much do you need? Keep your fat intake to less than 30 percent of your daily calorie count. In a 2,000-calorie diet, that would mean roughly 600 fat calories or about 65 grams of fat a day. When choosing fats, go for the good ones: unsaturated or saturated fats that have no cholesterol. You'll find them in vegetable oils such as canola oil and olive oil, and in plant foods such as avocados and nuts. Another healthy food choice that is rich in healthy fats? Oily fish such as salmon and tuna. They are full of omega-3 fatty acids, which improve cardiovascular health.

Try to limit animal fats, such as butter, lard, and the fat found in meats, poultry, and dairy products. These are saturated fats that contain cholesterol, which can contribute to heart disease. The fat to avoid at all costs is trans fat, also known as partially hydrogenated vegetable oil. It's used in baked goods, in convenience and packaged foods, and as the oil for deep frying—and it has been linked to obesity, diabetes, and heart disease. Fortunately, many food manufacturers and restaurant chains have wised up to the health risks and stopped using trans fat, but check food labels to be sure.

Fiber

Meet the calorie-counter's best friend. Dietary fiber is made up of all the parts of plant food that your body can't digest. Because it doesn't get broken down or absorbed, it passes right through your system—calorie-free. It gets even better: Fiber also makes you feel full. (Doctors agree, this does not involve magic.) Imagine eating six chocolate chip cookies in a row. All too easy, right? Now imagine eating six apples one after the other. Almost impossible, because just one or two apples would take a while to chew and would fill you up very quickly. Foods that are high in fiber tend to be low in calories—

there are 4 grams of fiber and only about 95 calories in a medium apple compared to 2 grams of fiber and 208 calories (108 of them from fat) in those six cookies. Because fiber sticks with you, eating a high-fiber snack in the late afternoon can keep you satisfied until supper. Similarly, starting your meal with a salad (use a low-calorie dressing) will help you avoid overeating later on.

Of course, fiber is also packed with healthy goodness. Apart from its famed ability to help prevent constipation and bowel problems such as hemorrhoids, fiber from foods like oatmeal, beans, peas, and bran can help lower your cholesterol and control your blood sugar.

You'd think we would all be gorging on this wonder food, yet most of us don't get the amount of dietary fiber that we need—studies show that only about 26 percent of all American adults eat 3 or more servings of vegetables each day. The Institute of Medicine suggests that women under age 50 should aim for 25 grams of daily fiber; for men the recommendation is 38 grams. Above age 50, women should aim for 21 grams daily, while men should aim for 30 grams.

Sugar

You don't have to have a sweet tooth to overload on the stuff: it's in almost every packaged food, including salad dressing and savory sauces—even pizza.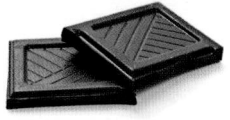
The USDA estimates that the average person consumes 32 teaspoons of sugar each day. There are 16 calories in one teaspoon, so that means you may be racking up 500 daily calories in sugar alone! According to the American Heart Association, women should be getting no more than

100 calories a day (about 6 teaspoons) from added sugar (as opposed to the natural sugar contained in whole foods like fruit); for men, it's 150 calories (about 9 teaspoons).

Clearly, there's plenty of opportunity to cut calories here. Simply skipping or eating smaller portions of sweet foods such as baked goods, fruit juice, and ice cream is a good start. Instead of adding sugar to your coffee or tea, try using a low-calorie sweetener. But beware of the sugar-free or reduced-sugar versions of sweet foods. Like low-fat alternatives, these may be just as high in calories as the regular version. The manufacturers simply bolster the flavor with other ingredients. Likewise, watch out for healthy-sounding sweeteners such as fruit juice concentrate; they have just as many calories as plain old sugar.

Salt

How can salt, which has no calories, be a big reason for excess weight? Because so many high-fat, high-calorie snack foods are salted. Take away the chips, pretzels, cheese curls, and other salty snacks, and you'll save a lot of calories. You'll also improve your health. Eating too much salt may raise your blood pressure, which in turn raises your risk of heart disease and stroke. The American Heart Association recommends taking in no more 1,500 milligrams of salt per day. That's just a bit more than half a teaspoon. The average American consumes about 3,500 milligrams a day, or close to 2 teaspoons.

Some of that comes from salt you add to food yourself, and about 12 percent comes from the salt that is naturally in food, but a whopping 77 percent of the salt in the

American diet comes from processed foods. That means salty snack foods and other products, such as tomato sauce, canned soups, and prepared mixes.

Because many doctors and health-related organizations recommend limiting salt, many food manufacturers offer low- or reduced-salt options. It's the sodium in salt that raises your blood pressure, which is why the package labels list sodium instead of salt. Read the label carefully. Some foods have less salt than the original version, but the total amount of sodium is still high.

Vitamins and Minerals

As long as you eat a wide variety of foods, you should get enough of all the essential nutrients your body needs. But on those days when you just can't manage to pull together a healthy or well-balanced meal, take a multivitamin with minerals.

As a calorie-counter, you should watch your calcium intake. Cutting back on full-fat dairy foods like cheese may keep you from getting the recommended 1000 milligrams a day of calcium. So be sure to swap those dairy calories for high-calcium, lower-calorie foods like low-fat dairy products, almonds, beans, spinach, and tofu. Check in with your doctor to see if you need a calcium supplement.

66 I lost 21 lbs in 21 weeks. And I'll continue to keep to my diet, using My Calorie Counter at EverydayHealth.com, eating more fresh veggies and fruit, exercising, and drinking a lot of water. I wouldn't be able to do it without this website. 99

ASHLEY H.

THE NUTRITIONAL LABEL, DECODED

Knowing how to read all those tiny numbers and unpronounceable ingredients will help you make better choices and avoid overeating by accident.

Serving Size: The package might *look* like just one serving, but is it? It pays to check. Many 20-ounce drinks, for example, contain 2.5 8-ounce servings. The calories and other info on the nutritional label are for less than half the bottle, so you may be consuming more calories than you think.

Nutrition Facts

Serving Size 3 oz. (85g)

Amount Per Serving	As Served
Calories 38	Calories from Fat 0

	% Daily Value
Total Fat 0g	0%
Saturated Fat 0g	0%
Cholesterol 0g	0%
Sodium 0g	2%
Total Carbohydrate 0g	3%
Dietary Fiber 0g	8%
Sugars 0g	
Protein 0g	

Vitamin A 270%	¥	Vitamin C 10%
Calcium 2%	¥	Iron 0%

Percent Daily Values are based on a 2,000 calorie diet. Your daily values may be higher or lower depending on your calorie needs:

	Calories	2,000	2,500
Total Fat	Less than	65g	80g
Sat Fat	Less than	20g	80g
Cholesterol	Less than	300mg	300mg
Sodium	Less than	2,400mg	2,400mg
Total Carbohydrate		300g	375g
Dietary Fiber		25g	30g

Calories: In general, less than 100 calories per serving is low, 100 to 400 calories per serving is moderate, and anything that's more than 400 calories per serving is high. Keep portions in mind—a couple servings of a low-calorie food still adds up.

The Daily Value Column: Use this as a rough guide. It's calculated for a 2,000-calorie diet. If your ideal calorie count is lower than that, adjust accordingly. In general, a DV of 5 percent or less is considered low for a particular ingredient. If the DV is 20 percent or more, it's considered high.

Fat/Trans Fats/Sodium: The lower the number and its DV the better. If a mid-morning snack promises to saddle you with 35 percent of your fat and sodium intake for the day, choose something else. Avoid trans fats altogether.

Dietary Fiber: The DV for fiber is 25 to 30 grams, though many experts feel this is on the low side and recommend more.

Sugar: Less is more—healthy, that is. (There is no DV for sugar.)

Ingredients: A good rule of thumb: the more ingredients a food has (especially unpronounceable ones), the more processed it is, and the more calories it contains. Ingredients are also listed by most to least, so make sure the first few are the healthiest.

It's All in the Portions

In a world where Super-Size is the new Regular, it's easy to undercount your calories. Here are some tips to help you recognize standard serving sizes, and keep your portions under control.

Spend a half an hour in your kitchen with some measuring cups and a scale. Using uncooked rice or something similar, measure out a cup (the standard portion for milk, pasta, beans, and other foods) or three ounces (standard for meat, poultry, and fish). Pour it onto a dinner plate, a salad plate, into a soup bowl, and a drinking glass. You might be surprised by how little space a correct portion actually occupies.

- **Try not to eat right out of containers.** Measure out a small portion of a snack food and put it on a plate.

- **Ditch the desktop candy bowl.** Who on Earth can keep track of how many pieces they munch on during the day? (Your colleagues will also thank you.)

- **Spoil your appetite with a nutritious snack**—celery sticks with peanut butter, for example—an hour before mealtime. You'll eat less and feel more satisfied later. A recent study found that people who eat no more than one ounce of nuts throughout the day tend not to overeat at meals.

- **Use smaller plates and bowls.** A healthy portion looks lean and lonesome on an oversize plate but looks just right if you shrink its surroundings.

- **Divide your (smaller) plate.** Fill one half of the plate with vegetables and salad greens, one quarter with starchy foods—such as rice, beans, or potatoes—and one quarter with protein foods such as meat, poultry, or fish.

- **Think of a tennis ball.** That's about the size of 1 cup of food. Compare the correct portion of foods you eat regularly with something that's easy to remember.

66 With the help of EverydayHealth.com, I set myself a daily calorie goal and began weighing and measuring portions. I have lost 50 lbs, and 9 inches off my hips alone. 99

KATHY S.

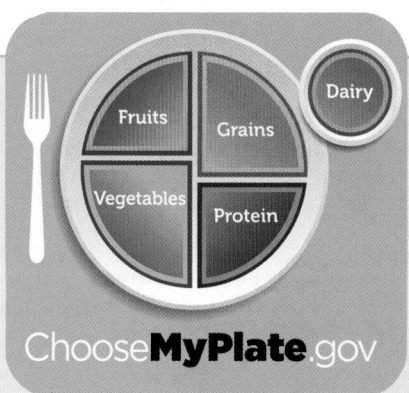

THE USDA MYPLATE DIETARY GUIDELINES

MyPlate reminds everyone to eat a balanced meal featuring the five different nutrient-rich food groups suggested for good health. A healthy plate contains the following proportions:

- 1/2 fruits and vegetables
- 1/4 protein
- 1/4 grains
- 1 serving dairy

Here are some additional tricks for a well-balanced meal:

- Vary your vegetables
- Eat lean protein
- Make at least half your grains whole grains
- Switch to fat-free or low-fat milk
- Choose food with low sodium
- Drink water instead of sugary drinks
- Avoid oversized portions
- Enjoy food, but eat less

If at First You Don't Succeed...

When you first start counting calories, you'll probably lose weight steadily. After a few weeks, however, your weight loss is likely to slow as your body adjusts to eating less. Plateaus and stalls are nearly inevitable, as is the occasional binge or indulgence. Get back on track with these ideas:

- **Find a weight-loss buddy.** Counting calories with a friend provides mutual support, encouragement, and an incentive to stick with it.

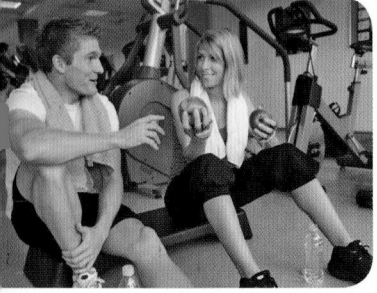

- **Eat more.** As in more low-calorie snacks between meals. It's hard to stay motivated when you're hungry. And healthy snacking helps you keep your mealtime choices and portions under control.

- **Plan ahead.** If you know you've got a busy week of deadlines coming up, stock up on healthy foods that are easy to prepare or can go in the microwave. You'll avoid the temptation to eat high-calorie fast food or take-out instead.

- **If you eat because you're bored**, find something else to do. Take up knitting, go for a walk, call a friend—anything that engages you and takes your mind off food.

- **If you're an emotional eater**, seek out other ways to cope with your feelings. Emotional eating is tough to overcome, but while you're working on it, surround yourself with low-calorie foods.

- **Enlist your family for support.** Explain that you want to lose weight to look and feel better and that you need their help. Ask them to understand your needs and not pressure you to eat more or eat foods you want to avoid.

- **Tap into a supportive weight-loss community.** As you learn to count calories and eat a healthier diet, you're bound to have lots of questions, moments to celebrate, and times when you need advice or some extra support. You can find all that and more on EverydayHealth.com.

Now, You're Ready to Start Counting

You've set your goals, learned about calories, healthy nutrition, and portion control, and picked up some tips on how to stay motivated. So let's get counting!

Use the *Everyday Health: My Calorie Counter* to plan your grocery shopping trips and check out restaurant menus in advance. You can't always plan ahead, of course, which is why this book is portable. Keep it in your handbag: it's a handy, discreet way to find and track the calories in the foods you eat over the course of the day.

In the charts on the following pages, you'll find some 1,800 common food items, listed alphabetically by types (cheese, fruits, vegetables, etc.) and then names, like artichoke to zucchini.

There are also thousands of brand names listed alphabetically, so if you like to start your morning with Post's Raisin Bran, just flip to Post to find the calorie count and nutritional content for your breakfast cereal.

Chances are you'll eat at least one meal away from home today—and that can be a real challenge when you're counting calories. So check out the Restaurant section that starts on page 175. Some 135 restaurants are listed alphabetically. Under each name, the menu items are then broken out alphabetically by category (salads, entrées, etc.) and then listed alphabetically by name.

For example:

Burger King
BK SALAD COLLECTION

Chicken Garden, Tendercrisp	1 salad	470	26	8	1170	26	2	31
Chicken Garden, Tendergrill	1 salad	290	12	6	1030	8	1	38
Garden, No Chicken	1 salad	130	8	5	200	6	1	8
BREAKFAST								
Biscuit, Bacon, Egg, & Cheese	1 sandwich	470	28	17	1420	33	1	17
Biscuit, Sausage, Egg, & Cheese	1 sandwich	570	37	19	1510	34	1	20
BK Wrapper, Cheesy Bacon	1 wrap	410	25	8	980	28	2	14
Breakfast Platter	1 platter	810	54	22	1790	57	4	25
Croissan'wich, Bacon, Egg, & Cheese	1 sandwich	380	22	8	890	26	0	15

Remember all the info you just read about carbs, fat, protein, and salt? Along with calories, the charts in this book show how much of each of these nutrients is contained in every listed food. Armed with these details, and the great tools at EverydayHealth.com, you can make smarter choices every time you eat.

So turn the page, visit EverydayHealth.com, and start your journey toward weight loss and better health.

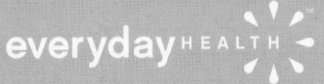

everyday HEALTH

common foods

common foods

Beverages
ALCOHOLS

	SERVING SIZE	CALORIES	TOTAL FAT (G)	SAT FAT (G)	SODIUM (MG)	CARBS (G)	FIBER (G)	PROTEIN (G)
Beer								
Beer, Light	12 fl oz	103	0	0	14	6	0	1
Beer, Regular	12 fl oz	153	0	0	14	13	0	2
Cocktails & Liqueurs								
Crème de Menthe, 72 Proof	1 fl oz	125	0	0	2	14	0	0
Daiquiri, Canned	8 fl oz	305	0	0	98	38	0	0
Daiquiri, Prepared From Recipe	8 fl oz	449	0	0	12	17	0	0
Liqueur, Coffee w/Cream, 34 Proof	1 fl oz	102	5	3	29	6	0	1
Liqueur, Coffee, 53 Proof	1 fl oz	113	0	0	3	16	0	0
Liqueur, Coffee, 63 Proof	1 fl oz	107	0	0	3	11	0	0
Pina Colada, Canned	8 fl oz	618	20	17	185	72	0	2
Pina Colada, Prepared From Recipe	8 fl oz	437	5	4	15	57	1	1
Tequila Sunrise, Canned	8 fl oz	274	0	0	142	28	0	1
Whiskey Sour, Canned	8 fl oz	293	0	0	108	33	0	0
Whiskey Sour, Prepared w/Whiskey, Water & Powder Mix	8 fl oz	386	0	0	111	37	0	0
Spirits								
Distilled, All 80 Proof (Gin, Rum, Vodka, Whiskey)	1 fl oz	64	0	0	0	0	0	0
Distilled, All 86 Proof	1 fl oz	70	0	0	0	0	0	0
Distilled, All 90 Proof	1 fl oz	73	0	0	0	0	0	0
Distilled, All 94 Proof	1 fl oz	76	0	0	0	0	0	0
Distilled, All 100 Proof	1 fl oz	82	0	0	0	0	0	0
Wine								
Cooking	1 fl oz	15	0	0	182	2	0	0
Dessert, Dry	3.5 fl oz	157	0	0	9	12	0	0
Dessert, Sweet	3.5 fl oz	165	0	0	9	14	0	0
Non-Alcoholic	5 fl oz	9	0	0	10	2	0	1
Red, All Varieties	5 fl oz	123	0	0	2	4	0	0
Sake	1 fl oz	39	0	0	1	1	0	0
White, All Varieties	5 fl oz	120	0	0	1	4	0	0
CARBONATED BEVERAGES								
Cola, w/Caffeine	12 fl oz	136	0	0	15	35	0	0
Cola, w/Higher Caffeine	12 fl oz	151	0	0	15	39	0	0
Cola, w/o Caffeine	12 fl oz	151	0	0	15	39	0	0

	SERVING SIZE	CALORIES	TOTAL FAT (G)	SAT FAT (G)	SODIUM (MG)	CARBS (G)	FIBER (G)	PROTEIN (G)
Ginger Ale	12 fl oz	124	0	0	26	32	0	0
Root Beer	12 fl oz	152	0	0	48	39	0	0
Soda, Chocolate-Flavored	12 fl oz	155	0	0	325	39	0	0
Soda, Club	12 fl oz	0	0	0	75	0	0	0
Soda, Cream	12 fl oz	189	0	0	44	49	0	0
Soda, Grape	12 fl oz	160	0	0	56	42	0	0
Soda, Lemon-Lime, w/Caffeine	12 fl oz	151	0	0	37	38	0	0
Soda, Orange	12 fl oz	179	0	0	45	46	0	0
Tonic Water	12 fl oz	124	0	0	44	32	0	0
COFFEES & TEAS								
Coffee, Brewed	8 fl oz	2	0	0	5	0	0	0
Coffee, Brewed, Decaffeinated	8 fl oz	0	0	0	5	0	0	0
Coffee, Brewed, Espresso	1 fl oz	1	0	0	4	0	0	0
Coffee, Brewed, Espresso, Decaffeinated	1 fl oz	0	0	0	4	0	0	0
Coffee, Instant, Prepared w/Water	8 fl oz	5	0	0	10	1	0	0
Coffee, Instant, Prepared w/Water, Decaffeinated	8 fl oz	5	0	0	10	1	0	0
Tea, Brewed	8 fl oz	2	0	0	7	1	0	0
Tea, Brewed, Decaffeinated	8 fl oz	2	0	0	7	1	0	0
DRINK MIXES								
Chocolate Malt Mix, Prepared w/Whole Milk	8 fl oz	225	9	5	159	30	1	9
Cocoa Mix, Prepared w/Water	8 fl oz	151	2	1	200	32	1	3
Cocoa Mix, w/Aspartame, Prepared w/Water	8 fl oz	74	1	0	184	14	2	3
JUICES & NECTARS								
Apple Juice, Unsweetened	8 fl oz	114	0	0	10	28	0	0
Blackberry Juice, Canned	8 fl oz	95	2	0	3	20	0	1
Carrot Juice, Canned	8 fl oz	94	0	0	156	22	2	2
Citrus Fruit Juice Drink, Frozen Concentrate, Prepared w/Water	8 fl oz	114	0	0	10	28	0	1
Clam & Tomato Juice, Canned	8 fl oz	116	0	0	875	26	1	1
Coconut Water, Fresh	8 fl oz	46	0	0	252	9	3	2
Cranberry Juice Cocktail, Bottled	8 fl oz	137	0	0	5	34	0	0
Cranberry Juice Cocktail, Bottled, Low Calorie	8 fl oz	45	0	0	7	11	0	0
Cranberry Juice Cocktail, Frozen Concentrate, Prepared w/Water	8 fl oz	111	0	0	9	28	0	0
Cranberry Juice, Unsweetened	8 fl oz	116	0	0	5	31	0	1

common foods

	SERVING SIZE	CALORIES	TOTAL FAT (G)	SAT FAT (G)	SODIUM (MG)	CARBS (G)	FIBER (G)	PROTEIN (G)
Cranberry-Apple Juice Drink	8 fl oz	154	0	0	5	39	0	0
Cranberry-Grape Juice Drink	8 fl oz	137	0	0	7	34	0	0
Fruit Flavored Drink, Less than 3% Fruit Juice	8 fl oz	152	0	0	86	38	0	0
Fruit Punch Drink, Frozen Concentrate, Prepared w/Water	8 fl oz	114	0	0	12	29	0	0
Grape Juice, Canned or Bottled, Unsweetened	8 fl oz	152	0	0	13	37	1	1
Grapefruit Juice, White or Pink, Fresh	8 fl oz	96	0	0	2	23	0	1
Grapefruit Juice, White, Canned, Sweetened	8 fl oz	115	0	0	5	28	0	1
Guava Nectar, Canned	8 fl oz	143	0	0	18	37	3	0
Lemon Juice, Canned or Bottled	1 tbsp	3	0	0	3	1	0	0
Lemonade, Frozen Concentrate, Pink, Prepared w/Water	8 fl oz	106	0	0	10	27	0	0
Lemonade, Frozen Concentrate, White, Prepared w/Water	8 fl oz	99	0	0	10	26	0	0
Limeade, Frozen Concentrate, Prepared w/Water	8 fl oz	128	0	0	7	34	0	0
Mango Nectar, Canned	8 fl oz	128	0	0	13	33	1	0
Orange Drink, Canned, w/Added Vitamin C	8 fl oz	122	0	0	7	31	0	0
Orange Juice, Canned, Unsweetened	8 fl oz	117	0	0	10	27	1	2
Orange-Strawberry-Banana Juice	8 fl oz	117	0	0	9	29	0	1
Papaya Nectar, Canned	8 fl oz	143	0	0	13	36	2	0
Peach Nectar, Canned	8 fl oz	134	0	0	17	35	1	1
Pineapple & Orange Juice Drink, Canned	8 fl oz	125	0	0	8	30	0	3
Pineapple Juice, Canned, Unsweetened	8 fl oz	133	0	0	5	32	1	1
Pomegranate Juice, Bottled	8 fl oz	134	1	0	22	33	0	0
Prune Juice, Canned	8 fl oz	182	0	0	10	45	3	2
Tomato Juice, Canned, w/Salt	8 fl oz	41	0	0	654	10	1	2
Tomato Juice, Canned, w/o Salt	8 fl oz	41	0	0	24	10	1	2
Vegetable & Fruit Juice Blend	8 fl oz	113	0	0	71	27	0	1
Vegetable Juice Cocktail, Canned	8 fl oz	46	0	0	479	11	2	2

Bread & Bread Products
BAGELS

	SERVING SIZE	CALORIES	TOTAL FAT (G)	SAT FAT (G)	SODIUM (MG)	CARBS (G)	FIBER (G)	PROTEIN (G)
Cinnamon-Raisin	1 whole, 3" dia	188	1	0	299	38	2	7

	SERVING SIZE	CALORIES	TOTAL FAT (G)	SAT FAT (G)	SODIUM (MG)	CARBS (G)	FIBER (G)	PROTEIN (G)
Egg	1 whole, 2-1/2" dia	72	1	0	131	14	1	3
Oat Bran	1 whole, 3" dia	176	1	0	407	37	2	7
Plain, Onion, Poppy, or Sesame	1 whole, 2-1/2" dia	72	0	0	139	14	1	3
BISCUITS								
Mixed Grain, Refrigerator Dough, Baked	1, 2-1/2" dia (44 g)	116	2	1	295	21	n/a	3)
Plain or Buttermilk, Dry Mix, Prepared	1, 2 oz (57 g)	190	7	2	541	27	1	4
Plain or Buttermilk, Homemade	1, 2-1/2" dia (60 g)	212	10	3	348	27	1	4
Plain or Buttermilk, Refrigerator Dough, Higher Fat, Baked	1, 2-1/2" dia (27 g)	95	4	1	292	13	0	2
Plain or Buttermilk, Refrigerator Dough, Lower Fat, Baked	1, 2-1/4" dia (21 g)	63	1	0	210	12	0	2
BREADS								
Banana, Homemade w/Margarine	1 slice (28 g)	92	3	1	86	15	0	1
Boston Brown, Canned	1 slice (45 g)	88	1	0	284	19	2	2
Bread Sticks, Plain	1, 4-1/4" long	21	0	0	33	3	0	1
Cheese	1 slice (48 g)	196	10	3	360	22	1	5
Cornbread, Dry Mix, Prepared	1 piece (60 g)	188	6	2	467	29	1	4
Cornbread, Homemade w/Reduced-Fat (2%) Milk	1 piece (65 g)	173	5	1	428	28	n/a	4
Cracked-Wheat	1 oz	74	1	0	153	14	2	2
Egg	1 slice (40 g)	113	2	1	165	19	1	4
Focaccia, Plain	1 piece (57 g)	142	4	0	320	20	1	5
French, Vienna, or Sourdough	1 slice (32 g)	92	1	0	164	18	1	4
Garlic, Frozen	1 slice (59 g)	207	10	3	321	25	1	5
Irish Soda, Homemade	1 oz	82	1	0	113	16	1	2
Italian	1 slice (30 g)	81	1	0	175	15	1	3
Multigrain (Includes Whole-Grain)	1 slice (26 g)	69	1	0	109	11	2	3
Oat Bran	1 slice (30 g)	71	1	0	122	12	1	3
Oat Bran, Reduced-Calorie	1 slice (23 g)	46	1	0	132	9	3	2
Oatmeal	1 slice (27 g)	73	1	0	127	13	1	2
Oatmeal, Reduced-Calorie	1 slice (23 g)	48	1	0	89	10	n/a	2
Pita, White	6-1/2" dia	165	1	0	322	33	1	5

common foods

	SERVING SIZE	CALORIES	TOTAL FAT (G)	SAT FAT (G)	SODIUM (MG)	CARBS (G)	FIBER (G)	PROTEIN (G)
Pita, Whole-Wheat	6-1/2" dia	170	2	0	340	35	5	6
Potato	1 slice (32 g)	85	1	0	120	15	2	4
Pumpernickel	1 slice (26 g)	65	1	0	174	12	2	2
Raisin	1 slice (32 g)	88	1	0	100	17	1	3
Rice Bran	1 slice (27 g)	66	1	0	82	12	1	2
Rye	1 slice (32 g)	83	1	0	211	15	2	3
Rye, Reduced-Calorie	1 slice (23 g)	47	1	0	118	9	3	2
Wheat	1 slice (29 g)	78	1	0	151	14	1	3
Wheat, Reduced-Calorie	1 slice (21 g)	46	1	0	70	9	2	3
White	1 slice (28 g)	74	1	0	137	14	1	3
White, Reduced-Calorie	1 slice (23 g)	48	1	0	104	10	2	2
Whole-Wheat, Homemade	1 slice (46 g)	128	2	0	159	24	3	4
BREAD CRUMBS & STUFFING								
Bread Crumbs, Plain	1 cup	427	6	1	791	78	5	14
Bread Crumbs, Seasoned	1 cup	460	7	2	2111	82	6	17
Bread Stuffing, Dry Mix, Prepared	1/2 cup	177	9	2	524	22	3	3
Cornbread Stuffing, Dry Mix, Prepared	1/2 cup	179	9	2	455	22	3	3
CRACKERS								
Cheese, Bite Size	1 cup	303	14	3	603	37	1	7
Cheese, Sandwich w/Cheese Filling	1 sandwich	32	2	0	57	4	0	1
Cheese, Sandwich w/Peanut Butter Filling	1 sandwich	32	2	0	59	4	0	1
Matzo, Egg	1 matzo	109	1	0	6	22	1	3
Matzo, Egg & Onion	1 matzo	109	1	0	80	22	1	3
Matzo, Plain	1 matzo	111	0	0	0	23	1	3
Matzo, Whole-Wheat	1 matzo	98	0	0	1	22	3	4
Melba Toast, Plain	1 toast	20	0	0	30	4	0	1
Melba Toast, Rye or Pumpernickel	1 toast	19	0	0	45	4	0	1
Melba Toast, Wheat	1 toast	19	0	0	42	4	0	1
Milk	1 cracker	50	2	0	65	8	0	1
Rusk Toast	1 rusk	41	1	0	25	7	n/a	1
Rye, Crispbread	1 crispbread	37	0	0	45	8	2	1
Rye, Sandwich w/Cheese Filling	1 sandwich	34	2	0	73	4	0	1
Rye, Wafers, Plain	1 cracker	84	0	0	139	20	6	2
Rye, Wafers, Seasoned	1 cracker	84	2	0	195	16	5	2
Saltines	1 cracker	13	0	0	33	2	0	0
Saltines, Unsalted Tops	1 cracker	13	0	0	23	2	0	0
Saltines, Whole-Wheat or Multigrain	1 cracker	56	1	0	170	10	0	0

	SERVING SIZE	CALORIES	TOTAL FAT (G)	SAT FAT (G)	SODIUM (MG)	CARBS (G)	FIBER (G)	PROTEIN (G)
Wheat, Sandwich w/Cheese Filling	1 sandwich	35	2	0	64	4	0	1
Wheat, Sandwich w/Peanut Butter Filling	1 sandwich	35	2	0	56	4	0	1
Whole-Wheat	1 cracker	20	1	0	33	3	0	0
Whole-Wheat, Reduced-Fat	1 cracker	17	0	0	31	3	0	0
ENGLISH MUFFINS								
Mixed-Grain or Granola	1 muffin	155	1	0	220	31	2	6
Plain or Sourdough	1 muffin	129	1	0	206	25	2	5
Raisin- or Apple-Cinnamon	1 muffin	137	1	0	158	27	1	5
Wheat	1 muffin	127	1	0	218	26	3	5
Whole-Wheat	1 muffin	134	1	0	240	27	4	6
FRENCH TOAST								
French Toast, Frozen, Reheated	1 slice (59 g)	126	4	1	292	19	1	4
French Toast, Homemade w/Reduced-Fat (2%) Milk	1 slice (65 g)	149	7	2	311	16	n/a	5
MUFFINS								
Blueberry	1 mini	67	3	1	59	8	0	1
Blueberry, Homemade w/Reduced-Fat (2%) Milk	1 muffin	162	6	1	251	23	n/a	4
Blueberry, Low-Fat	1 small	181	3	1	293	36	3	3
Corn	1 mini	52	1	0	109	9	1	1
Corn, Homemade w/Reduced-Fat (2%) Milk	1 muffin	180	7	1	333	25	n/a	4
Oat Bran	1 mini	46	1	0	67	8	1	1
OTHER BREAD PRODUCTS								
Croutons, Plain	1 cup	122	2	0	209	22	2	4
Croutons, Seasoned	1 cup	186	7	2	436	25	2	4
Phyllo Dough	1 sheet	57	1	0	92	10	0	1
Taco Shells, Baked	1 large	98	4	1	82	13	1	1
Tortillas, Ready-To-Bake/Fry, Corn	1 tortilla	41	1	0	9	8	1	1
Tortillas, Ready-To-Bake/Fry, Flour	1 tortilla	146	4	1	364	24	1	4
Tostada Shells, Corn	1 shell	58	3	1	81	8	1	1
Wonton or Egg-Roll Wrappers	1 wrapper	93	0	0	183	19	1	3
PANCAKES								
Blueberry, Homemade	4" dia	84	3	1	157	11	n/a	2
Buttermilk, Homemade	4" dia	86	4	1	198	11	n/a	3
Plain or Buttermilk, Frozen, Ready-to-Heat	1 pancake	91	2	0	215	16	1	2

common foods	SERVING SIZE	CALORIES	TOTAL FAT (G)	SAT FAT (G)	SODIUM (MG)	CARBS (G)	FIBER (G)	PROTEIN (G)
Plain, Dry Mix, Prepared	4" dia	74	1	0	239	14	0	2
Plain, Homemade	4" dia	86	4	1	167	11	n/a	2
Whole-Wheat, Dry Mix, Prepared	4" dia	92	3	1	252	13	1	4
ROLLS								
Dinner, Egg	1 roll	107	2	1	161	18	1	3
Dinner, Oat Bran	1 roll	78	2	0	136	13	1	3
Dinner, Plain	1 roll	87	2	0	150	15	1	3
Dinner, Plain, Homemade w/Reduced-Fat (2%) Milk	1 large	136	3	1	178	23	1	4
Dinner, Rye	1 medium	103	1	0	234	19	2	4
Dinner, Wheat	1 roll	76	2	0	136	13	1	2
Dinner, Whole-Wheat	1 roll	74	1	0	112	14	2	2
French	1 roll	105	2	0	193	19	1	3
Hamburger or Hotdog, Mixed-Grain	1 roll	113	3	1	197	19	2	4
Hamburger or Hotdog, Plain	1 roll	117	2	0	210	21	1	4
Hamburger or Hotdog, Reduced-Calorie	1 roll	84	1	0	190	18	3	4
Hard or Kaiser	1 roll	167	2	0	310	30	1	6
Pumpernickel	1 medium	100	1	0	255	19	2	4
WAFFLES								
Buttermilk, Frozen, Ready-To-Heat, Microwaved	1 waffle	101	3	1	232	15	1	2
Chocolate Chip, Frozen, Ready-To-Heat	1 waffle	98	4	1	190	15	0	2
Plain, Frozen, Ready-To-Heat	1 waffle	99	3	1	230	15	1	2
Plain, Homemade	1 waffle	218	11	2	383	25	n/a	6
Cereals								
HOT CEREALS, COOKED W/WATER								
Corn Grits, White, Regular & Quick, w/Salt	1 cup	182	1	0	573	38	2	4
Corn Grits, Yellow, Regular & Quick, w/Salt	1 cup	151	1	0	520	32	2	3
Cream of Rice, w/Salt	1 cup	127	0	0	422	28	0	2
Cream of Wheat (10 Minute), w/Salt	1 cup	126	1	0	324	27	1	4
Cream of Wheat, Instant, w/Salt	1 cup	149	1	0	364	32	1	4
Farina, w/Salt	1 cup	123	1	0	294	25	2	4
Oats, Instant, Plain	1 cup	159	3	1	115	27	4	6
Oats, Instant, w/Cinnamon & Spices	1 cup	257	3	1	324	52	4	6
Oats, Instant, w/Raisins & Spices	1 cup	240	3	0	362	49	4	5

	SERVING SIZE	CALORIES	TOTAL FAT (G)	SAT FAT (G)	SODIUM (MG)	CARBS (G)	FIBER (G)	PROTEIN (G)
READY-TO-EAT								
Bran Flakes	3/4 cup	96	1	0	220	24	5	3
Corn Flakes, Low-Sodium	1 cup	100	0	0	3	22	0	2
Granola, Homemade	1 cup	597	29	5	31	65	11	18
Mini Wheats, Apple Cinnamon	3/4 cup	182	1	0	20	44	5	4
Muesli, Dried Fruit & Nuts	1 cup	289	4	1	196	66	6	8
Puffed Corn, Chocolate-Flavored, Frosted	1 cup	122	1	0	201	26	1	1
Rice, Puffed	1 cup	56	0	0	0	13	0	1
Wheat Germ, Toasted, Plain	1 cup	432	12	2	5	56	17	33
Wheat, Puffed	1 cup	44	0	0	0	10	1	2
Wheat, Shredded, Plain, Sugar- & Salt-Free	2, 23-g biscuits	155	1	0	3	36	6	5

Condiments, Gravies & Sauces

CONDIMENTS

	SERVING SIZE	CALORIES	TOTAL FAT (G)	SAT FAT (G)	SODIUM (MG)	CARBS (G)	FIBER (G)	PROTEIN (G)
Apple Butter	1 tbsp	29	0	0	3	7	0	0
Bacon Bits	1 tbsp	33	2	0	124	2	1	2
Chocolate-Flavored Hazelnut Spread	1 tbsp	100	6	5	8	11	1	1
Cocoa Powder, Unsweetened	1 tbsp	12	1	0	1	3	2	1
Cranberry Sauce, Canned, Sweetened	1 slice	86	0	0	17	22	1	0
Cranberry-Orange Relish, Canned	1 cup	490	0	0	88	127	0	1
Horseradish	1 tbsp	7	0	0	47	2	0	0
Hummus, Ready-to-Serve	1 tbsp	26	1	0	47	3	1	1
Jams & Preserves, No Added Sugar, Any Flavor	1 tbsp	18	0	0	0	8	0	0
Jams, Jellies & Preserves	1 tbsp	56	0	0	6	14	0	0
Ketchup	1 tbsp	15	0	0	167	4	0	0
Mayonnaise	1 tbsp	57	5	1	105	4	0	0
Mayonnaise, Light	1 tbsp	49	5	1	101	1	0	0
Mayonnaise, Low-Sodium, Low-Calorie	1 tbsp	32	3	0	15	2	0	0
Mayonnaise, Made w/Tofu	1 tbsp	48	5	0	116	0	0	1
Mayonnaise, No Cholesterol	1 tbsp	103	12	2	73	0	0	0
Miso	1 tbsp	34	1	0	641	5	1	2
Mustard, Yellow	1 tsp	3	0	0	57	0	0	0
Olives, Black, Canned, Jumbo	1 olive	7	1	0	61	0	0	0
Olives, Black, Canned, Large	1 olive	5	0	0	32	0	0	0
Olives, Green, Pickled, Canned or Bottled	1 olive	4	0	0	42	0	0	0

common foods

	SERVING SIZE	CALORIES	TOTAL FAT (G)	SAT FAT (G)	SODIUM (MG)	CARBS (G)	FIBER (G)	PROTEIN (G)
Pickles, Dill or Kosher Dill	1 spear	4	0	0	306	1	0	0
Pickles, Sweet	1 spear	32	0	0	160	7	0	0
Pimento, Canned	1 tbsp	3	0	0	2	1	0	0
Relish, Hamburger (Ketchup-Based)	1 tbsp	19	0	0	164	5	0	0
Relish, Hot Dog (Mustard-Based)	1 tbsp	14	0	0	164	4	0	0
Relish, Sweet	1 tbsp	20	0	0	122	5	0	0
Salsa, Ready-to-Serve	1 tbsp	4	0	0	96	1	0	0
Sauerkraut, Canned	1 cup	27	0	0	939	6	4	1
Soy Sauce (Tamari)	1 tbsp	11	0	0	1005	1	0	2
Soy Sauce, Low-Sodium	1 tbsp	8	0	0	533	1	0	1
Vanilla Extract	1 tbsp	37	0	0	1	2	0	0
Vanilla Extract, Imitation, w/Alcohol	1 tbsp	31	0	0	1	0	0	0
Vanilla Extract, Imitation, w/o Alcohol	1 tbsp	7	0	0	0	2	0	0
Vinegar, Balsamic	1 tbsp	14	0	0	4	3	0	0
Vinegar, Cider	1 tbsp	3	0	0	1	0	0	0
Vinegar, Distilled	1 tbsp	3	0	0	0	0	0	0
Vinegar, Red Wine	1 tbsp	3	0	0	1	0	0	0
GRAVIES								
Au Jus, Canned	1 cup	38	0	0	119	6	0	3
Beef, Canned, Ready-to-Serve	1 cup	123	5	3	1305	11	1	9
Chicken, Canned, Ready-to-Serve	1 cup	188	14	3	1009	13	1	5
Meat or Poultry, Low-Sodium, Prepared	1 cup	125	6	2	42	15	1	9
Mushroom, Canned	1 cup	119	6	1	1357	13	1	3
Turkey, Canned, Ready-to-Serve	1 cup	121	5	1	1373	12	1	6
SAUCES								
Barbecue Sauce	2 tbsp	47	0	0	265	11	0	0
Cheese Sauce, Ready-to-Serve	2 tbsp	55	4	2	261	2	0	2
Cocktail Sauce	2 tbsp	37	0	0	295	8	1	0
Duck Sauce	2 tbsp	81	0	0	150	20	0	0
Fish Sauce	2 tbsp	13	0	0	2826	1	0	2
Hoisin Sauce	2 tbsp	70	1	0	517	14	1	1
Hot Sauce, Pepper	1 tsp	1	0	0	124	0	0	0
Oyster Sauce	2 tbsp	18	0	0	984	4	0	0
Pasta, Spaghetti/Marinara Sauce	1/2 cup	65	2	0	553	10	2	2
Pizza Sauce, Canned	1/2 cup	68	1	1	233	11	3	3
Plum Sauce	2 tbsp	70	0	0	204	16	0	0
Steak Sauce	2 tbsp	32	0	0	560	7	1	0

	SERVING SIZE	CALORIES	TOTAL FAT (G)	SAT FAT (G)	SODIUM (MG)	CARBS (G)	FIBER (G)	PROTEIN (G)
Sweet & Sour Sauce	2 tbsp	52	0	0	130	13	0	0
Tartar Sauce, Ready-to-Serve	2 tbsp	63	5	1	200	3	0	0
Teriyaki Sauce	2 tbsp	32	0	0	1380	6	0	2
Worcestershire Sauce	2 tbsp	27	0	0	333	7	0	0

Dairy & Dairy Alternatives

CHEESES

	SERVING SIZE	CALORIES	TOTAL FAT (G)	SAT FAT (G)	SODIUM (MG)	CARBS (G)	FIBER (G)	PROTEIN (G)
American	1 slice (21 g)	69	5	3	270	2	0	4
American or Cheddar, Fat-Free	1 slice (21 g)	31	0	0	321	3	0	5
American, Reduced-Fat	1 slice (21 g)	50	3	2	333	2	0	4
American, Spread	1 oz	82	6	4	461	2	0	5
Blue	1 oz	100	8	5	395	1	0	6
Blue	1/4 cup	119	10	6	471	1	0	7
Brick	1 slice (28 g)	104	8	5	157	1	0	7
Brie	1 oz	95	8	5	178	0	0	6
Camembert	1 cup	738	60	38	2071	1	0	49
Camembert	1 oz	85	7	4	239	0	0	6
Caraway	1 oz	107	8	5	196	1	0	7
Cheddar	1 slice (28 g)	114	9	6	176	0	0	7
Cheddar or Colby, Low-Fat, Shredded	1 cup	195	8	5	692	2	0	28
Cheddar, Imitation	1 slice	50	3	2	282	2	0	4
Cheddar, Shredded	1 cup	455	37	24	702	1	0	28
Cheshire	1 oz	110	9	6	198	1	0	7
Colby	1 slice (28 g)	110	9	6	169	1	0	7
Colby, Shredded	1 cup	445	36	23	683	3	0	27
Cottage, Low-Fat, 1% Milk	1 cup	163	2	1	918	6	0	28
Cottage, Nonfat	1 cup	104	0	0	479	10	0	15
Cottage, Reduced-Fat, 2% Milk	1 cup	194	6	2	746	8	0	27
Cottage, w/Fruit	1 cup	219	9	5	777	10	0	24
Cream Cheese	1 cup	793	79	45	745	9	0	14
Cream Cheese	1 tbsp	50	5	3	47	1	0	1
Cream Cheese, Fat-Free	1 cup	207	3	2	2022	22	0	45
Cream Cheese, Fat-Free	1 tbsp	19	0	0	126	1	0	3
Cream Cheese, Low-Fat	1 cup	482	37	22	1128	20	0	19
Cream Cheese, Low-Fat	1 tbsp	30	2	1	71	1	0	1
Edam	1 oz	101	8	5	274	0	0	7
Feta	1 oz	75	6	4	316	1	0	4

	SERVING SIZE	CALORIES	TOTAL FAT (G)	SAT FAT (G)	SODIUM (MG)	CARBS (G)	FIBER (G)	PROTEIN (G)
Feta, Crumbled	1/4 cup	99	8	6	419	2	0	5
Fondue	1/2 cup	247	15	9	143	4	0	15
Fontina	1 oz	110	9	5	227	0	0	7
Fontina, Shredded	1 cup	420	34	21	864	2	0	28
Goat, Hard	1 oz	128	10	7	98	1	0	9
Goat, Semisoft	1 oz	103	8	6	146	1	0	6
Goat, Soft	1 oz	76	6	4	104	0	0	5
Gouda	1 oz	101	8	5	232	1	0	7
Gruyere	1 oz	117	9	5	95	0	0	8
Gruyere, Shredded	1 cup	446	35	20	363	0	0	32
Limburger	1 oz	93	8	5	227	0	0	6
Mexican Blend, Shredded	1 cup	401	32	19	780	2	0	26
Monterey, Low-Fat, Shredded	1 cup	350	24	16	637	1	0	32
Monterey, Shredded	1 cup	421	34	22	606	1	0	28
Mozzarella	1 oz	90	7	4	118	1	0	6
Mozzarella, Nonfat, Shredded	1 cup	159	0	0	840	4	2	36
Mozzarella, Part-Skim	1 oz	72	5	3	175	1	0	7
Mozzarella, Part-Skim, Shredded	1 cup	341	23	12	737	4	0	29
Mozzarella, Shredded	1 cup	336	25	15	702	2	0	25
Muenster	1 slice	104	9	5	178	0	0	7
Muenster, Shredded	1 cup	416	34	22	710	1	0	26
Muenster, Low-Fat, Shredded	1 cup	306	20	12	678	4	0	28
Neufchatel	1 oz	72	6	4	95	1	0	3
Parmesan, Grated	1 cup	431	29	17	1529	4	0	38
Parmesan, Grated	1 tbsp	22	1	1	76	0	0	2
Parmesan, Hard	1 oz	111	7	5	454	1	0	10
Parmesan, Reduced-Fat, Grated	1 cup	265	20	13	1529	1	0	20
Parmesan, Reduced-Fat, Grated	1 tbsp	13	1	1	76	0	0	1
Pimiento	1 slice	79	7	4	300	0	0	5
Port du Salut, Diced	1 oz	100	8	5	151	0	0	7
Provolone	1 slice	98	7	5	245	1	0	7
Provolone, Reduced-Fat	1 slice	77	5	3	245	1	0	7
Queso Anejo	1 oz	106	8	5	321	1	0	6
Queso Anejo, Crumbled	1 cup	492	40	25	1493	6	0	28
Ricotta, Part-Skim	1 cup	339	19	12	308	13	0	28
Ricotta, Part-Skim	1 cup	339	19	12	308	13	0	28
Ricotta, Whole	1 cup	428	32	20	207	7	0	28

	SERVING SIZE	CALORIES	TOTAL FAT (G)	SAT FAT (G)	SODIUM (MG)	CARBS (G)	FIBER (G)	PROTEIN (G)
Romano	1 oz	110	8	5	340	1	0	9
Roquefort	1 oz	105	9	5	513	1	0	6
Swiss	1 slice	92	7	4	440	1	0	6
Swiss, Low-Fat, Shredded	1 cup	187	6	4	281	4	0	31
Swiss, Shredded	1 cup	410	30	19	207	6	0	29
MILK								
Buttermilk	1 cup	152	8	5	257	12	0	8
Buttermilk, Low-Fat	1 cup	98	2	1	257	12	0	8
Buttermilk, Whole	1 cup	152	8	5	257	12	0	8
Chocolate	1 cup	208	8	5	150	26	2	8
Chocolate, Low-Fat (1%)	1 cup	158	3	2	153	26	1	8
Chocolate, Reduced-Fat (2%)	1 cup	190	5	3	165	30	2	7
Chocolate, Whole	1 cup	208	8	5	150	26	2	8
Condensed, Sweetened	1 cup	982	27	17	389	166	0	24
Cream, Half & Half	2 tbsp	39	3	2	12	1	0	1
Cream, Half & Half, Fat-Free	2 tbsp	17	0	0	29	3	0	1
Cream, Heavy Whipping, Fluid	1 cup	821	88	55	90	7	0	5
Cream, Light	2 tbsp	59	6	4	12	1	0	1
Cream, Light Whipping, Fluid	1 cup	698	74	46	81	7	0	5
Eggnog	1 cup	224	11	7	137	20	0	12
Evaporated, Nonfat	1 cup	200	1	0	294	29	0	19
Evaporated, Whole	1 cup	338	19	12	267	25	0	17
Milk, Cow Low-Fat (1%)	1 cup	102	2	2	107	12	0	8
Milk, Nonfat (Fat-Free/Skim)	1 cup	83	0	0	103	12	0	8
Milk, Reduced-Fat (2%)	1 cup	122	5	3	115	12	0	8
Milk, Whole (3.25%)	1 cup	149	8	5	105	12	0	8
Milk, Goat	1 cup	168	10	7	122	11	0	9
Powdered	1 cup	635	34	21	475	49	0	34
Powdered, Nonfat, Instant	1/3 cup	82	0	0	126	12	0	8
Powdered, Whole	1 cup	635	34	21	475	49	0	34
MILKSHAKES								
Chocolate, Thick	8 fl oz	270	6	4	252	48	1	7
Vanilla, Thick	8 fl oz	254	7	4	216	40	0	9
SOUR CREAMS								
Fat-Free	1 tbsp	9	0	0	17	2	0	0
Reduced-Fat	1 tbsp	22	2	1	8	1	0	1
Regular	1 tbsp	23	2	1	10	0	0	0

common foods

	SERVING SIZE	CALORIES	TOTAL FAT (G)	SAT FAT (G)	SODIUM (MG)	CARBS (G)	FIBER (G)	PROTEIN (G)
YOGURT								
Fruit, Low-Fat	1 cup	238	3	2	148	42	0	11
Fruit, Nonfat	1 cup	233	0	0	142	47	0	11
Plain, Low-Fat	1 cup	154	4	2	172	17	0	13
Plain, Nonfat (Skim)	1 cup	137	0	0	189	19	0	14
Plain, Whole	1 cup	149	8	5	113	11	0	9
Vanilla, Low-Fat	1 cup	208	3	2	162	34	0	12
DAIRY ALTERNATIVES								
Coconut Milk, Canned	1 cup	445	48	43	29	6	n/a	5
Creamer, Liquid	1 tbsp	38	2	0	12	5	0	0
Creamer, Powdered	1 tbsp	45	2	2	18	7	0	0
Mozzarella Substitute	1 slice	70	3	1	194	7	0	3
Mozzarella Substitute, Shredded	1 cup	280	14	4	774	27	0	13
Rice Drink, Unsweetened	8 fl oz	113	2	0	94	22	1	1
Sour Cream, Imitation, Cultured	2 tbsp	60	6	5	29	2	0	1
Soymilk, All Flavors	1 cup	109	5	1	122	8	1	7
Soymilk, All Flavors, Low-Fat	1 cup	104	2	0	90	17	2	4
Soymilk, All Flavors, Nonfat	1 cup	68	0	0	139	10	0	6
Soymilk, All Flavors, Unsweetened	1 cup	80	4	1	90	4	1	7
## Desserts								
CAKES								
Angel Food	1 piece (28 g)	72	0	0	210	16	0	2
Boston Cream Pie	1 piece (92 g)	232	8	2	234	39	1	2
Cheesecake	1 piece (80 g)	257	18	8	166	20	0	4
Chocolate, w/Chocolate Frosting	1 piece (138 g)	537	28	8	480	73	4	5
Chocolate, w/o Frosting, Homemade	1 piece (95 g)	352	14	5	299	51	2	5
Coffeecake, Cheese	1 piece (76 g)	258	12	4	258	34	1	5
Coffeecake, Cinnamon, w/Crumb Topping	1 piece (63 g)	263	15	4	221	29	1	4
Fruitcake	1 piece (43 g)	139	4	0	138	26	2	1

	SERVING SIZE	CALORIES	TOTAL FAT (G)	SAT FAT (G)	SODIUM (MG)	CARBS (G)	FIBER (G)	PROTEIN (G)
Gingerbread	1 piece (74 g)	263	12	3	242	36	n/a	3
Pineapple Upside-Down, Homemade	1 piece (115 g)	367	14	3	367	58	1	4
Pound	1 piece (30 g)	116	6	3	119	15	0	2
Pound, Fat-Free	1 piece (34 g)	96	0	0	116	21	0	2
Shortcake, Biscuit-Type, Homemade	1 oz	98	4	1	143	14	n/a	2
Sponge	1 piece (38 g)	110	1	0	54	23	0	2
White, w/Coconut Frosting, Homemade	1 piece (112 g)	399	12	4	318	71	1	5
White, w/o Frosting, Homemade	1 piece (74 g)	264	9	2	242	42	1	4
Yellow, w/Chocolate Frosting	1 piece (144 g)	546	26	8	446	80	n/a	5
Yellow, w/Vanilla Frosting	1 piece (64 g)	239	9	2	220	38	0	2
Yellow, w/o Frosting, Homemade	1 piece (68 g)	245	10	3	233	36	0	4
COOKIES & BARS								
Brownies	2-3/4" x 7/8" sq	227	9	2	144	36	1	3
Butter	1 cookie	23	1	1	12	3	0	0
Chocolate Chip	1 cookie	48	2	1	32	7	0	1
Chocolate Sandwich, w/Crème Filing	1 cookie	54	2	1	58	8	0	1
Chocolate Wafers	1 wafer	26	1	0	41	4	0	0
Coconut Macaroons	1 cookie	97	3	3	59	17	0	1
Fig Bars	1 cookie	56	1	0	56	11	1	1
Fortune	1 cookie	30	0	0	22	7	0	0
Fudge, Cake-Type	1 cookie	73	1	0	40	16	1	1
Gingersnaps	1 cookie	29	1	0	39	5	0	0
Marshmallow, Chocolate-Coated	1 cookie	118	5	1	47	19	1	1
Molasses	1 cookie	138	4	1	147	24	0	2
Oatmeal	1 cookie	67	3	1	90	10	n/a	1
Oatmeal, w/Raisins	1 cookie	65	2	0	81	10	n/a	1

common foods

	SERVING SIZE	CALORIES	TOTAL FAT (G)	SAT FAT (G)	SODIUM (MG)	CARBS (G)	FIBER (G)	PROTEIN (G)
Peanut Butter	1 cookie	95	5	1	104	12	n/a	2
Peanut Butter Sandwich	1 cookie	67	3	1	52	9	0	1
Shortbread, Plain	1 cookie	40	2	0	36	5	0	0
Sugar Wafers, w/Crème Filling	1 wafer	51	2	1	10	7	0	0
Vanilla Wafers	1 wafer	28	1	0	18	4	0	0
DOUGHNUTS								
Cake-Type, Chocolate	1 doughnut	250	12	3	238	34	1	3
Cake-Type, Plain	1 doughnut	297	17	5	395	32	1	4
Cake-Type, Plain, Chocolate Frosted	1 mini	81	5	2	59	9	0	1
Crème Filled	1 doughnut	307	21	5	263	26	1	5
French Crullers, Glazed	1 cruller	169	8	2	141	24	0	1
Glazed	1 hole	52	2	1	41	7	0	1
Jelly Filled	1 doughnut	289	16	4	204	33	1	5
Raised, Sugared or Glazed	1 doughnut	192	10	3	181	23	1	2
FROZEN NOVELTIES								
Creamsicle, No Sugar Added	1 pop	25	0	0	18	6	0	1
Creamsicle, Sugar-Free	1 pop	20	1	1	2	5	3	1
Fruit & Juice Bars	1 bar	33	0	0	2	8	0	0
Fudgesicle Bars, Fat-Free	1 bar	65	0	0	48	14	1	3
Fudgesicle Pops, No Sugar Added	1 pop	88	1	0	86	19	1	3
Ice Cream Bar, Chocolate Covered	1 bar	166	12	7	34	12	0	2
Ice Cream Cone, Chocolate Covered, w/Nuts	1 cone	340	21	11	90	33	1	5
Ice Cream Sandwich, Light Ice Cream, Vanilla	1 serving	130	2	1	102	28	0	3
Italian Ice	1/2 cup	61	0	0	5	16	0	0
Popsicle	1 pop	41	0	0	4	10	0	0
Popsicle, Sugar-Free, Orange, Cherry, or Grape	1 pop	12	0	0	6	3	0	0
GELATINS, PUDDINGS & CUSTARDS								
Egg Custard, Baked	1/2 cup	147	6	3	86	16	0	7
Flan, Caramel Custard	1/2 cup	222	6	3	81	35	0	7
Gelatin, Prepared w/Water	1/2 cup	84	0	0	101	19	0	2
Gelatin, Reduced-Calorie, Prepared w/Water	1/2 cup	23	0	0	56	5	0	1
Mousse, Chocolate	1/2 cup	455	32	18	77	32	1	8
Pudding, Chocolate, Dry Mix, Instant, Prepared w/Whole Milk	1/2 cup	163	5	3	417	28	1	5

	SERVING SIZE	CALORIES	TOTAL FAT (G)	SAT FAT (G)	SODIUM (MG)	CARBS (G)	FIBER (G)	PROTEIN (G)
Pudding, Coconut, Dry Mix, Instant, Prepared w/Whole Milk	1/2 cup	172	5	3	362	28	0	4
Pudding, Lemon, Dry Mix, Instant, Prepared w/Whole Milk	1/2 cup	169	4	3	392	30	0	4
Pudding, Vanilla, Dry Mix, Instant, Prepared w/Whole Milk	1/2 cup	162	4	2	406	28	0	4
ICE CREAMS & SHERBETS								
Chocolate	1/2 cup	143	7	4	50	19	1	3
Chocolate, Light, No Sugar Added	1/2 cup	125	4	3	54	19	1	3
Chocolate or French Vanilla, Soft-Serve	1/2 cup	191	11	6	52	19	1	4
Sherbet, Orange	1/2 cup	107	1	1	34	22	1	1
Strawberry	1/2 cup	127	6	3	40	18	1	2
Vanilla	1/2 cup	137	7	4	53	16	0	2
Vanilla, Fat-Free	1/2 cup	92	0	0	65	20	1	3
Vanilla, Light	1/2 cup	137	4	2	56	22	0	4
Vanilla, Light, No Sugar Added	1/2 cup	115	5	3	65	15	0	3
Vanilla, Light, Soft-Serve	1/2 cup	111	2	1	62	19	0	4
PASTRIES								
Cinnamon or Honey Buns, Frosted	1 bun	283	16	8	198	32	1	3
Cream Puffs, w/Custard Filling	1 cream puff	335	20	5	443	30	1	9
Croissants, Apple	1 medium (57 g)	145	5	3	156	21	1	4
Croissants, Butter	1 medium (57 g)	231	12	7	198	26	2	5
Croissants, Cheese	1 medium (57 g)	236	12	6	206	27	2	5
Danish, Cheese	1 pastry	266	16	5	229	26	1	6
Danish, Fruit	1 large	527	26	7	503	68	3	8
Éclairs, Custard-Filled w/Chocolate Glaze	1 éclair	293	18	5	377	27	1	7
Puff Pastry, Frozen, Baked	1 shell (40 g)	223	15	2	101	18	1	3
Strudel, Apple	1 piece	195	8	1	111	29	2	2
Sweet Roll, Cheese	1 roll	238	12	4	236	29	1	5
Sweet Rolls, Cinnamon w/Raisins	1 large	309	14	3	252	42	2	5
Toaster Pastry, Fruit, Toasted	1 pastry	209	6	1	181	37	1	2
PIES, CRISPS, CRUSTS & FILLINGS								
Apple Crisp	1/2 cup	227	5	1	495	43	2	2

common foods

	SERVING SIZE	CALORIES	TOTAL FAT (G)	SAT FAT (G)	SODIUM (MG)	CARBS (G)	FIBER (G)	PROTEIN (G)
Apple Pie	1 slice	411	19	5	327	58	n/a	4
Banana Crème Pie, No Bake Mix	1 slice	231	12	6	267	29	1	3
Blueberry Pie	1 slice	360	17	4	272	49	n/a	4
Cherry Pie	1 slice	486	22	5	344	69	n/a	5
Chocolate Crème Pie	1 slice	301	19	5	135	33	2	3
Crust, Cookie-Type, Chocolate, Ready Crust	1 crust (182 g)	881	41	9	915	117	5	11
Crust, Cookie-Type, Graham Cracker, Ready Crust	1 crust (183 g)	917	45	9	604	118	3	9
Crust, Standard-Type, Baked	1 crust (154 g)	782	44	14	719	87	5	10
Crust, Standard-Type, Baked	1 piece (23 g)	121	8	2	125	11	0	1
Dutch Apple Pie	1 slice	397	16	3	274	61	2	3
Egg Custard Pie	1 slice	221	12	2	158	22	2	6
Fillings, Apple, Canned	21 oz	595	1	0	280	155	6	1
Fillings, Blueberry, Canned	1 cup	474	1	0	31	116	7	1
Fillings, Cherry, Canned	21 oz	684	0	0	107	167	4	2
Fillings, Pumpkin Pie Mix, Canned	1 cup	281	0	0	562	71	22	3
Fried Pies, Fruit	5" pie	404	21	3	479	55	3	4
Lemon Meringue Pie	1 slice	362	16	4	307	50	n/a	5
Mince Pie	1 slice	477	18	4	419	79	4	4
Peach Pie	1 slice	261	12	2	227	38	1	2
Pecan Pie	1 slice	503	27	5	320	64	n/a	6
Pumpkin Pie	1 slice	316	14	4	349	41	n/a	7
TOPPINGS								
Butterscotch or Caramel	2 tbsp	103	0	0	143	27	0	1
Chocolate, Fudge-Type	2 tbsp	133	3	2	131	24	1	2
Frosting, Chocolate, Creamy, Ready-to-Eat	2 tbsp	163	7	2	75	26	0	0
Frosting, Cream Cheese-Flavor, Creamy, Ready-to-Eat	2 tbsp	137	6	1	63	22	0	0
Marshmallow Cream	1 oz	91	0	0	23	22	0	0
Nuts in Syrup	2 tbsp	184	9	1	17	24	1	2
Pineapple	2 tbsp	106	0	0	18	28	0	0
Strawberry	2 tbsp	107	0	0	9	28	0	0
Whipped Cream, Imitation, Pressurized, Canned	1/4 cup	46	4	3	11	3	0	0

	SERVING SIZE	CALORIES	TOTAL FAT (G)	SAT FAT (G)	SODIUM (MG)	CARBS (G)	FIBER (G)	PROTEIN (G)
Whipped Cream, Imitation, Semisolid, Frozen	1/4 cup	60	5	4	5	4	0	0
Whipped Cream, Pressurized, Canned	1/4 cup	39	3	2	1	2	0	0

Eggs

	SERVING SIZE	CALORIES	TOTAL FAT (G)	SAT FAT (G)	SODIUM (MG)	CARBS (G)	FIBER (G)	PROTEIN (G)
Substitute, Liquid or Frozen, Fat-Free	1/4 cup	29	0	0	119	1	0	6
White, Fresh	1 large	17	0	0	55	0	0	4
Whole, Fresh	1 large	72	5	2	71	0	0	6
Whole, Fried	1 large	90	7	2	95	0	0	6
Whole, Hard-Boiled	1 large	78	5	2	62	1	0	6
Whole, Poached	1 large	72	5	2	149	0	0	6
Whole, Scrambled	1/2 cup	164	12	4	145	2	0	11
Yolk, Fresh	1 large	55	5	2	8	1	0	3
NON-CHICKEN EGGS								
Duck, Whole, Fresh	1 egg	130	10	3	102	1	0	9
Goose, Whole, Fresh	1 egg	266	19	5	199	2	0	20
Quail, Whole, Fresh	1 egg	14	1	0	13	0	0	1
Turkey, Whole, Fresh	1 egg	135	9	3	119	1	0	11

Fats, Oils, Spreads & Dressings

	SERVING SIZE	CALORIES	TOTAL FAT (G)	SAT FAT (G)	SODIUM (MG)	CARBS (G)	FIBER (G)	PROTEIN (G)
BUTTER								
Salted	1 tbsp	102	12	7	101	0	0	0
Unsalted	1 tbsp	102	12	7	2	0	0	0
Whipped, w/Salt	1 tbsp	67	8	5	78	0	0	0
DRESSINGS								
Blue or Roquefort Cheese	2 tbsp	143	15	2	312	1	0	0
Blue or Roquefort Cheese, Fat-Free	2 tbsp	39	0	0	277	9	1	1
Blue or Roquefort Cheese, Light	2 tbsp	28	1	0	300	4	0	1
Buttermilk, Light	2 tbsp	61	4	0	336	6	0	0
Caesar	2 tbsp	159	17	3	355	1	0	1
Caesar, Fat-Free	2 tbsp	45	0	0	430	10	0	0
Caesar, Low Calorie	2 tbsp	33	1	0	344	6	0	0
Coleslaw	2 tbsp	125	11	2	227	8	0	0
Coleslaw, Reduced-Fat	2 tbsp	112	7	1	544	14	0	0
Creamy, Made w/Sour Cream &/or Buttermilk, Reduced-Calorie	2 tbsp	48	4	1	336	2	0	0
Creamy, Made w/Sour Cream &/or Buttermilk, Reduced-Calorie, Fat-Free	2 tbsp	36	1	0	305	7	0	0

common foods

	SERVING SIZE	CALORIES	TOTAL FAT (G)	SAT FAT (G)	SODIUM (MG)	CARBS (G)	FIBER (G)	PROTEIN (G)
French	2 tbsp	146	14	2	268	5	0	0
French, Fat-Free	2 tbsp	42	0	0	273	10	1	0
French, Reduced-Calorie	2 tbsp	64	4	1	268	9	0	0
French, Reduced-Fat	2 tbsp	71	4	0	268	10	0	0
Honey Mustard	2 tbsp	139	12	2	195	7	0	0
Honey Mustard, Reduced-Calorie	2 tbsp	62	3	0	270	9	0	0
Italian	2 tbsp	86	8	1	299	3	0	0
Italian, Fat-Free	2 tbsp	13	0	0	316	2	0	0
Italian, Reduced-Calorie	2 tbsp	56	6	1	301	2	0	0
Italian, Reduced-Fat	2 tbsp	23	2	0	322	1	0	0
Peppercorn	2 tbsp	151	16	3	296	1	0	0
Ranch	2 tbsp	145	15	2	328	2	0	0
Ranch, Fat-Free	2 tbsp	33	1	0	251	7	0	0
Ranch, Reduced-Fat	2 tbsp	59	4	0	336	6	0	0
Russian	2 tbsp	107	8	1	340	10	0	0
Russian, Reduced-Calorie	2 tbsp	45	1	0	278	9	0	0
Spray-Style, Assorted Flavors	approx. 10 sprays	13	1	0	88	1	0	0
Thousand Island	2 tbsp	118	11	2	276	5	0	0
Thousand Island, Fat-Free	2 tbsp	42	0	0	252	9	1	0
Thousand Island, Reduced-Fat	2 tbsp	59	3	0	287	7	0	0
FATS & SHORTENINGS								
Bacon Grease	1 tbsp	116	13	5	19	0	0	0
Beef Tallow	1 tbsp	115	13	6	0	0	0	0
Chicken Fat	1 tbsp	115	13	4	0	0	0	0
Duck Fat	1 tbsp	113	13	4	0	0	0	0
Goose Fat	1 tbsp	115	13	4	0	0	0	0
Lard	1 tbsp	115	13	5	0	0	0	0
Mutton Tallow	1 tbsp	115	13	6	0	0	0	0
Turkey Fat	1 tbsp	115	13	4	0	0	0	0
Vegetable Shortening	1 tbsp	113	13	3	0	0	0	0
Vegetable Shortening	1 cup	1812	205	51	0	0	0	0
MARGARINES & MARGARINE SUBSTITUTES								
Butter-Margarine Blend	1 tbsp	101	11	2	89	0	0	0
Margarine, Stick, w/Salt	1 tbsp	100	11	2	105	0	0	0
Margarine, Stick, w/o Salt	1 tbsp	102	11	2	0	0	0	0
Margarine-Like Spread w/Yogurt	1 tbsp	88	10	2	83	0	0	0

	SERVING SIZE	CALORIES	TOTAL FAT (G)	SAT FAT (G)	SODIUM (MG)	CARBS (G)	FIBER (G)	PROTEIN (G)
Margarine-Like Spread w/Yogurt, Light	1 tbsp	46	5	1	88	0	0	0
Margarine-Like Vegetable-Oil Spread, Fat-Free, Tub	1 tbsp	6	0	0	85	1	0	0
Margarine-Like Vegetable-Oil Spread, Light, w/Salt	1 tbsp	26	3	0	110	0	0	0
Margarine-Like Vegetable-Oil Spread, Light, w/o Salt	1 tbsp	22	2	0	0	0	0	0
Margarine-Like Vegetable-Oil Spread, Stick/Tub/Bottle, w/Salt	1 tbsp	75	8	1	100	0	0	0
Tub Margarine, Light	1 tbsp	59	7	1	90	0	0	0
Tub Margarine, w/Salt	1 tbsp	101	11	2	93	0	0	0
Tub Margarine, w/o Salt	1 tbsp	101	11	2	4	0	0	0
OILS								
Almond	1 tbsp	120	14	1	0	0	0	0
Avocado	1 tbsp	124	14	2	0	0	0	0
Canola	1 tbsp	124	14	1	0	0	0	0
Cocoa Butter	1 tbsp	120	14	8	0	0	0	0
Coconut	1 tbsp	117	14	12	0	0	0	0
Cottonseed, Salad or Cooking	1 tbsp	120	14	4	0	0	0	0
Flaxseed	1 tbsp	120	14	1	0	0	0	0
Grapeseed	1 tbsp	120	14	1	0	0	0	0
Hazelnut	1 tbsp	120	14	1	0	0	0	0
Olive, Salad or Cooking	1 tbsp	119	14	2	0	0	0	0
Palm	1 tbsp	120	14	7	0	0	0	0
Peanut, Salad or Cooking	1 tbsp	119	14	2	0	0	0	0
Safflower, Salad or Cooking, High Oleic	1 tbsp	120	14	1	0	0	0	0
Sesame, Salad or Cooking	1 tbsp	120	14	2	0	0	0	0
Soybean, Salad or Cooking	1 tbsp	120	14	2	0	0	0	0
Sunflower	1 tbsp	120	14	1	0	0	0	0
Vegetable	1 tbsp	124	14	1	0	0	0	0
Walnut	1 tbsp	120	14	1	0	0	0	0
Wheat Germ	1 tbsp	120	14	3	0	0	0	0
Flours, Grains & Pasta								
FLOURS								
Arrowroot	1 cup	457	0	0	3	113	4	0
Barley	1 cup	511	2	0	6	110	15	16
Buckwheat, Whole-Groat	1 cup	402	4	1	13	85	12	15

common foods

	SERVING SIZE	CALORIES	TOTAL FAT (G)	SAT FAT (G)	SODIUM (MG)	CARBS (G)	FIBER (G)	PROTEIN (G)
Corn, Whole-Grain	1 cup	422	5	1	6	90	9	8
Cornmeal	1 cup	581	3	0	11	125	6	11
Cornmeal, Whole-Grain	1 cup	442	4	1	43	94	9	10
Millet	1 cup	444	5	1	5	87	4	13
Rice, Brown	1 cup	574	4	1	13	121	7	11
Rice, White	1 cup	578	2	1	0	127	4	9
Rye, Dark	1 cup	416	3	0	3	88	30	20
Rye, Light	1 cup	364	1	0	2	78	8	10
Rye, Medium	1 cup	356	2	0	2	77	12	11
Semolina	1 cup	601	2	0	2	122	7	21
Sesame, Low-Fat	1 oz	94	0	0	11	10	n/a	14
Sesame, Partially Defatted	1 oz	108	3	0	12	10	n/a	11
Sorghum	1 cup	437	4	1	5	94	8	10
Soy, Defatted	1 cup	347	1	0	21	40	18	49
Soy, Full-Fat	1 cup	366	17	3	11	30	8	29
Soy, Low-Fat	1 cup	330	8	1	8	31	14	40
Sunflower Seed, Partially Defatted	1 cup	209	1	0	2	23	3	31
Triticale, Whole-Grain	1 cup	439	2	0	3	95	19	17
Wheat, White, All-Purpose	1 cup	455	1	0	3	95	3	13
Wheat, White, Bread	1 cup	495	2	0	3	99	3	16
Wheat, White, Cake	1 cup	496	1	0	3	107	2	11
Wheat, Whole-Grain	1 cup	408	3	1	2	86	13	16
GRAINS								
Amaranth, Cooked	1 cup	251	4	n/a	15	46	5	9
Amaranth, Dry	1/2 cup	358	7	1	4	63	6	13
Barley, Hulled, Dry	1/2 cup	326	2	0	11	68	16	11
Barley, Pearled, Cooked	1 cup	193	1	0	5	44	6	4
Barley, Pearled, Dry	1/2 cup	352	1	0	9	78	16	10
Buckwheat, Dry	1/2 cup	292	3	1	1	61	9	11
Buckwheat, Groats, Roasted, (Kasha), Cooked	1 cup	155	1	0	7	33	5	6
Buckwheat, Groats, Roasted, (Kasha), Dry	1/2 cup	284	2	0	9	61	8	10
Bulgur, Cooked	1 cup	151	0	0	9	34	8	6
Bulgur, Dry	1/2 cup	239	1	0	12	53	13	9
Kamut, Cooked	1 cup	251	2	n/a	10	52	7	11
Kamut, Dry	1/2 cup	313	2	0	6	65	8	14

	SERVING SIZE	CALORIES	TOTAL FAT (G)	SAT FAT (G)	SODIUM (MG)	CARBS (G)	FIBER (G)	PROTEIN (G)
Millet, Cooked	1 cup	207	2	0	3	41	2	6
Millet, Dry	1/2 cup	378	4	1	5	73	9	11
Oat Bran, Cooked	1 cup	88	2	0	2	25	6	7
Oat Bran, Dry	1/4 cup	58	2	0	1	16	4	4
Oats, Dry	1/2 cup	303	5	1	2	52	8	13
Oats, Regular & Quick, Cooked	1 cup	166	4	1	9	28	4	6
Quinoa, Cooked	1 cup	222	4	n/a	13	39	5	8
Quinoa, Dry	1/2 cup	313	5	1	4	55	6	12
PASTA								
Couscous, Cooked	1 cup	176	0	0	8	36	2	6
Couscous, Dry	1/2 cup	325	1	0	9	67	4	11
Macaroni, Elbow, Cooked	1 cup	221	1	0	1	43	3	8
Macaroni, Elbow, Dry	1/2 cup	195	1	0	3	39	2	7
Macaroni, Vegetable, Spiral, Cooked	1 cup	172	0	0	8	36	6	6
Macaroni, Vegetable, Spiral, Dry	1/2 cup	154	0	0	18	31	2	6
Macaroni, Whole-Wheat, Elbow, Cooked	1 cup	174	1	0	4	37	4	7
Macaroni, Whole-Wheat, Elbow, Dry	1/2 cup	183	1	0	4	39	4	8
Noodles, Chinese, Cellophane or Long Rice, Dry	1/2 cup	246	0	0	7	60	0	0
Noodles, Chinese, Chow Mein	1 cup	237	14	2	198	26	2	4
Noodles, Egg, Cooked w/o Salt	1 cup	221	3	1	8	40	2	7
Noodles, Egg, Cooked w/Salt	1 cup	221	3	1	264	40	2	7
Noodles, Egg, Spinach, Cooked	1 cup	211	3	1	19	39	4	8
Noodles, Flat, Crunchy, Chinese Restaurant	1 cup	234	14	2	170	23	1	5
Noodles, Japanese, Soba, Cooked	1 cup	113	0	0	68	24	n/a	6
Noodles, Japanese, Somen, Cooked	1 cup	231	0	0	283	48	n/a	7
Pasta w/Meatballs in Tomato Sauce, Canned	1 cup	273	13	5	742	28	7	11
Pasta w/Sliced Franks in Tomato Sauce, Canned	1 cup	227	6	2	600	32	4	11
Pasta w/Tomato Sauce, Canned	1 cup	167	1	0	647	34	2	5
Pasta, Corn, Cooked	1 cup	176	1	0	0	39	7	4
Pasta, Corn, Dry	1/2 cup	187	1	0	2	42	6	4
Pasta, Fresh, Refrigerated	4.5 oz	369	3	0	33	70	n/a	14
Pasta, Fresh, Refrigerated, Cooked	2 oz	75	1	0	3	14	n/a	3
Pasta, Fresh, Refrigerated, Spinach	4.5 oz	370	3	1	35	71	n/a	14

common foods

	SERVING SIZE	CALORIES	TOTAL FAT (G)	SAT FAT (G)	SODIUM (MG)	CARBS (G)	FIBER (G)	PROTEIN (G)
Pasta, Fresh, Refrigerated, Spinach, Cooked	2 oz	74	1	0	3	14	n/a	3
Pasta, Homemade, w/Egg, Cooked	2 oz	74	1	0	47	13	n/a	3
Pasta, Homemade, w/o Egg, Cooked	2 oz	71	1	0	42	14	n/a	2
Ravioli, Cheese-Filled, Canned	1 cup	191	4	2	741	33	3	6
Ravioli, Meat-Filled, w/Tomato or Meat Sauce, Canned	1 cup	259	9	4	927	36	4	9
Rice Noodles, Cooked	1 cup	192	0	0	33	44	2	2
Spaghetti, Cooked w/Salt	1 cup	220	1	0	183	43	3	8
Spaghetti, Cooked w/o Salt	1 cup	221	1	0	1	43	3	8
Spaghetti, Spinach, Cooked	1 cup	182	1	0	20	37	n/a	6
Spaghetti, Whole-Wheat, Cooked	1 cup	174	1	0	4	37	6	7
Tortellini, w/Cheese Filling, Fresh	1 cup	332	8	4	665	51	2	15
RICE								
Long-Grain, Brown, Cooked	1 cup	216	2	0	10	45	4	5
Long-Grain, Instant, White, Cooked	1 cup	193	1	0	7	41	1	4
Long-Grain, Instant, White, Dry	1/2 cup	181	0	0	5	39	1	4
Long-Grain, Parboiled, White, Cooked	1 cup	194	1	0	3	41	1	5
Long-Grain, Parboiled, White, Dry	1/2 cup	346	1	0	2	75	2	7
Long-Grain, White, Cooked	1 cup	205	0	0	2	45	1	4
Long-Grain, White, Dry	1/2 cup	338	1	0	5	74	1	7
Medium-Grain, Brown, Cooked	1 cup	218	2	0	2	46	4	5
Medium-Grain, Brown, Dry	1/2 cup	344	3	1	4	72	3	7
Medium-Grain, White, Cooked	1 cup	242	0	0	0	53	1	4
Medium-Grain, White, Dry	1/2 cup	351	1	0	1	77	1	6
Short-Grain, White, Cooked	1 cup	242	0	0	0	53	n/a	4
Short-Grain, White, Dry	1/2 cup	358	1	0	1	79	3	7
Sticky (Sweet/Glutinous), White, Cooked	1 cup	169	0	0	9	37	2	4
Sticky (Sweet/Glutinous), White, Dry	1/2 cup	342	1	0	6	76	3	6
Wild Rice, Cooked	1 cup	166	1	0	5	35	3	7
Wild Rice, Dry	1/2 cup	286	1	0	6	60	5	12
Rye, Dry	1/2 cup	286	1	0	2	64	13	9
Spelt, Cooked	1 cup	246	2	n/a	10	51	8	11
Spelt, Dry	1/2 cup	294	2	0	7	61	9	13
Teff, Cooked	1 cup	255	2	n/a	20	50	7	10
Teff, Dry	1/2 cup	354	2	0	12	71	8	13
Triticale, Dry	1/2 cup	323	2	0	5	69	n/a	13

	SERVING SIZE	CALORIES	TOTAL FAT (G)	SAT FAT (G)	SODIUM (MG)	CARBS (G)	FIBER (G)	PROTEIN (G)
Wheat, Bran	1/4 cup	31	1	0	0	9	6	2
Wheat, Durum, Dry	1/2 cup	325	2	0	2	68	n/a	13
Wheat, Germ	1/4 cup	104	3	0	3	15	4	7
Wheat, Sprouted	1 cup	214	1	0	17	46	1	8
Wheat Berries, Hard Red Spring, Dry	1/2 cup	316	2	0	2	65	12	15
Wheat Berries, Hard Red Winter, Dry	1/2 cup	314	1	0	2	68	12	12
Wheat Berries, Hard White, Dry	1/2 cup	328	2	0	2	73	12	11
Wheat Berries, Soft Red Winter, Dry	1/2 cup	278	1	0	2	62	11	9
Wheat Berries, Soft White, Dry	1/2 cup	286	2	0	2	63	11	9

Fruit

	SERVING SIZE	CALORIES	TOTAL FAT (G)	SAT FAT (G)	SODIUM (MG)	CARBS (G)	FIBER (G)	PROTEIN (G)
Apples, Canned, Sweetened, Slices	1 cup	137	1	0	6	34	4	0
Apples, Dried	1/2 cup	104	0	0	37	28	4	0
Apples, Dried	1 ring	16	0	0	6	4	1	0
Apples, w/Skin	1 medium	95	0	0	2	25	4	0
Apples, w/Skin, Quartered or Chopped	1 cup	65	0	0	1	17	3	0
Apples, w/Skin, Sliced	1 cup	57	0	0	1	15	3	0
Apples, w/o Skin	1 medium	77	0	0	0	21	2	0
Apples, w/o Skin, Sliced, Cooked	1 cup	91	1	0	2	23	4	0
Applesauce, Sweetened	1 cup	194	0	0	71	51	3	0
Applesauce, Unsweetened	1 cup	102	0	0	5	27	3	0
Apricots, Canned in Heavy Syrup, Halved	1 cup	214	0	0	10	55	4	1
Apricots, Canned in Heavy Syrup, Halved, Drained	1 cup	182	0	0	9	47	6	1
Apricots, Canned in Juice, Halved	1 cup	117	0	0	10	30	4	2
Apricots, Canned in Light Syrup, Halved	1 cup	159	0	0	10	42	4	1
Apricots, Canned in Water, Halved	1 cup	66	0	0	7	16	4	2
Apricots, Dried	1/2 cup	157	0	0	7	41	5	2
Apricots, Dried	1 piece	17	0	0	1	4	1	0
Apricots, Fresh	1 whole	17	0	0	0	4	1	0
Bananas	1 medium	105	0	0	1	27	3	1
Bananas, Chips	1/2 cup	173	1	0	2	44	5	2
Bananas, Sliced	1 cup	134	0	0	2	34	4	2
Blackberries	1 cup	62	1	0	1	14	8	2
Blackberries, Canned in Heavy Syrup	1 cup	236	0	0	8	59	9	3
Blackberries, Frozen, Unsweetened	1 cup	97	1	0	2	24	8	2
Blueberries	1 cup	84	0	0	1	21	4	1
Blueberries, Canned in Heavy Syrup	1 cup	225	1	0	8	56	4	2

common foods

	SERVING SIZE	CALORIES	TOTAL FAT (G)	SAT FAT (G)	SODIUM (MG)	CARBS (G)	FIBER (G)	PROTEIN (G)
Blueberries, Canned in Light Syrup, Drained	1 cup	215	1	0	7	55	6	3
Blueberries, Frozen, Sweetened	1 cup	196	0	0	2	50	5	1
Blueberries, Frozen, Unsweetened	1 cup	79	1	0	2	19	4	1
Boysenberries, Canned in Heavy Syrup	1 cup	225	0	0	8	57	7	3
Boysenberries, Frozen, Unsweetened	1 cup	66	0	0	1	16	7	1
Cherries, Maraschino, Canned, Drained	1 cherry	8	0	0	0	2	0	0
Cherries, Sour	1 cup	78	0	0	5	19	2	2
Cherries, Sour, Frozen, Unsweetened	1 cup	71	1	0	2	17	2	1
Cherries, Sweet	1 cup	97	0	0	0	25	3	2
Cherries, Sweet, Canned in Juice	1 cup	135	0	0	8	35	4	2
Cherries, Sweet, Frozen, Sweetened	1 cup	231	0	0	3	58	5	3
Clementines	1 fruit	35	0	n/a	1	9	1	1
Coconut, Dried, Sweetened, Flaked	1 cup	388	24	22	242	44	8	3
Coconut, Dried, Toasted	1 oz	168	13	12	10	13	n/a	2
Coconut, Dried, Unsweetened	1 oz	187	18	16	10	7	5	2
Coconut, Shredded	1 cup	283	27	24	16	12	7	3
Cranberries, Dried, Sweetened	1/3 cup	123	1	0	1	33	2	0
Cranberries, Whole	1 cup	46	0	0	2	12	5	0
Currants, Red & White	1 cup	63	0	0	1	15	5	2
Dates, Pitted	1 date	20	0	0	0	5	1	0
Elderberries	1 cup	106	1	0	9	27	10	1
Figs, Dried	1/4 cup	93	0	0	4	24	4	1
Figs, Medium	1 fig	37	0	0	1	10	1	0
Fruit Cocktail, Canned in Heavy Syrup	1 cup	181	0	0	15	47	2	1
Fruit Cocktail, Canned in Juice	1 cup	109	0	0	9	28	2	1
Fruit Cocktail, Canned in Light Syrup	1 cup	138	0	0	15	36	2	1
Gooseberries	1 cup	66	1	0	2	15	6	1
Grapefruit, Pink & Red, Sections, w/Juice	1 cup	69	0	0	0	17	3	1
Grapefruit, Pink, Red, White	1/2 large	53	0	0	0	13	2	1
Grapefruit, Sections, Canned in Juice	1 cup	92	0	0	17	23	1	2
Grapefruit, Sections, Canned in Light Syrup	1 cup	152	0	0	5	39	1	1
Grapefruit, Sections, Canned in Water	1 cup	88	0	0	5	22	1	1
Grapes, Green or Red	1 cup	62	0	0	2	16	1	1
Grapes, Green or Red	10 grapes	34	0	0	1	9	0	0
Grapes, Seedless, Canned in Heavy Syrup	1 cup	195	0	0	13	50	2	1

	SERVING SIZE	CALORIES	TOTAL FAT (G)	SAT FAT (G)	SODIUM (MG)	CARBS (G)	FIBER (G)	PROTEIN (G)
Grapes, Seedless, Canned in Water	1 cup	98	0	0	15	25	1	1
Guavas	1 cup	112	2	0	3	24	9	4
Guavas	1 fruit	37	1	0	1	8	3	1
Kiwi	1 fruit	42	0	0	2	10	2	1
Kumquats	1 fruit	13	0	0	2	3	1	0
Lemon	1 fruit	17	0	0	1	5	2	1
Lime	1 fruit	20	0	0	1	7	2	0
Loganberries, Frozen	1 cup	81	0	0	1	19	8	2
Lychee	1 fruit	6	0	0	0	2	0	0
Lychee, Dried	1 fruit	7	0	0	0	2	0	0
Mandarin Oranges, Canned in Juice	1 cup	92	0	0	12	24	2	2
Mandarin Oranges, Canned in Juice, Drained	1 cup	72	0	0	9	18	2	1
Mandarin Oranges, Canned in Light Syrup	1 cup	154	0	0	15	41	2	1
Mangoes	1 fruit	202	1	0	3	50	5	3
Mangoes, Sliced	1 cup	99	1	0	2	25	3	1
Melon Balls, Frozen	1 cup	57	0	0	54	14	1	1
Melon, Cantaloupe, Cubed	1 cup	54	0	0	26	13	1	1
Melon, Casaba, Cubed	1 cup	48	0	0	15	11	2	2
Melon, Honeydew, Diced	1 cup	61	0	0	31	15	1	1
Melon, Watermelon, Diced	1 cup	46	0	0	2	11	1	1
Mulberries	1 cup	60	1	0	14	14	2	2
Nectarines	1 medium	62	0	0	0	15	2	2
Oranges	1 large	86	0	0	0	22	4	2
Papayas, Cubed	1 cup	62	0	0	12	16	2	1
Passion-Fruit, Purple	1 fruit	17	0	0	5	4	2	0
Peaches	1 medium	58	0	0	0	14	2	1
Peaches, Canned in Heavy Syrup	1 cup	194	0	0	16	52	3	1
Peaches, Canned in Heavy Syrup, Drained	1 cup	160	0	0	13	41	3	1
Peaches, Canned in Juice	1 cup	110	0	0	10	29	3	2
Peaches, Canned in Light Syrup, Halved or Sliced	1 cup	136	0	0	13	37	3	1
Peaches, Canned in Water, Halved or Sliced	1 cup	59	0	0	7	15	3	1
Peaches, Dried	1/2 cup	191	1	0	6	49	7	3
Peaches, Dried	1 half	31	0	0	1	8	1	0

common foods

	SERVING SIZE	CALORIES	TOTAL FAT (G)	SAT FAT (G)	SODIUM (MG)	CARBS (G)	FIBER (G)	PROTEIN (G)
Peaches, Frozen, Sliced, Sweetened	1 cup	235	0	0	15	60	5	2
Pears, Asian	1 medium	116	1	0	0	29	10	1
Pears, Canned in Heavy Syrup	1 cup	197	0	0	13	51	4	1
Pears, Canned in Juice, Halved	1 cup	124	0	0	10	32	4	1
Pears, Canned in Light Syrup, Halved	1 cup	143	0	0	13	38	4	0
Pears, Canned in Water, Halved	1 cup	71	0	0	5	19	4	0
Pears, Dried	1 half	47	0	0	1	13	1	0
Pears, Medium	1 fruit	103	0	0	2	28	6	1
Persimmons, Japanese	1 fruit	118	0	0	2	31	6	1
Persimmons, Japanese, Dried	1 fruit	93	0	n/a	1	25	5	0
Pineapple	1 cup	83	0	0	2	22	2	1
Pineapple, Canned in Heavy Syrup, Crushed, Sliced, or Chunked	1 cup	198	0	0	3	51	2	1
Pineapple, Canned in Juice, Crushed, Sliced, or Chunked	1 cup	149	0	0	2	39	2	1
Pineapple, Canned in Juice, Drained, Crushed or Chunked	1 cup	113	0	0	2	29	2	1
Pineapple, Canned in Water, Crushed, Sliced, or Chunked	1 cup	79	0	0	2	20	2	1
Plantains	1 medium	218	1	0	7	57	4	2
Plantains, Cooked, Mashed	1 cup	232	0	0	10	62	5	2
Plantains, Green, Fried	1 cup	365	14	4	2	58	4	2
Plantains, Yellow, Fried	1 cup	399	13	3	10	69	5	2
Plums	1 fruit	30	0	0	0	8	1	0
Plums, Canned in Heavy Syrup, Drained	1 cup	163	0	0	35	42	3	1
Plums, Canned in Heavy Syrup, Pitted	1 cup	230	0	0	49	60	2	1
Plums, Canned in Juice, Pitted	1 cup	146	0	0	3	38	2	1
Plums, Canned in Light Syrup, Pitted	1 cup	159	0	0	50	41	2	1
Plums, Canned in Water, Pitted	1 cup	102	0	0	2	27	2	1
Pomegranates	1/2 cup	72	1	0	3	16	3	1
Prickly Pears	1 fruit	42	1	0	5	10	4	1
Prunes	1/2 cup	209	0	0	2	56	6	2
Prunes, Canned in Heavy Syrup	1 cup	246	0	0	7	65	9	2
Pummelo, Sectioned	1 cup	72	0	n/a	2	18	2	1
Quinces	1 fruit	52	0	0	4	14	2	0
Raisins, Seedless	1/2 cup	247	0	0	9	65	3	3
Raspberries	1 cup	64	1	0	1	15	8	1

	SERVING SIZE	CALORIES	TOTAL FAT (G)	SAT FAT (G)	SODIUM (MG)	CARBS (G)	FIBER (G)	PROTEIN (G)
Raspberries, Canned in Heavy Syrup	1 cup	233	0	0	8	60	8	2
Raspberries, Frozen, Sweetened	1 cup	258	0	0	3	65	11	2
Starfruit, Sliced	1 cup	33	0	0	2	7	3	1
Strawberries, Frozen, Sweetened, Sliced	1 cup	245	0	0	8	66	5	1
Strawberries, Frozen, Sweetened, Whole	1 cup	199	0	0	3	54	5	1
Strawberries, Frozen, Unsweetened	1 cup	77	0	0	4	20	5	1
Strawberries, Halved	1 cup	49	0	0	2	12	3	1
Tangerines	1 medium	47	0	0	2	12	2	1

Herbs & Spices

	SERVING SIZE	CALORIES	TOTAL FAT (G)	SAT FAT (G)	SODIUM (MG)	CARBS (G)	FIBER (G)	PROTEIN (G)
Allspice, Ground	1 tbsp	16	1	0	5	4	1	0
Basil, Dried	1 tbsp	5	0	0	2	1	1	0
Basil, Fresh, Chopped	1 tbsp	1	0	0	0	0	0	0
Bay Leaf, Crumbled	1 tbsp	6	0	0	0	1	0	0
Cardamom, Ground	1 tbsp	18	0	0	1	4	2	1
Chili Powder	1 tbsp	23	1	0	131	4	3	1
Cinnamon, Ground	1 tbsp	20	0	0	1	6	4	0
Cloves, Ground	1 tbsp	18	1	0	18	4	2	0
Curry Powder	1 tbsp	20	1	0	3	4	2	1
Dill, Dried	1 tbsp	8	0	0	6	2	0	1
Garlic Powder	1 tbsp	32	0	0	6	7	1	2
Ginger, Ground	1 tbsp	17	0	0	1	4	1	0
Mustard, Ground	1 tbsp	32	2	0	1	2	1	2
Nutmeg, Ground	1 tbsp	37	3	2	1	3	1	0
Onion Powder	1 tbsp	24	0	0	5	5	1	1
Oregano, Dried	1 tbsp	8	0	0	1	2	1	0
Paprika	1 tbsp	19	1	0	5	4	2	1
Parsley, Dried	1 tbsp	5	0	0	7	1	0	0
Pepper, Black, Ground	1 tbsp	17	0	0	1	4	2	1
Pepper, Red or Cayenne	1 tbsp	17	1	0	2	3	1	1
Pepper, White, Ground	1 tbsp	21	0	0	0	5	2	1
Peppermint, Fresh	1 tbsp	1	0	0	0	0	0	0
Poultry Seasoning	1 tbsp	14	0	0	1	3	0	0
Pumpkin Pie Spice	1 tbsp	19	1	0	3	4	1	0
Rosemary, Dried	1 tbsp	11	1	0	2	2	1	0
Rosemary, Fresh	1 tbsp	2	0	0	0	0	0	0
Saffron	1 tbsp	7	0	0	3	1	0	0
Sage, Ground	1 tbsp	6	0	0	0	1	1	0

	SERVING SIZE	CALORIES	TOTAL FAT (G)	SAT FAT (G)	SODIUM (MG)	CARBS (G)	FIBER (G)	PROTEIN (G)
Salt, Table	1 tbsp	0	0	0	6976	0	0	0
Spearmint, Dried	1 tbsp	5	0	0	6	1	0	0
Spearmint, Fresh	1 tbsp	3	0	0	2	0	0	0
Tarragon, Dried	1 tbsp	5	0	0	1	1	0	0
Thyme, Dried	1 tbsp	7	0	0	1	2	1	0
Thyme, Fresh	1 tbsp	2	0	0	0	1	0	0
Turmeric, Ground	1 tbsp	24	1	0	3	4	1	1

Meat
BEEF
Cured

	SERVING SIZE	CALORIES	TOTAL FAT (G)	SAT FAT (G)	SODIUM (MG)	CARBS (G)	FIBER (G)	PROTEIN (G)
Chopped Beef, Smoked	1 oz	37	1	1	352	1	0	6
Corned Beef, Brisket, Cooked	3 oz	213	16	5	964	0	0	15
Corned Beef, Canned	3 oz	213	13	5	856	0	0	23
Dried Beef	10 slices	43	1	0	781	1	0	9

Ground, Cooked

	SERVING SIZE	CALORIES	TOTAL FAT (G)	SAT FAT (G)	SODIUM (MG)	CARBS (G)	FIBER (G)	PROTEIN (G)
75% Lean Meat / 25% Fat	3 oz	236	16	6	73	0	0	22
80% Lean Meat / 20% Fat	3 oz	231	15	6	71	0	0	22
85% Lean Meat / 15% Fat	3 oz	215	13	5	68	0	0	23
90% Lean Meat / 10% Fat	3 oz	190	10	4	66	0	0	23
95% Lean Meat / 5% Fat	3 oz	155	6	3	64	0	0	24

Ribs, 1/8" Fat Trim, Average of All Grades, Cooked

	SERVING SIZE	CALORIES	TOTAL FAT (G)	SAT FAT (G)	SODIUM (MG)	CARBS (G)	FIBER (G)	PROTEIN (G)
Large End	3 oz	302	24	10	54	0	0	20
Small End	3 oz	290	23	9	54	0	0	19
Whole	3 oz	298	24	10	54	0	0	19

Roasts, 1/8" Fat Trim, Average of All Grades, Cooked

	SERVING SIZE	CALORIES	TOTAL FAT (G)	SAT FAT (G)	SODIUM (MG)	CARBS (G)	FIBER (G)	PROTEIN (G)
Brisket, Flat Half	3 oz	246	16	6	41	0	0	24
Brisket, Point Half	3 oz	297	23	9	59	0	0	21
Brisket, Whole	3 oz	281	21	8	54	0	0	22
Chuck, Blade Roast	3 oz	290	21	9	55	0	0	23
Chuck, Pot Roast	3 oz	257	16	6	43	0	0	26
Round, Bottom Round	3 oz	185	10	4	30	0	0	22
Round, Eye Round	3 oz	177	8	3	31	0	0	24
Round, Full Cut	3 oz	193	10	4	53	0	0	23
Round, Tip Round	3 oz	186	10	4	54	0	0	23
Round, Top Round	3 oz	202	9	3	38	0	0	29

	SERVING SIZE	CALORIES	TOTAL FAT (G)	SAT FAT (G)	SODIUM (MG)	CARBS (G)	FIBER (G)	PROTEIN (G)
Tenderloin	3 oz	275	21	8	48	0	0	20
Steaks, 1/8" Fat Trim, Average of All Grades, Cooked								
Filet, Top Loin, Boneless	3 oz	203	12	4	79	1	0	23
Flank, Choice, 0" Fat	3 oz	224	14	6	60	0	0	23
NY Strip/Top Loin	3 oz	224	14	6	46	0	0	22
Porterhouse	3 oz	252	19	7	54	0	0	20
Ribeye, Boneless	3 oz	247	19	8	46	0	0	20
Round, Bottom Round	3 oz	210	10	4	37	0	0	28
Round, Top Round	3 oz	173	8	3	35	0	0	26
Skirt, 0" Fat	3 oz	181	10	4	64	0	0	22
T-Bone	3 oz	238	17	6	56	0	0	21
Tenderloin	3 oz	227	15	6	46	0	0	22
Top Sirloin	3 oz	207	12	5	48	0	0	23
DELI MEATS								
Beef, Thin Sliced	3 oz	100	3	1	450	3	0	15
Bologna, Beef	3 oz	265	24	9	919	3	0	9
Bologna, Beef, Low-Fat	3 oz	174	13	5	1004	4	0	10
Bologna, Beef & Pork	3 oz	264	21	8	823	5	0	13
Bologna, Beef & Pork, Low-Fat	3 oz	196	16	6	942	2	0	10
Bologna, Chicken & Pork	3 oz	286	26	8	1055	4	0	9
Bologna, Chicken, Pork & Beef	3 oz	231	19	6	953	5	0	10
Bologna, Chicken, Turkey & Pork	3 oz	253	22	7	784	5	0	8
Bologna, Pork	3 oz	207	17	6	995	1	0	13
Bologna, Pork & Turkey, Light	3 oz	177	13	5	601	3	0	11
Bologna, Pork, Turkey & Beef	3 oz	286	25	10	897	6	0	10
Bologna, Turkey	3 oz	176	13	4	900	4	0	10
Chicken Breast, Oven-Roasted, Fat-Free, Sliced	3 oz	67	0	0	925	2	0	14
Chicken Breast Roll, Oven-Roasted	3 oz	113	6	2	742	2	0	12
Chicken Roll, Light Meat	3 oz	94	2	1	901	4	0	14
Ham, Sliced	3 oz	139	7	2	1109	3	1	14
Ham, Sliced, Prepackaged, 96% Fat-Free	3 oz	89	3	1	1023	1	0	14
Ham & Cheese Loaf or Roll	3 oz	202	16	6	907	3	0	11
Headcheese, Pork	3 oz	132	9	3	697	0	0	12
Olive Loaf	3 oz	197	14	5	1247	8	0	10
Pastrami, Beef, 98% Fat-Free	3 oz	81	1	0	859	1	0	17

common foods

	SERVING SIZE	CALORIES	TOTAL FAT (G)	SAT FAT (G)	SODIUM (MG)	CARBS (G)	FIBER (G)	PROTEIN (G)
Pastrami, Beef, Cured	3 oz	125	5	2	754	0	0	19
Pastrami, Turkey	3 oz	113	5	1	835	2	0	14
Pepperoni	3 oz	415	37	12	1389	0	0	19
Salami, Beef	3 oz	222	19	8	970	2	0	11
Salami, Beef & Pork	3 oz	286	22	8	1232	2	0	19
Salami, Dry or Hard, Pork	3 oz	345	29	10	1915	1	0	19
Salami, Dry or Hard, Pork & Beef	3 oz	323	25	9	1688	3	0	19
Salami, Italian Pork	3 oz	357	31	11	1588	1	0	18
Salami, Italian, Pork & Beef, 50% Less Sodium	3 oz	298	22	8	796	5	0	19
Salami, Pork & Beef, Less Sodium	3 oz	337	26	9	530	13	0	13
Salami, Turkey	3 oz	146	8	2	854	1	0	16
Turkey Ham, Cured Thigh Meat	3 oz	106	4	1	936	2	0	15
Turkey Ham, Sliced, Extra Lean	3 oz	105	3	1	883	2	0	17
Turkey Roll, Light & Dark Meat	3 oz	127	6	2	498	2	0	15
Turkey, Breast	3 oz	87	1	0	853	4	0	14
Turkey, Breast, Low-Salt	3 oz	99	1	0	657	4	0	19
Turkey, Breast, Smoked, Lemon Pepper Flavor, 97% Fat-Free	3 oz	81	1	0	987	1	0	18
Turkey, White Rotisserie, Deli Cut	3 oz	95	3	0	1022	7	0	12
GAME MEAT								
Bear, Cooked	3 oz	220	11	3	60	0	0	28
Beefalo, Cooked	3 oz	160	5	2	70	0	0	26
Bison, Chuck, Shoulder Roast, Cooked	3 oz	164	5	2	48	0	0	29
Bison, Ground, Cooked	3 oz	202	13	5	62	0	0	20
Bison, Ground, Grass-Fed, Cooked	3 oz	152	7	3	65	0	0	22
Bison, Ribeye 1" Steak, Cooked	3 oz	150	5	2	44	0	0	25
Bison, Top Round, 1" Steak, Cooked	3 oz	148	4	2	35	0	0	26
Bison, Top Sirloin, 1" Steak, Cooked	3 oz	145	5	2	45	0	0	24
Caribou, Cooked	3 oz	142	4	1	51	0	0	25
Elk, Cooked	3 oz	124	2	1	52	0	0	26
Goat, Cooked	3 oz	122	3	1	73	0	0	23
Moose, Cooked	3 oz	114	1	0	59	0	0	25
Rabbit, Domesticated, Cooked	3 oz	167	7	2	40	0	0	25
Rabbit, Wild, Cooked	3 oz	147	3	1	38	0	0	28
Venison, Cooked	3 oz	134	3	1	46	0	0	26
Venison, Ground, Cooked	3 oz	159	7	3	66	0	0	22

	SERVING SIZE	CALORIES	TOTAL FAT (G)	SAT FAT (G)	SODIUM (MG)	CARBS (G)	FIBER (G)	PROTEIN (G)
Venison, Loin, Cooked	3 oz	128	2	1	48	0	0	26
Venison, Shoulder Roast, Cooked	3 oz	162	3	2	44	0	0	31
Venison, Tenderloin Roast, Cooked	3 oz	127	2	1	48	0	0	25
Venison, Top Round, 1" Steak, Cooked	3 oz	129	2	1	38	0	0	27
HOT DOGS & SAUSAGES								
Beef, Fresh, Cooked	3 oz	282	24	9	555	0	0	15
Berliner, Pork & Beef	3 oz	196	15	5	1103	2	0	13
Blood Sausage	3 oz	322	29	11	578	1	0	12
Bratwurst, Beef & Pork, Smoked	3 oz	253	22	5	721	2	0	10
Bratwurst, Chicken, Cooked	3 oz	150	9	n/a	61	0	0	17
Bratwurst, Pork, Beef & Turkey, Light, Smoked	3 oz	158	12	n/a	835	1	0	12
Bratwurst, Pork, Cooked	3 oz	283	25	8	719	2	0	12
Bratwurst, Veal, Cooked	3 oz	286	27	13	50	0	0	12
Chicken & Beef, Smoked	3 oz	251	20	6	867	0	0	16
Chicken, Beef & Pork, Skinless, Smoked	3 oz	184	12	4	879	7	0	12
Chorizo, Pork & Beef	1 oz	129	11	4	350	1	0	7
Corn Dogs, Frozen	1 corn dog	208	10	3	490	23	1	6
Frankfurter, Beef	1 frank	155	14	6	409	1	0	6
Frankfurter, Beef, Low-Fat	1 frank	131	11	5	593	1	0	7
Frankfurter, Beef & Pork	1 frank	137	12	5	504	1	0	5
Frankfurter, Beef & Pork, Low-Fat	1 frank	87	6	2	716	3	0	6
Frankfurter, Beef, Pork & Turkey, Fat-Free	1 frank	62	1	0	502	6	0	7
Frankfurter, Chicken	1 frank	100	7	2	380	1	0	7
Frankfurter, Pork	1 frank	204	18	7	620	0	0	10
Frankfurter, Turkey	1 frank	100	8	2	485	2	0	6
Italian, Pork, Cooked	3 oz	293	23	8	1027	4	0	16
Italian, Sweet	3 oz	125	7	3	479	2	0	14
Italian, Turkey, Smoked	3 oz	133	7	3	780	4	1	13
Kielbasa, Polish, Turkey & Beef, Smoked	3 oz	190	15	5	1008	3	0	11
Knackwurst, Pork & Beef	3 oz	261	24	9	791	3	0	9
Polish, Pork	3 oz	277	24	9	745	1	0	12
Polish, Pork & Beef, Smoked	3 oz	257	23	8	724	2	0	10
Pork & Beef, w/Cheddar Cheese, Smoked	3 oz	253	22	8	726	2	0	11
Pork & Beef, Fresh, Cooked	3 oz	337	31	11	685	2	0	12
Pork & Turkey, Precooked	3 oz	291	26	8	745	3	0	10
Pork, Fresh, Cooked	3 oz	288	24	8	637	0	0	17

common foods

	SERVING SIZE	CALORIES	TOTAL FAT (G)	SAT FAT (G)	SODIUM (MG)	CARBS (G)	FIBER (G)	PROTEIN (G)
Pork, Smoked	3 oz	261	24	8	703	0	0	10
Turkey, Breakfast, Mild	2 oz	132	10	2	328	1	0	9
Turkey, Fresh, Cooked	3 oz	167	9	2	566	0	0	20
Turkey, Hot, Smoked	3 oz	133	7	3	780	4	1	13
Vienna, Chicken, Beef & Pork, Canned	3 oz	196	16	6	824	2	0	9
LAMB, 1/8" FAT TRIM								
Foreshank, Cooked	3 oz	207	11	5	61	0	0	24
Ground	3 oz	241	17	7	69	0	0	21
Leg, Shank Half, Cooked	3 oz	184	10	4	55	0	0	23
Leg, Sirloin Half, Cooked	3 oz	241	17	7	58	0	0	21
Leg, Whole (Shank & Sirloin), Cooked	3 oz	206	12	5	57	0	0	22
Loin, Cooked	3 oz	247	18	8	54	0	0	20
Rib, Cooked	3 oz	290	23	10	63	0	0	19
Shoulder, Arm, Cooked	3 oz	227	16	7	55	0	0	19
Shoulder, Blade, Cooked	3 oz	230	16	7	57	0	0	19
Shoulder, Whole (Arm & Blade), Cooked	3 oz	229	16	7	56	0	0	19
Sirloin Chop, Boneless, Cooked	3 oz	160	7	3	56	0	n/a	23
PORK								
Chops								
Center Loin, Bone-In, Cooked	3 oz	178	9	3	47	0	0	22
Loin, Blade, Bone-In, Cooked	3 oz	196	12	4	63	0	0	20
Loin, Blade, Boneless, Cooked	3 oz	172	9	3	49	1	0	21
Loin, Center-Rib, Bone-In, Cooked	3 oz	189	11	4	47	0	0	21
Loin, Center-Rib, Boneless, Cooked	3 oz	221	13	5	53	0	0	23
Sirloin, Bone-In, Cooked	3 oz	189	10	3	73	0	0	23
Sirloin, Boneless, Cooked	3 oz	145	5	2	55	0	0	24
Top Loin, Boneless, Cooked	3 oz	167	8	3	37	0	0	23
Ground								
72% Lean, Cooked	3 oz	333	28	10	80	1	0	19
84% Lean, Cooked	3 oz	246	17	6	76	0	0	23
96% Lean, Cooked	3 oz	159	6	2	71	0	0	26
Ham, Cured								
Boneless, Low-Sodium, Cooked	3 oz	146	7	2	824	0	0	19
Boneless, Regular (Approx. 11% Fat), Cooked	3 oz	151	8	3	1275	0	0	19
Canned, Extra Lean (Approx. 4% Fat), Cooked	3 oz	116	4	1	965	0	0	18

	SERVING SIZE	CALORIES	TOTAL FAT (G)	SAT FAT (G)	SODIUM (MG)	CARBS (G)	FIBER (G)	PROTEIN (G)
Canned, Regular (Approx. 13% Fat), Cooked	3 oz	192	13	4	800	0	0	17
Center, Sliced, Unheated	3 oz	173	11	4	1179	0	0	17
Ham Steak, Boneless, Extra Lean, Unheated	3 oz	104	4	1	1079	0	0	17
Honey Smoked, Cooked	3 oz	101	2	1	743	6	0	15
Patties, Cooked	1 patty	205	19	7	638	1	0	8
Rump, Bone-In, Cooked	3 oz	150	8	3	715	1	0	19
Shank, Bone-In, Cooked	3 oz	162	9	3	681	0	0	19
Shoulder, Arm, Picnic, Cooked	3 oz	238	18	7	911	0	0	17
Shoulder, Blade Roll, Cooked	3 oz	244	20	7	827	0	0	15
Spiral Sliced, Boneless, Cooked	3 oz	116	4	0	830	0	0	19
Whole, Boneless, Cooked	3 oz	97	3	1	1002	1	0	17
Whole, Cooked	3 oz	207	14	5	1009	0	0	18
Ham, Fresh								
Rump Half, Cooked	3 oz	178	9	3	65	0	0	23
Shank Half, Cooked	3 oz	197	11	4	69	0	0	22
Whole, Cooked	3 oz	232	15	5	51	0	0	23
Other Cured Pork								
Bacon, Cooked	1 slice	43	3	1	185	0	0	3
Canadian-Style Bacon, Cooked	2 slices	87	4	1	727	1	0	11
Other Pork Products								
Pig's Feet, Pickled	1 oz	40	3	1	159	0	0	3
Pulled Pork in Barbecue Sauce	1 cup	418	11	4	1658	47	3	33
Scrapple, Pork, Cooked	3 oz	160	10	4	494	11	0	6
Ribs								
Back Ribs, Cooked	3 oz	243	18	7	80	0	0	20
Country-Style, Cooked	3 oz	232	15	5	49	0	0	23
Spareribs, Cooked	3 oz	337	26	9	79	0	0	25
Roasts								
Center Loin, Bone-In, Cooked	3 oz	196	11	4	71	0	0	23
Leg Sirloin, Tip Roast, Boneless, Cooked	3 oz	133	2	1	37	0	0	26
Loin, Blade, Bone-In, Cooked	3 oz	216	14	5	65	0	0	21
Loin, Center Rib Roast, Bone-In, Cooked	3 oz	211	12	5	77	0	0	23
Loin, Center Rib Roast, Boneless, Cooked	3 oz	214	13	5	41	0	0	23
Loin, Whole, Cooked	3 oz	211	12	5	50	0	0	23
Picnic (Shoulder), Cooked	3 oz	200	12	4	82	0	0	21
Shoulder, Arm Picnic, Cooked	3 oz	269	20	7	60	0	0	20
Shoulder, Whole, Cooked	3 oz	248	18	7	58	0	0	20

common foods

	SERVING SIZE	CALORIES	TOTAL FAT (G)	SAT FAT (G)	SODIUM (MG)	CARBS (G)	FIBER (G)	PROTEIN (G)
Sirloin, Bone-In, Cooked	3 oz	196	11	3	48	0	0	23
Sirloin, Boneless, Cooked	3 oz	163	6	2	56	0	0	25
Tenderloin, Cooked	3 oz	125	3	1	48	0	0	22
Top Loin, Boneless, Cooked	3 oz	163	7	2	39	0	0	22
VEAL								
Breast, Point Half, Boneless, Cooked	3 oz	211	12	5	56	0	n/a	24
Breast, Whole, Boneless, Cooked	3 oz	226	14	6	55	0	n/a	23
Ground, Cooked	3 oz	146	6	3	71	0	0	21
Leg, Top Round, Breaded, Fried	3 oz	202	8	3	386	8	0	23
Leg, Top Round, Fried	3 oz	179	7	3	65	0	0	27
Leg, Top Round, Roasted	3 oz	136	4	2	58	0	0	24
Loin, Cooked	3 oz	184	10	4	79	0	0	21
Rib, Cooked	3 oz	194	12	5	78	0	0	20
Shank, (Fore & Hind), Cooked	3 oz	162	5	2	79	0	n/a	27
Shoulder, Arm, Cooked	3 oz	156	7	3	77	0	0	22
Shoulder, Blade, Cooked	3 oz	158	7	3	85	0	0	21
Shoulder, Whole, (Arm & Blade), Cooked	3 oz	156	7	3	82	0	0	22
Sirloin, Cooked	3 oz	172	9	4	71	0	0	21
Meat Alternatives								
Bacon, Meatless, Cooked	1 oz	50	5	1	234	1	0	2
Chicken, Meatless	1 cup	376	21	3	1191	6	6	40
Frankfurter, Meatless	1 frankfurter	163	10	1	330	5	3	14
Sausage, Meatless	1 link	64	5	1	222	2	1	5
Veggie Burger or Soy Burger, Unprepared	1 patty	124	4	1	398	10	3	11
TEMPEH & TOFU								
Tempeh	1 cup	320	18	4	15	16	n/a	31
Tofu, Extra Firm	1/5 block	83	5	0	7	2	0	9
Tofu, Firm	1/2 cup	88	5	1	15	2	1	10
Tofu, Fried	1 oz	77	6	1	5	3	1	5
Tofu, Salted & Fermented	1 block	13	1	0	316	1	n/a	1
Tofu, Soft	1/2 cup	76	5	1	10	2	0	8
Poultry								
CHICKEN								
Average of All Dark Meat								
Skinless, Fried	3 oz	203	10	3	82	2	0	25
Skinless, Roasted, Chopped or Diced	3 oz	174	8	2	79	0	0	23
Skinless, Stewed, Chopped or Diced	3 oz	163	8	2	63	0	0	22

	SERVING SIZE	CALORIES	TOTAL FAT (G)	SAT FAT (G)	SODIUM (MG)	CARBS (G)	FIBER (G)	PROTEIN (G)
w/Skin, Battered, Fried	3 oz	253	16	4	251	8	n/a	19
w/Skin, Floured, Fried	3 oz	242	14	4	76	3	0	23
w/Skin, Roasted	3 oz	215	13	4	74	0	0	22
w/Skin, Stewed	3 oz	198	12	3	60	0	0	20
Average of All Light Meat								
Skinless, Fried	3 oz	163	5	1	69	0	0	28
Skinless, Roasted, Chopped, or Diced	3 oz	147	4	1	65	0	0	26
Skinless, Stewed, Chopped or Diced	3 oz	135	3	1	55	0	0	25
w/Skin, Battered, Fried	3 oz	236	13	4	244	8	n/a	20
w/Skin, Floured, Fried	3 oz	209	10	3	65	2	0	26
w/Skin, Roasted	3 oz	189	9	3	64	0	0	25
w/Skin, Stewed	3 oz	171	8	2	54	0	0	22
Breast								
Skinless, Fried, Boneless	3 oz	159	4	1	67	0	0	28
Skinless, Roasted, Chopped or Diced	3 oz	140	3	1	63	0	0	26
Skinless, Rotisserie, Boneless	3 oz	126	3	1	290	0	0	25
Skinless, Stewed, Chopped or Diced	3 oz	128	3	1	54	0	0	25
w/Skin, Battered, Fried, Boneless	3 oz	221	11	3	234	8	0	21
w/Skin, Floured, Fried, Boneless	3 oz	189	8	2	65	1	0	27
w/Skin, Roasted, Chopped or Diced	3 oz	167	7	2	60	0	0	25
w/Skin, Rotisserie, Boneless	3 oz	156	7	2	295	0	0	23
w/Skin, Stewed, Chopped or Diced	3 oz	156	6	2	53	0	0	23
Chicken Products								
Nuggets, Frozen, Cooked	5 pieces	296	20	4	557	14	2	15
Paté, Canned	1 oz	57	4	1	109	2	0	4
Patty, Frozen, Cooked	1 patty	172	12	2	319	8	0	9
Spread	1 oz	45	5	1	205	1	0	5
Tenders, Baked	3 oz	249	15	3	389	14	1	13
Tenders, Microwaved	3 oz	214	11	3	379	15	0	14
Wings, Frozen, Barbecue-Flavored, Baked	3 oz	206	13	3	475	3	0	19
Drumsticks								
Skinless, Fried	1 drumstick	82	3	1	40	0	0	12
Skinless, Rotisserie	1 drumstick	93	4	1	221	0	0	15
Skinless, Stewed, Chopped or Diced	1 cup	270	9	2	128	0	0	44
w/Skin, Fried, Battered	1 drumstick	193	11	3	194	6	0	16
w/Skin, Fried, Floured	1 drumstick	120	7	2	44	1	0	13
w/Skin, Roasted	1 drumstick	195	10	3	120	0	0	24

common foods	SERVING SIZE	CALORIES	TOTAL FAT (G)	SAT FAT (G)	SODIUM (MG)	CARBS (G)	FIBER (G)	PROTEIN (G)
w/Skin, Rotisserie	1 drumstick	114	6	2	218	0	0	14
w/Skin, Stewed, Chopped or Diced	1 cup	286	15	4	106	0	0	35
Legs (Drumstick and Thigh)								
Skinless, Fried	1 leg	196	9	2	90	1	0	27
Skinless, Roasted	1 leg	346	16	4	197	0	0	48
Skinless, Stewed, Chopped or Diced	1 cup	296	13	4	125	0	0	42
w/Skin, Fried, Battered	1 leg	431	26	7	441	14	0	34
w/Skin, Fried, Floured	1 leg	284	16	4	99	3	0	30
w/Skin, Roasted	1 leg	475	23	6	253	0	0	62
w/Skin, Stewed, Chopped or Diced	1 cup	308	18	5	102	0	0	34
Offal								
Giblets, Fried, Chopped or Diced	1 cup	402	20	6	164	6	0	47
Giblets, Simmered, Chopped or Diced	1 cup	228	7	2	97	0	0	39
Other								
Canned, No Broth	5 oz	231	10	3	603	1	0	32
Canned, w/Broth	5 oz	234	11	3	714	0	0	31
Ground, Pan-Browned	3 oz	161	9	3	64	0	0	20
Thighs								
Skinless, Fried	1 thigh	113	5	1	49	1	0	15
Skinless, Roasted	1 thigh	205	10	3	101	0	0	28
Skinless, Rotisserie	1 thigh	174	10	3	300	0	0	21
Skinless, Stewed	1 thigh	107	5	1	41	0	0	14
w/Skin, Fried, Battered	1 thigh	238	14	4	248	8	0	19
w/Skin, Fried, Floured	1 thigh	162	9	3	55	2	0	17
w/Skin, Roasted	1 thigh	309	20	6	116	0	0	31
w/Skin, Rotisserie	1 thigh	207	14	4	307	0	0	20
w/Skin, Stewed	1 thigh	158	10	3	48	0	0	16
Wings								
Fried, Skin Removed	1 wing	42	2	1	18	0	0	6
Roasted, Skin Removed	1 wing	43	2	0	19	0	0	6
Skinless, Rotisserie	1 wing	104	5	1	384	0	0	15
Skinless, Stewed, Chopped or Diced	1 cup	253	10	3	102	0	0	38
w/Skin, Fried, Battered	1 wing	159	11	3	157	5	0	10
w/Skin, Fried, Floured	1 wing	103	7	2	25	1	0	8
w/Skin, Roasted, Chopped or Diced	1 cup	406	27	8	115	0	0	38
w/Skin, Rotisserie	1 wing	141	10	3	323	0	0	13
w/Skin, Stewed, Chopped or Diced	1 cup	349	24	7	94	0	0	32

	SERVING SIZE	CALORIES	TOTAL FAT (G)	SAT FAT (G)	SODIUM (MG)	CARBS (G)	FIBER (G)	PROTEIN (G)
DUCK								
Domesticated, Skinless, Roasted	3 oz	171	10	3	55	0	0	20
Domesticated, w/Skin, Roasted	3 oz	287	24	8	50	0	0	16
Pekin (Long Island), Breast, Boneless, Cooked w/o Skin	3 oz	119	2	0	89	0	n/a	23
Pekin (Long Island), Breast, Boneless, w/Skin, Roasted	3 oz	172	9	2	71	0	n/a	21
Pekin (Long Island), Leg, Bone-In, Cooked w/o Skin	3 oz	151	5	1	92	0	n/a	25
Pekin (Long Island), Leg, Bone-In, w/Skin, Roasted	3 oz	185	10	3	94	0	n/a	23
GAME POULTRY								
Emu, Fan Fillet, Cooked	3 oz	131	2	0	45	0	0	27
Emu, Full Rump, Cooked	3 oz	143	2	1	94	0	0	29
Emu, Ground, Cooked	3 oz	139	4	1	55	0	0	24
Emu, Inside Drums, Cooked	3 oz	133	2	1	100	0	0	28
Emu, Top Loin, Cooked	3 oz	129	3	1	49	0	0	25
Ostrich, Ground, Cooked	3 oz	149	6	2	68	0	0	22
Ostrich, Inside Strip, Cooked	3 oz	139	4	1	62	0	0	25
Ostrich, Outside Strip, Cooked	3 oz	133	3	1	61	0	0	24
Ostrich, Tip, Cooked	3 oz	123	2	1	68	0	0	24
Ostrich, Top Loin, Cooked	3 oz	132	3	1	65	0	0	24
Pheasant, Cooked	3 oz	203	10	3	37	0	0	28
Quail, Cooked	3 oz	193	12	3	44	0	0	21
GOOSE								
Domesticated, Skinless, Roasted	3 oz	202	11	4	65	0	0	25
Domesticated, w/Skin, Roasted	3 oz	259	19	6	60	0	0	21
Pâté de Foie Gras, Canned, Smoked	1 tbsp	60	6	2	91	1	0	1
TURKEY								
Average of All Dark Meat								
All Classes, Skinless, Roasted	3 oz	160	6	2	67	0	0	24
All Classes, w/Skin, Roasted	3 oz	188	10	3	65	0	0	23
Average of All Light Meat								
All Classes, Skinless, Roasted	3 oz	134	3	1	54	0	0	25
All Classes, w/Skin, Roasted	3 oz	168	7	2	54	0	0	24
Breast								
Fryer-Roaster, Skinless, Roasted	3 oz	115	1	0	44	0	0	26

common foods

	SERVING SIZE	CALORIES	TOTAL FAT (G)	SAT FAT (G)	SODIUM (MG)	CARBS (G)	FIBER (G)	PROTEIN (G)
Fryer-Roaster, w/Skin, Roasted	3 oz	130	3	1	45	0	0	25
All Classes, w/Skin, Pre-Basted, Roasted	3 oz	107	3	1	338	0	0	19
All Classes, w/Skin, Roasted	3 oz	161	6	2	54	0	0	24
Ground								
85% Lean, Cooked	3 oz	219	15	4	72	0	0	21
93% Lean, Cooked	3 oz	181	10	3	77	0	0	23
Fat-Free, Cooked	3 oz	128	2	1	52	0	0	27
Legs								
Fryer-Roaster, Skinless, Roasted	1 leg	356	8	3	181	0	0	65
Fryer-Roaster, w/Skin, Roasted	1 leg	417	13	4	196	0	0	70
Other								
Bacon, Cooked	1 oz	107	8	2	640	1	0	8
Giblets, Simmered, Some Giblet Fat, Chopped or Diced	1 cup	289	17	6	93	1	0	30
Canned, Meat, w/Broth	1 cup	228	9	3	630	2	0	32
Patties, Breaded or Battered, Fried	3 oz	241	15	4	482	13	0	12
Wings								
Fryer-Roaster, Skinless, Roasted	1 wing	98	2	1	47	0	0	19
Fryer-Roaster, w/Skin, Roasted	1 wing	186	9	2	66	0	0	25
WHOLE BIRDS								
Cornish Game Hens								
Skinless, Roasted	1 bird	295	9	2	139	0	0	51
w/Skin, Roasted	1 bird	666	47	13	164	0	0	57
Roasting Chicken								
Dark Meat, Skinless, Roasted	3 oz	151	7	2	81	0	0	20
Giblets, Simmered, Chopped or Diced	1 cup	239	8	2	87	1	0	39
Light Meat, Skinless, Roasted	3 oz	130	3	1	43	0	0	23
w/Skin, Roasted	3 oz	190	11	3	62	0	0	20
Stewing Chicken								
Dark Meat, Skinless, Stewed	3 oz	219	13	3	81	0	0	24
Giblets, Simmered, Chopped or Diced	1 cup	281	13	4	81	0	0	37
Light Meat, Skinless, Stewed	3 oz	181	7	2	49	0	0	28
w/Skin, Stewed	3 oz	242	16	4	62	0	0	23
## Seafood								
FISH								
Anchovies, Raw	1 oz	37	1	0	29	0	0	6
Anchovies, Canned in Oil, Boneless, Drained	1 oz	60	3	1	1040	0	0	8

	SERVING SIZE	CALORIES	TOTAL FAT (G)	SAT FAT (G)	SODIUM (MG)	CARBS (G)	FIBER (G)	PROTEIN (G)
Bass, Freshwater, Cooked	3 oz	124	4	1	77	0	0	21
Bass, Striped, Cooked	3 oz	105	3	1	75	0	0	19
Bluefish, Cooked	3 oz	135	5	1	65	0	0	22
Carp, Cooked	3 oz	138	6	1	54	0	0	19
Catfish, Channel, Breaded & Fried	3 oz	195	11	3	238	7	1	15
Catfish, Channel, Farmed, Cooked	3 oz	122	6	1	101	0	0	16
Catfish, Channel, Wild, Cooked	3 oz	89	2	1	43	0	0	16
Cod, Atlantic, Cooked	3 oz	89	1	0	66	0	0	19
Cod, Atlantic, Dried & Salted	1 oz	82	1	0	1992	0	0	18
Cod, Pacific, Cooked	3 oz	72	0	0	316	0	0	16
Flounder & Sole (Flatfish), Cooked	3 oz	73	2	0	309	0	0	13
Grouper, Cooked	3 oz	100	1	0	45	0	0	21
Haddock, Cooked	3 oz	77	0	0	222	0	0	17
Haddock, Smoked, Boneless	1 oz	33	0	0	216	0	0	7
Halibut, Atlantic & Pacific, Cooked	3 oz	94	1	0	70	0	0	19
Halibut, Greenland, Cooked	3 oz	203	15	3	88	0	0	16
Herring, Atlantic, Cooked	3 oz	173	10	2	98	0	0	20
Herring, Atlantic, Kippered, Boneless	1 oz	62	4	1	260	0	0	7
Herring, Atlantic, Pickled, Boneless	1 oz	74	5	1	247	3	0	4
Herring, Pacific, Cooked	3 oz	213	15	4	81	0	0	18
Mackerel, Atlantic, Cooked	3 oz	223	15	4	71	0	0	20
Mackerel, Jack, Canned, Drained	1 oz	44	2	1	107	0	0	7
Mackerel, King, Cooked	3 oz	114	2	0	173	0	0	22
Mackerel, Pacific & Jack, Cooked, Boneless	1 oz	57	3	1	31	0	0	7
Mackerel, Spanish, Cooked	3 oz	134	5	2	56	0	0	20
Monkfish, Cooked	3 oz	82	2	n/a	20	0	0	16
Ocean Perch, Atlantic, Cooked	3 oz	82	2	0	295	0	0	16
Orange Roughy, Cooked	3 oz	89	1	0	59	0	0	19
Perch, Cooked	3 oz	99	1	0	67	0	0	21
Pike, Northern, Cooked	3 oz	96	1	0	42	0	0	21
Pike, Walleye, Cooked	3 oz	101	1	0	55	0	0	21
Pollock, Walleye, Cooked	3 oz	94	1	0	356	0	0	20
Rockfish, Pacific, Cooked	3 oz	93	1	0	76	0	0	19
Salmon, Atlantic, Farmed, Cooked	3 oz	175	10	2	52	0	0	19
Salmon, Atlantic, Wild, Cooked	3 oz	155	7	1	48	0	0	22
Salmon, Smoked (Lox)	3 oz	99	4	1	1700	0	0	16
Salmon, Sockeye (Red), Canned, Drained	3 oz	142	6	1	347	0	0	20

common foods

	SERVING SIZE	CALORIES	TOTAL FAT (G)	SAT FAT (G)	SODIUM (MG)	CARBS (G)	FIBER (G)	PROTEIN (G)
Salmon, Sockeye (Red), Canned, w/Bones, w/o Salt, Drained	3 oz	130	6	1	64	0	0	17
Salmon, Sockeye (Red), Canned, w/o Skin or Bones, Drained	3 oz	134	5	1	328	0	0	22
Salmon, Sockeye (Red), Cooked	3 oz	144	6	1	114	0	0	22
Salmon, Sockeye (Red), Kippered	3 oz	120	4	1	391	0	0	21
Salmon, Sockeye (Red), Raw, Boneless	1 oz	40	2	0	32	0	0	6
Salmon, Sockeye (Red), Smoked, Canned	3 oz	175	6	1	510	0	0	30
Sardine, Atlantic, Canned in Oil, w/Bone, Drained	1 oz	59	3	0	143	0	0	7
Sardine, Pacific, Canned in Tomato Sauce, w/Bone, Drained	1 oz	52	3	1	117	0	0	6
Sea Bass, Cooked	3 oz	105	2	1	74	0	0	20
Sea Trout, Cooked	3 oz	113	4	1	63	0	0	18
Shad, American, Cooked	3 oz	214	15	0	55	0	0	18
Smelt, Cooked	3 oz	105	3	0	65	0	0	19
Snapper, Cooked	3 oz	109	1	0	48	0	0	22
Sturgeon, Cooked, Boneless	1 oz	38	1	0	20	0	0	6
Sturgeon, Smoked	3 oz	147	4	1	628	0	0	27
Sunfish, Pumpkin Seed, Cooked	3 oz	97	1	0	88	0	0	21
Swordfish, Cooked	3 oz	146	7	2	82	0	0	20
Tilapia, Cooked	3 oz	109	2	1	48	0	0	22
Tilefish, Cooked	3 oz	125	4	1	50	0	0	21
Trout, Cooked	3 oz	162	7	1	57	0	0	23
Trout, Rainbow, Farmed, Cooked	3 oz	143	6	1	52	0	0	20
Trout, Rainbow, Wild, Cooked	3 oz	128	5	1	48	0	0	19
Tuna, Blue Fin, Cooked	3 oz	156	5	1	43	0	0	25
Tuna, Blue Fin, Raw	3 oz	122	4	1	33	0	0	20
Tuna, Light, Canned in Oil, w/o Salt, Drained	3 oz	168	7	1	43	0	0	25
Tuna, Light, Canned in Water, w/o Salt, Drained	3 oz	99	1	0	43	0	0	22
Tuna, Skipjack, Cooked	3 oz	112	1	0	40	0	0	24
Tuna, White, Canned in Oil, Drained	3 oz	158	7	1	337	0	0	23
Tuna, White, Canned in Water, w/o Salt, Drained	3 oz	109	3	1	43	0	0	20
Tuna, Yellowfin, Cooked	3 oz	111	1	0	46	0	0	25
Tuna, Yellowfin, Raw, Boneless	1 oz	31	0	0	13	0	0	7

	SERVING SIZE	CALORIES	TOTAL FAT (G)	SAT FAT (G)	SODIUM (MG)	CARBS (G)	FIBER (G)	PROTEIN (G)
Whitefish, Cooked	3 oz	146	6	1	55	0	0	21
Whitefish, Raw	3 oz	114	5	1	43	0	0	16
Whitefish, Smoked, Boneless	1 oz	31	0	0	289	0	0	7
Yellowtail, Cooked	3 oz	159	6	n/a	43	0	0	25
Yellowtail, Raw	3 oz	124	4	1	33	0	0	20
OTHER SEAFOOD								
Calamari (Squid), Fried	3 oz	149	6	2	260	7	0	15
Caviar, Black & Red, Granular	1 tbsp	42	3	1	240	1	0	4
Eel, Cooked	1 oz	67	4	1	18	0	0	7
Gefilte Fish	1 piece	35	1	0	220	3	0	4
Octopus, Cooked	3 oz	139	2	0	391	4	0	25
Surimi	3 oz	84	1	0	122	6	0	13
SHELLFISH & MOLLUSKS								
Abalone, Fried	3 oz	161	6	1	502	9	0	17
Clam, Breaded & Fried	3 oz	172	9	2	309	9	n/a	12
Clam, Canned, Drained	3 oz	121	1	0	95	5	0	21
Clam, Cooked	3 oz	126	2	0	1022	4	0	22
Clam, Raw	1 large	17	0	0	120	1	0	3
Crab, Alaska King, Cooked	3 oz	82	1	0	911	0	0	16
Crab, Alaska King, Imitation, Made from Surimi	3 oz	81	0	0	715	13	0	6
Crab, Blue, Cake	1 cake	93	5	1	198	0	0	12
Crab, Blue, Canned	1 oz	24	0	0	112	0	0	5
Crab, Blue, Cooked	3 oz	71	1	0	336	0	0	15
Crab, Dungeness, Cooked	3 oz	94	1	0	321	1	0	19
Crab, Queen, Cooked	3 oz	98	1	0	587	0	0	20
Crayfish, Farmed, Cooked	3 oz	74	1	0	82	0	0	15
Crayfish, Wild, Cooked	3 oz	70	1	0	80	0	0	14
Lobster, Northern, Cooked	3 oz	76	1	0	413	0	0	16
Lobster, Spiny, Cooked	3 oz	122	2	0	193	3	0	22
Mussel, Blue, Cooked	3 oz	146	4	1	314	6	0	20
Oyster, Eastern, Breaded & Fried	3 oz	169	11	3	354	10	n/a	7
Oyster, Eastern, Canned, Drained	3 oz	58	2	1	95	3	0	6
Oyster, Eastern, Farmed, Cooked	3 oz	67	2	1	139	6	0	6
Oyster, Eastern, Farmed, Raw	3 oz	50	1	0	151	5	0	4
Oyster, Eastern, Wild, Cooked, Dry Heat	3 oz	67	2	1	112	4	0	8
Oyster, Eastern, Wild, Cooked, Moist Heat	3 oz	87	3	1	141	5	0	10

common foods

	SERVING SIZE	CALORIES	TOTAL FAT (G)	SAT FAT (G)	SODIUM (MG)	CARBS (G)	FIBER (G)	PROTEIN (G)
Oyster, Eastern, Wild, Raw	6 medium	43	1	0	71	2	0	5
Oyster, Pacific, Cooked	3 oz	139	4	1	180	8	0	16
Oyster, Pacific, Raw	3 oz	69	2	0	90	4	0	8
Scallop, Bay & Sea, Cooked	3 oz	94	1	0	567	5	0	17
Scallop, Breaded & Fried	2 large	67	3	1	144	3	n/a	6
Scallop, Imitation, Made from Surimi	3 oz	84	0	0	676	9	0	11
Scallop, Raw	3 oz	59	0	0	333	3	0	10
Shrimp, Breaded & Fried	3 oz	206	10	2	292	10	0	18
Shrimp, Canned	1 oz	28	0	0	220	0	0	6
Shrimp, Cooked	3 oz	101	1	0	805	1	0	19
Shrimp, Imitation, Made From Surimi	3 oz	86	1	0	599	8	0	11

Nuts, Nut Butters & Seeds

NUTS

	SERVING SIZE	CALORIES	TOTAL FAT (G)	SAT FAT (G)	SODIUM (MG)	CARBS (G)	FIBER (G)	PROTEIN (G)
Almonds, Blanched	1/4 cup	215	19	1	7	7	4	8
Almonds, Dry-Roasted, w/Salt	1/4 cup	205	18	1	117	7	4	7
Almonds, Dry-Roasted, w/o Salt	1/4 cup	205	18	1	1	7	4	7
Almonds, Honey-Roasted	1/4 cup	214	18	2	47	10	5	7
Almonds, Oil-Roasted, w/Salt	1/4 cup	238	22	2	133	7	4	8
Almonds, Oil-Roasted, w/o Salt	1/4 cup	238	22	2	0	7	4	8
Almonds, Sliced	1/4 cup	132	11	1	0	5	3	5
Brazil Nuts, Dried	1/4 cup	218	22	5	1	4	3	5
Cashews, Dry-Roasted, w/Salt	1/4 cup	197	16	3	219	11	1	5
Cashews, Dry-Roasted, w/o Salt	1/4 cup	197	16	3	5	11	1	5
Cashews, Oil-Roasted, w/Salt	1/4 cup	187	15	3	99	10	1	5
Cashews, Oil-Roasted, w/o Salt	1/4 cup	187	15	3	4	10	1	5
Cashews, Raw	1/4 cup	187	15	3	4	10	1	5
Chestnuts, Boiled & Steamed	1 oz	37	0	0	8	8	n/a	1
Chestnuts, Roasted	1/2 cup	175	2	0	1	38	4	2
Hazelnuts (Filberts), Chopped	1/4 cup	181	17	1	0	5	3	4
Hazelnuts (Filberts), Blanched	1 oz	178	17	1	0	5	3	4
Hazelnuts (Filberts), Dry-Roasted	1 oz	183	18	1	0	5	3	4
Macadamia Nuts, Dry-Roasted, w/Salt	1/4 cup	236	25	4	87	4	3	3
Macadamia Nuts, Dry-Roasted, w/o Salt	1/4 cup	237	25	n/a	1	4	3	3
Macadamia Nuts, Raw	1/4 cup	241	25	4	2	5	3	3
Mixed Nuts, Dry-Roasted, w/Peanuts, w/Salt	1/4 cup	203	18	2	229	9	3	6

	SERVING SIZE	CALORIES	TOTAL FAT (G)	SAT FAT (G)	SODIUM (MG)	CARBS (G)	FIBER (G)	PROTEIN (G)
Mixed Nuts, Dry-Roasted, w/Peanuts, w/o Salt	1/4 cup	203	18	2	4	9	3	6
Mixed Nuts, Oil-Roasted, w/Peanuts, w/Salt	1/4 cup	203	18	3	91	7	2	7
Mixed Nuts, Oil-Roasted, w/Peanuts, w/o Salt	1/4 cup	203	18	2	2	7	2	7
Mixed Nuts, Oil-Roasted, w/o Peanuts, w/Salt	1/4 cup	221	20	3	110	8	2	6
Mixed Nuts, Oil-Roasted, w/o Peanuts, w/o Salt	1/4 cup	221	20	3	4	8	2	6
Peanuts, Boiled, w/Salt, in Shell	1 cup	200	14	2	473	13	6	9
Peanuts, Dry-Roasted, w/Salt	1/4 cup	214	18	3	248	8	3	9
Peanuts, Dry-Roasted, w/o Salt	1/4 cup	214	18	3	2	8	3	9
Peanuts, Oil-Roasted, Chopped, w/Salt	1/4 cup	216	19	3	151	5	3	10
Peanuts, Oil-Roasted, Chopped, w/o Salt	1/4 cup	193	16	2	2	6	2	9
Peanuts, Raw	1/4 cup	207	18	2	7	6	3	9
Pecans, Dry-Roasted, w/Salt	1/4 cup	176	18	2	95	3	2	2
Pecans, Dry-Roasted, w/o Salt	1/4 cup	176	18	2	0	3	2	2
Pecans, Halved	1/4 cup	171	18	2	0	3	2	2
Pecans, Oil-Roasted, w/Salt	1/4 cup	197	21	2	108	4	3	3
Pecans, Oil-Roasted, w/o Salt	1/4 cup	197	21	2	0	4	3	3
Pili Nuts, Dried	1/4 cup	216	24	9	1	1	n/a	3
Pine Nuts (Pinyon), Dried	10 nuts	6	1	0	1	0	0	0
Pistachios, Dry-Roasted, w/Salt	1/4 cup	173	14	2	132	9	3	6
Pistachios, Dry-Roasted, w/o Salt	1/4 cup	174	14	2	2	9	3	6
Pistachios, Raw	1/4 cup	173	14	2	0	8	3	6
Walnuts, Black, Dried, Chopped	1/4 cup	193	18	1	1	3	2	8
Walnuts, English, Chopped	1/4 cup	191	19	2	1	4	2	4
NUT BUTTERS								
Almond, w/Salt	2 tbsp	196	18	1	69	6	3	7
Almond, w/o Salt	2 tbsp	196	18	1	2	6	3	7
Cashew, w/Salt	2 tbsp	188	16	3	196	9	1	6
Cashew, w/o Salt	2 tbsp	188	16	3	5	9	1	6
Peanut, Chunky, w/Salt	2 tbsp	188	16	2	156	7	3	8
Peanut, Chunky, w/o Salt	2 tbsp	188	16	2	5	7	3	8
Peanut, Smooth, Reduced-Fat, w/Salt	2 tbsp	187	12	2	194	13	2	9
Peanut, Smooth, w/Omega-3, w/Salt	2 tbsp	195	17	3	114	5	2	8
Peanut, Smooth, w/Salt	2 tbsp	188	16	3	147	6	2	8

common foods

	SERVING SIZE	CALORIES	TOTAL FAT (G)	SAT FAT (G)	SODIUM (MG)	CARBS (G)	FIBER (G)	PROTEIN (G)
Peanut, Smooth, w/o Salt	2 tbsp	188	16	3	5	6	2	8
Sunflower, w/Salt	2 tbsp	197	18	1	106	7	2	6
Sunflower, w/o Salt	2 tbsp	197	18	1	1	7	2	6
SEEDS								
Flax, Whole	1 tbsp	55	4	0	3	3	3	2
Pumpkin & Squash, Roasted, w/Salt	1/4 cup	71	3	1	407	9	3	3
Pumpkin & Squash, Roasted, w/o Salt	1/4 cup	71	3	1	3	9	3	3
Sesame, Dried	1 tbsp	52	4	2	1	2	1	2
Sesame, Roasted	1 oz	160	14	2	3	7	4	5
Sesame, Tahini	2 tbsp	179	16	2	35	6	3	5
Sunflower, Whole, Dried	1/4 cup	67	6	1	1	2	1	2
Sunflower, Dry-Roasted, w/Salt	1/4 cup	186	16	2	131	8	3	6
Sunflower, Dry-Roasted, w/o Salt	1/4 cup	186	16	2	1	8	4	6
Sunflower, Oil-Roasted, w/Salt	1/4 cup	200	17	2	138	8	4	7
Sunflower, Oil-Roasted, w/o Salt	1/4 cup	200	17	2	1	8	4	7
Sunflower, Toasted, w/Salt	1/4 cup	207	19	2	205	7	4	6
Sunflower, Toasted, w/o Salt	1/4 cup	207	19	2	1	7	4	6
Snacks								
Animal Crackers	1 cookie	11	0	0	12	2	0*	0
Bagel Chips, Plain	1 oz	128	4	2	66	19	1	3
Beef Jerky	1 oz	116	7	3	590	3	1	9
Beef Sticks, Smoked	1 oz	156	14	6	434	2	n/a	6
Cheese Puffs & Twists, Baked	1 oz	122	3	1	240	21	3	2
Corn Nuts, Barbecue-Flavored	1 oz	124	4	1	170	20	2	3
Corn Nuts, Plain	1 oz	126	4	1	180	20	2	2
Fruit Leather, Rolls	1 large	78	1	0	67	18	0	0
Graham Crackers, Chocolate-Coated	1 square	68	3	2	36	9	0	1
Graham Crackers, Plain, Honey, or Cinnamon	1 square	30	1	0	33	5	0	0
Plantain Chips, Salted	1 oz	151	8	2	57	18	1	1
Pork Skins, Barbecue-Flavored	1 oz	153	9	3	756	0	n/a	16
Pork Skins, Plain	1 oz	154	9	3	515	0	0	17
Rice Cakes, Brown, Plain	1 cake	35	0	0	29	7	0	1
CANDIES & CHOCOLATES								
Butterscotch Candy	1 piece	21	0	0	21	5	0	0
Caramel	1 piece	39	1	0	25	8	0	0
Carob, Unsweetened	1 oz	153	9	8	30	16	1	2

	SERVING SIZE	CALORIES	TOTAL FAT (G)	SAT FAT (G)	SODIUM (MG)	CARBS (G)	FIBER (G)	PROTEIN (G)
Chocolate, Baking, Unsweetened, Squares	1 square	145	15	9	7	9	5	4
Chocolate Chips, Milk	1 cup	899	50	31	133	100	6	13
Chocolate Chips, Semisweet	1 cup	806	50	30	18	107	10	7
Chocolate, Dark, 45–50% Cacao	1 oz	155	9	5	7	17	2	1
Chocolate, Dark, 60–69% Cacao	1 oz	164	11	6	3	15	2	2
Chocolate, Dark, 70–85% Cacao	1 oz	170	12	7	6	13	3	2
Coffee Beans, Dark Chocolate–Covered	28 pieces	216	12	6	10	24	3	3
Fudge, Vanilla, w/Nuts	1 oz	123	4	1	12	21	0	1
Gumdrops	10 pieces	143	0	0	16	36	0	0
Gumdrops, Sugar-Free	10 pieces	81	0	0	4	44	9	0
Hard Candies	1 piece	24	0	0	2	6	0	0
Hard Candies, Sugar-Free	1 piece	12	0	0	0	3	0	0
Jelly Beans	10 small	41	0	0	6	10	0	0
Marshmallows	10 miniature	22	0	0	6	6	0	0
Peanut Brittle	1 oz	138	5	1	126	20	1	2
Peanuts, Milk Chocolate–Covered	10 pieces	208	13	6	16	20	2	5
Raisins, Milk Chocolate–Covered	10 pieces	39	1	1	4	7	0	0
GRANOLA BARS								
Fruit-Filled, Nonfat	1 oz	97	0	0	7	22	2	2
Hard, Chocolate Chip	1 oz	124	5	3	98	20	1	2
Soft, Nut & Raisin	1 oz	127	6	3	71	18	2	2
Soft, Peanut-Butter Filling, Chocolate-Coated	1 oz	152	9	5	55	15	1	3
POPCORN								
Air-Popped	1 cup	31	0	0	1	6	1	1
Caramel-Coated, w/Peanuts	1 cup	170	3	0	125	34	2	3
Cheese-Flavored	1 cup	58	4	1	98	6	1	1
Microwave, Butter-Flavored	1 cup	42	2	0	61	4	1	1
Oil-Popped	1 cup	64	5	1	116	5	1	1
Popcorn Cakes	1 cake	38	0	0	29	8	0	1
POTATO CHIPS								
Barbecue-Flavored	1 oz	139	9	2	213	15	1	2
Cheese-Flavored	1 oz	141	8	2	130	16	1	2
Fat-Free	1 oz	78	0	0	157	18	2	2
Light, Unsalted	1 oz	138	6	1	2	19	2	2
Plain, Salted	1 oz	154	10	1	136	14	1	2
Plain, Unsalted	1 oz	152	10	3	2	15	1	2

common foods

	SERVING SIZE	CALORIES	TOTAL FAT (G)	SAT FAT (G)	SODIUM (MG)	CARBS (G)	FIBER (G)	PROTEIN (G)
Potato Sticks	1 oz	148	10	3	179	15	1	2
Sour-Cream-and-Onion-Flavored	1 oz	151	10	3	156	15	1	2
Soy Chips or Crisps, Salted	1 oz	109	2	0	239	15	1	8
Sweet-Potato Chips, Unsalted	1 oz	151	9	1	10	16	2	1
PRETZELS								
Hard, Chocolate-Flavor-Coated	1 oz	130	5	2	161	20	0	2
Hard, Plain, Salted	1 oz	108	1	0	385	23	1	3
Hard, Whole-Wheat	1 oz	103	1	0	58	23	2	3
Soft	1 large	483	4	1	1151	99	2	12
TORTILLA CHIPS								
Light	1 oz	132	4	1	243	21	2	2
Low-Fat, Baked	1 oz	118	2	0	119	23	2	3
Nacho Cheese-Flavored	1 oz	146	7	1	174	18	1	2
Ranch-Flavored	1 oz	142	7	1	147	18	1	2
Taco-Flavored	1 oz	136	7	1	223	18	2	2
White Corn, Unsalted	1 oz	143	7	1	4	19	2	2
Yellow Corn, Salted	1 oz	141	6	1	86	19	1	2
TRAIL MIXES								
Regular	1/2 cup	347	22	4	172	34	n/a	10
Tropical	1/2 cup	285	12	6	7	46	n/a	4
w/Chocolate Chips, Nuts & Seeds, Salted	1/2 cup	353	23	4	88	33	n/a	10
Soups, Stews & Chilis								
BEAN								
Bean w/Bacon, Dry Mix, Prepared w/Water	1 cup	106	2	1	928	16	9	5
Bean w/Frankfurters, Canned, Prepared w/Water	1 cup	106	7	2	1093	22	0	10
Bean w/Ham, Chunky, Canned, Ready-to-Serve	1 cup	231	9	3	972	27	11	13
Bean w/Pork, Canned, Prepared w/Water	1 cup	168	6	1	930	22	8	8
Black Bean, Canned, Prepared w/Water	1 cup	114	2	0	1203	19	8	6
Black Turtle, Canned	1 cup	218	1	0	922	40	17	14
Black Turtle, Cooked, w/Salt	1 cup	241	1	0	442	45	15	15
Lentil w/Ham, Canned, Ready-to-Serve	1 cup	139	3	1	1319	20	0	9
BEEF								
Beef & Mushroom, Low-Sodium, Chunky	1 cup	173	6	4	63	24	1	11
Beef & Vegetable, Canned, Ready-to-Serve	1 cup	118	3	0	753	15	3	8

	SERVING SIZE	CALORIES	TOTAL FAT (G)	SAT FAT (G)	SODIUM (MG)	CARBS (G)	FIBER (G)	PROTEIN (G)
Beef Mushroom, Canned, Prepared w/Water	1 cup	73	3	1	942	6	0	6
Beef Noodle, Canned, Prepared w/Water	1 cup	83	3	1	930	9	1	5
Broth, Bouillon, Consommé, Prepared w/Water	1 cup	29	0	0	636	2	0	5
Broth or Bouillon, Canned, Ready-to-Serve	1 cup	17	1	0	893	0	0	3
Broth or Bouillon, Prepared w/Water	1 cup	7	0	0	917	1	0	1
Stew, Canned	1 cup	194	11	4	760	15	2	9
Stock, Homemade	1 cup	31	0	0	475	3	0	5
Stroganoff, Chunky, Canned, Ready-to-Serve	1 cup	235	11	6	1044	22	1	12
CHILE								
Canned, Prepared w/Water	1 cup	149	3	2	1013	24	3	6
w/Beans, Canned	1 cup	259	8	3	1087	32	8	14
w/o Beans, Canned	1 cup	283	17	5	934	15	0	18
CHICKEN								
Broth, Canned, Prepared w/Water	1 cup	39	1	0	747	1	0	5
Broth or Bouillon, Prepared w/Water	1 cup	10	1	0	966	1	0	1
Chicken Chili w/Beans, Canned	1 cup	287	14	6	1336	30	11	15
Chicken Mushroom, Canned, Prepared w/Water	1 cup	132	9	2	798	9	0	4
Chicken Noodle, Canned, Prepared w/Water	1 cup	25	1	0	349	3	0	1
Chicken Noodle, Dry-Mix, Prepared w/Water	1 cup	56	1	0	561	9	0	2
Chicken Noodle, Reduced-Sodium, Canned, Ready-to-Serve	1 cup	100	3	0	456	9	2	8
Chicken Rice, Canned, Prepared w/Water	1 cup	24	1	0	238	3	0	1
Chicken Rice, Chunky, Canned, Ready-to-Serve	1 cup	127	3	1	888	13	1	12
Chicken Rice, Dry Mix, Prepared w/Water	1 cup	58	1	0	931	9	1	2
Chicken Vegetable, Canned, Prepared w/Water	1 cup	77	3	1	972	9	1	4
Chicken Vegetable, Chunky, Canned, Ready-to-Serve	1 cup	166	5	1	833	19	0	12
Chicken w/Dumplings, Canned, Prepared w/Water	1 cup	96	6	1	735	6	0	6

common foods

	SERVING SIZE	CALORIES	TOTAL FAT (G)	SAT FAT (G)	SODIUM (MG)	CARBS (G)	FIBER (G)	PROTEIN (G)
Cream of Chicken, Canned, Prepared w/Milk	1 cup	191	11	5	898	15	0	7
Cream of Chicken, Canned, Prepared w/Water	1 cup	117	7	2	847	9	0	3
Cream of Chicken, Dry Mix, Prepared w/Water	1 cup	107	5	3	1185	13	0	2
Stock, Homemade	1 cup	86	3	1	343	8	0	6
SEAFOOD								
Clam Chowder, Manhattan, Canned, Chunky, Ready-to-Serve	1 cup	134	3	2	1001	19	3	7
Clam Chowder, Manhattan, Canned, Prepared w/Water	1 cup	75	2	0	562	12	1	2
Clam Chowder, New England, Canned, Prepared w/Water	1 cup	87	3	1	630	13	1	4
Clam Chowder, New England, Canned, Ready-to-Serve	1 cup	201	10	0	871	21	3	7
Fish Broth	1 cup	39	1	0	776	1	0	5
Fish Stock, Homemade	1 cup	40	2	0	363	0	0	5
SPLIT PEA								
w/Ham, Canned, Prepared w/Water	1 cup	190	4	2	1007	28	2	10
w/Ham, Chunky, Canned, Ready-to-Serve	1 cup	185	4	2	722	27	4	11
TOMATO								
Bisque, Canned, Prepared w/Milk	1 cup	198	7	3	1109	29	1	6
Bisque, Canned, Prepared w/Water	1 cup	124	3	1	1047	24	0	2
Canned, Prepared w/Milk	1 cup	139	3	2	529	23	2	6
Canned, Prepared w/Water	1 cup	74	1	0	471	16	1	2
Tomato Rice, Canned, Prepared w/Water	1 cup	116	3	1	788	21	2	2
TURKEY								
Turkey, Chunky, Canned, Ready-to-Serve	1 cup	135	4	1	923	14	0	10
Turkey Noodle, Canned, Prepared w/Water	1 cup	68	2	1	815	9	1	4
Turkey Vegetable, Canned, Prepared w/Water	1 cup	72	3	1	906	9	0	3
VEGETABLE								
Cream of Asparagus, Canned, Prepared w/Milk	1 cup	161	8	3	1042	16	1	6
Cream of Asparagus, Canned, Prepared w/Water	1 cup	85	4	1	981	11	0	2

	SERVING SIZE	CALORIES	TOTAL FAT (G)	SAT FAT (G)	SODIUM (MG)	CARBS (G)	FIBER (G)	PROTEIN (G)
Cream of Celery, Canned, Prepared w/Milk	1 cup	164	10	4	675	15	1	6
Cream of Celery, Canned, Prepared w/Water	1 cup	92	6	1	630	9	1	2
Cream of Mushroom, Canned, Prepared w/Milk	1 cup	169	10	3	844	14	0	6
Cream of Mushroom, Canned, Prepared w/Water	1 cup	104	7	2	789	8	0	2
Cream of Mushroom, Low-Sodium, Canned, Ready-to-Serve	1 cup	129	9	2	49	11	0	2
Gazpacho, Canned, Ready-to-Serve	1 cup	46	0	0	739	4	0	7
Minestrone, Canned, Prepared w/Water	1 cup	82	3	1	612	11	1	4
Minestrone, Chunky, Canned, Ready-to-Serve	1 cup	127	3	1	691	21	6	5
Minestrone, Reduced-Sodium, Ready-to-Serve	1 cup	122	2	0	527	22	6	5
Vegetable, Chunky, Canned, Ready-to-Serve	1 cup	125	4	1	880	19	1	4
Vegetable Beef, Canned, Prepared w/Water	1 cup	76	2	1	852	10	2	5
Vegetarian Vegetable, Canned, Prepared w/Water	1 cup	67	2	0	815	12	1	2

Sugars

Brown, Packed	1 cup	836	0	0	62	216	0	0
Cane, Natural (Turbinado)	1 tsp	18	0	0	0	5	0	0
Granulated	1 tsp	16	0	0	0	4	0	0
Granulated	1 cup	774	0	0	2	200	0	0
Honey	1 tbsp	64	0	0	1	17	0	0
Molasses	1 tbsp	58	0	0	7	15	0	0
Powdered, Unsifted	1 cup	467	0	0	2	120	0	0

Syrups

Chocolate Syrup	1 tbsp	54	0	0	14	13	1	0
Corn Syrup, Dark	1 tbsp	57	0	0	31	16	0	0
Corn Syrup, High-Fructose	1 tbsp	53	0	0	0	14	0	0
Corn Syrup, Light	1 tbsp	62	0	0	14	17	0	0
Malt Syrup	1 tbsp	67	0	0	7	15	0	1
Maple Syrup	1 tbsp	52	0	0	2	13	0	0
Pancake Syrup	1 tbsp	47	0	0	16	12	0	0
Pancake Syrup, Reduced-Calorie	1 tbsp	25	0	0	27	7	0	0

common foods	SERVING SIZE	CALORIES	TOTAL FAT (G)	SAT FAT (G)	SODIUM (MG)	CARBS (G)	FIBER (G)	PROTEIN (G)
Pancake Syrup, w/Butter	1 tbsp	59	0	0	20	15	0	0
Pancake Syrup, w/2% Maple	1 tbsp	53	0	0	12	14	0	0
Sorghum Syrup	1 tbsp	61	0	0	2	16	0	0

Vegetables

	SERVING SIZE	CALORIES	TOTAL FAT (G)	SAT FAT (G)	SODIUM (MG)	CARBS (G)	FIBER (G)	PROTEIN (G)
Artichoke	1 medium	60	0	0	120	13	7	4
Artichoke, Cooked, w/Salt	1 medium	61	0	0	355	14	10	3
Artichoke, Frozen, Cooked, w/Salt	1/2 cup	38	0	0	243	8	4	3
Asparagus	1/2 cup	13	0	0	1	3	1	1
Asparagus, Canned	1/2 cup	23	1	0	347	3	2	3
Asparagus, Cooked	1/2 cup	20	0	0	13	4	2	2
Asparagus, Frozen, Cooked, w/Salt	1/2 cup	16	0	0	216	2	1	3
Avocado, All Common Varieties, Cubed	1/2 cup	120	11	2	5	6	5	2
Avocado, California, w/o Skin & Seeds	1 medium	227	21	3	11	12	9	3
Avocado, Florida, w/o Skin & Seeds	1 medium	365	31	6	6	24	17	7
BEANS & OTHER LEGUMES								
Adzuki, Canned, Sweetened	1/2 cup	351	0	0	323	81	0	6
Adzuki, Cooked, w/Salt	1/2 cup	147	0	0	281	28	8	9
Baked Beans, Canned, No Salt	1/2 cup	133	1	0	1	26	7	6
Baked Beans, Canned, Plain or Vegetarian	1/2 cup	119	0	0	436	27	5	6
Baked Beans, Canned, w/Beef	1/2 cup	161	5	2	632	22	0	8
Baked Beans, Canned, w/Franks	1/2 cup	184	9	3	557	20	9	9
Baked Beans, Canned, w/Pork	1/2 cup	134	2	1	524	25	7	7
Baked Beans, Canned, w/Pork & Sweet Sauce	1/2 cup	142	2	1	423	27	5	7
Baked Beans, Canned, w/Pork & Tomato Sauce	1/2 cup	116	1	0	538	23	5	6
Baked Beans, Home Prepared	1/2 cup	196	7	2	534	27	7	7
Black Beans, Cooked, w/Salt	1/2 cup	114	0	0	204	20	7	8
Black-Eyed Peas (Cowpeas), Canned w/Pork	1/2 cup	100	2	1	420	20	4	3
Black-Eyed Peas (Cowpeas), Canned, Plain	1/2 cup	92	1	0	359	16	4	6
Black-Eyed Peas (Cowpeas), Cooked, w/Salt	1/2 cup	99	0	0	205	18	6	7
Black-Eyed Peas (Cowpeas), Cooked, w/o Salt	1/2 cup	99	0	0	3	18	6	7
Broad (Fava) Beans, Canned	1/2 cup	91	0	0	580	16	5	7
Broad (Fava) Beans, Cooked, w/Salt	1/2 cup	94	0	0	205	17	5	6

	SERVING SIZE	CALORIES	TOTAL FAT (G)	SAT FAT (G)	SODIUM (MG)	CARBS (G)	FIBER (G)	PROTEIN (G)
Chickpeas (Garbanzo Beans), Canned	1/2 cup	106	2	0	334	16	5	6
Chickpeas (Garbanzo Beans), Cooked, w/Salt	1/2 cup	134	2	0	199	22	6	7
Cranberry (Roman) Beans, Canned	1/2 cup	108	0	0	432	20	8	7
Cranberry (Roman) Beans, Cooked, w/Salt	1/2 cup	120	0	0	210	22	9	8
Great Northern Beans, Canned	1/2 cup	149	1	0	5	28	6	10
Great Northern Beans, Cooked, w/Salt	1/2 cup	104	0	0	211	19	6	7
Kidney Beans, All Types, Canned	1/2 cup	105	1	0	379	19	7	7
Kidney Beans, All Types, Cooked, w/Salt	1/2 cup	112	0	0	211	20	6	8
Green (Snap/String) Beans	1/2 cup	16	0	0	3	3	1	1
Green (Snap/String) Beans, Canned	1/2 cup	16	0	0	2	3	2	1
Green (Snap/String) Beans, Cooked, w/Salt	1/2 cup	22	0	0	149	5	2	1
Green (Snap/String) Beans, Frozen, Cooked, w/Salt	1/2 cup	18	0	0	165	4	2	1
Green (Snap/String) Beans, Frozen, Cooked, w/o Salt	1/2 cup	19	0	0	1	4	2	1
Lentils, Cooked, w/Salt	1/2 cup	113	0	0	236	19	8	9
Lima Beans, Baby, Cooked, w/Salt	1/2 cup	115	0	0	217	21	7	7
Lima Beans, Canned	1/2 cup	88	0	0	5	17	4	5
Lima Beans, Cooked, w/Salt	1/2 cup	105	0	0	215	20	5	6
Lima Beans, Frozen, Baby, Cooked, w/Salt	1/2 cup	95	0	0	239	18	5	6
Lima Beans, Large, Canned	1/2 cup	95	0	0	405	18	6	6
Lima Beans, Large, Cooked, w/Salt	1/2 cup	108	0	0	224	20	7	7
Mung Beans, Cooked, w/Salt	1/2 cup	106	0	0	240	19	8	7
Navy Beans, Canned	1/2 cup	148	1	0	587	27	7	10
Navy Beans, Cooked, w/Salt	1/2 cup	127	1	0	216	24	10	7
Peapods, Cooked, w/Salt	1/2 cup	32	0	0	192	5	2	3
Peapods, Fresh	1 cup	26	0	0	3	5	2	2
Peapods, Frozen	1 cup	60	0	0	6	10	4	4
Peapods, Frozen, Cooked, w/Salt	1 cup	80	1	0	386	13	5	6
Peas, Green	1 cup	117	1	0	7	21	7	8
Peas, Green, Canned	1/2 cup	72	0	0	229	13	4	4
Peas, Green, Cooked, w/Salt	1/2 cup	67	0	0	191	13	4	4
Peas, Green, Frozen	1 cup	103	1	0	145	18	6	7
Peas, Green, Frozen, Cooked, w/Salt	1/2 cup	62	0	0	258	11	4	4
Pigeon Peas, Cooked, w/Salt	1/2 cup	102	0	0	202	20	6	6

common foods

	SERVING SIZE	CALORIES	TOTAL FAT (G)	SAT FAT (G)	SODIUM (MG)	CARBS (G)	FIBER (G)	PROTEIN (G)
Pink Beans, Cooked, w/Salt	1/2 cup	126	0	0	201	24	4	8
Pinto Beans, Canned	1/2 cup	98	1	0	322	18	6	6
Pinto Beans, Canned, Drained & Rinsed	1/2 cup	99	1	0	179	18	0	6
Pinto Beans, Cooked, w/Salt	1/2 cup	122	1	0	203	22	8	8
Refried Beans, Canned, Fat-Free	1/2 cup	91	1	0	506	16	5	6
Refried Beans, Canned, Traditional-Style	1/2 cup	108	1	0	534	18	6	6
Refried Beans, Canned, Vegetarian	1/2 cup	100	1	0	520	16	6	6
Soybeans, Cooked, w/Salt	1/2 cup	149	8	1	204	9	5	14
Soybeans, Dry-Roasted	1/2 cup	388	19	3	2	28	7	34
Soybeans, Roasted, Salted	1/2 cup	405	22	3	140	29	15	30
Split Peas, Cooked, w/Salt	1/2 cup	114	0	0	233	20	8	8
Yellow Wax (Butter) Beans	1/2 cup	16	0	0	3	4	2	1
Yellow Wax (Butter) Beans, Canned	1/2 cup	15	0	0	2	3	1	1
Yellow Wax (Butter) Beans, Cooked	1/2 cup	22	0	0	2	5	2	1
Yellow Wax (Butter) Beans, Frozen, Cooked, w/Salt	1/2 cup	18	0	0	165	4	2	1
Beets	1 cup	58	0	0	106	13	4	2
Beets, Canned	1 cup	74	0	0	352	18	3	2
Beets, Cooked, Sliced	1 cup	75	0	0	131	17	3	3
Beets, Harvard, Canned, Sliced	1 cup	180	0	0	399	45	6	2
Beets, Pickled, Sliced	1 cup	148	0	0	599	37	6	2
Bok Choi, Cooked, w/Salt, Shredded	1/2 cup	20	0	0	459	3	2	3
Bok Choi, Cooked, w/o Salt, Shredded	1/2 cup	20	0	0	58	3	2	3
Broccoli	1 stalk	32	0	0	31	6	0	3
Broccoli, Chinese, Cooked	1 cup	19	1	0	6	3	2	1
Broccoli, Chopped	1 cup	31	0	0	30	6	2	3
Broccoli, Cooked, w/o Salt, Chopped	1/2 cup	27	0	0	32	6	3	2
Broccoli, Florets	1 cup	20	0	0	19	4	0	2
Broccoli, Frozen, Cooked, w/Salt, Chopped	1/2 cup	26	0	0	239	5	3	3
Broccoli, Frozen, Cooked, w/Salt, Spears	1/2 cup	26	0	0	239	5	3	3
Broccoli Raab, Chopped	1 cup	9	0	0	13	1	1	1
Broccoli Raab, Cooked	3 oz	28	0	0	48	3	2	3
Brussels Sprouts	1 cup	38	0	0	22	8	3	3
Brussels Sprouts, Cooked, w/Salt	1/2 cup	28	0	0	200	6	2	2
Brussels Sprouts, Frozen, Cooked, w/o Salt	1/2 cup	33	0	0	12	6	3	3
Cabbage, Chopped	1 cup	22	0	0	16	5	2	1

	SERVING SIZE	CALORIES	TOTAL FAT (G)	SAT FAT (G)	SODIUM (MG)	CARBS (G)	FIBER (G)	PROTEIN (G)
Cabbage, Cooked, w/Salt, Shredded	1/2 cup	17	0	0	191	4	1	1
Cabbage, Japanese Style, Pickled	1 cup	45	0	0	416	9	5	2
Cabbage, Mustard, Salted	1 cup	36	0	0	918	7	4	1
Cabbage, Napa, Cooked	1/2 cup	7	0	0	6	1	0	1
Cabbage, Red, Cooked, w/Salt, Shredded	1/2 cup	22	0	0	183	5	2	1
Cabbage, Red, Shredded	1 cup	22	0	0	19	5	1	1
Cabbage, Savoy, Cooked, w/Salt, Shredded	1/2 cup	17	0	0	189	4	2	1
Cabbage, Savoy, Shredded	1 cup	19	0	0	20	4	2	1
Cabbage, Shredded	1/2 cup	8	0	0	6	2	1	0
Carrots, Baby	1 large	5	0	0	12	1	0	0
Carrots, Canned, Sliced	1 cup	37	0	0	61	8	2	1
Carrots, Chopped	1 cup	52	0	0	88	12	4	1
Carrots, Cooked, w/Salt, Sliced	1/2 cup	27	0	0	236	6	2	1
Carrots, Frozen, Cooked, w/Salt, Sliced	1 cup	54	1	0	431	11	5	1
Carrots, Frozen, Sliced	1/2 cup	23	0	0	44	5	2	1
Cassava	1 cup	330	1	0	29	78	4	3
Cauliflower, Chopped	1 cup	27	0	0	32	5	2	2
Cauliflower, Cooked, w/Salt	1/2 cup	14	0	0	150	3	1	1
Cauliflower, Frozen	10 ounces	68	1	0	68	13	7	6
Cauliflower, Frozen, Cooked, w/Salt	1/2 cup	15	0	0	229	3	2	1
Cauliflower, Green	1 cup	20	0	0	15	4	2	2
Cauliflower, Green, Cooked, w/Salt	1/2 cup	20	0	0	161	4	2	2
Celeriac	1 cup	66	0	0	156	14	3	2
Celeriac, Cooked, w/Salt	1/2 cup	21	0	0	230	5	0	1
Celery, Chopped	1 cup	16	0	0	81	3	2	1
Celery, Cooked, w/Salt, Diced	1/2 cup	14	0	0	245	3	1	1
Corn, Sweet, White	1 small ear	63	1	0	11	14	2	2
Corn, Sweet, White, Canned, Cream-Style	1 cup	184	1	0	730	46	3	4
Corn, Sweet, White, Canned, Whole Kernels	1 cup	133	2	0	530	30	3	4
Corn, Sweet, White, Cooked, w/Salt	1 small ear	86	1	0	225	19	2	3
Corn, Sweet, White, Frozen, Kernels	1 cup	145	1	0	5	34	4	5
Corn, Sweet, White, Frozen, Kernels on Cob	1 ear	123	1	0	6	29	4	4
Corn, Sweet, White, Frozen, Kernels on Cob, Cooked, w/Salt	1 ear	59	0	0	151	14	2	2

common foods

	SERVING SIZE	CALORIES	TOTAL FAT (G)	SAT FAT (G)	SODIUM (MG)	CARBS (G)	FIBER (G)	PROTEIN (G)
Corn, Sweet, White, Frozen, Kernels, Cooked, w/Salt	1/2 cup	66	0	0	202	16	2	2
Corn, Sweet, Yellow	1 cup	125	2	0	22	27	3	5
Corn, Sweet, Yellow, Canned, Cream Style	1 cup	184	1	0	730	46	3	4
Corn, Sweet, Yellow, Canned, Whole Kernels	1 cup	130	2	0	305	29	3	4
Corn, Sweet, Yellow, Cooked, w/Salt	1 small ear	85	1	0	225	19	2	3
Corn, Sweet, Yellow, Frozen, Kernels	1 cup	120	1	0	4	28	3	4
Corn, Sweet, Yellow, Frozen, Kernels, Cooked, w/Salt	1 cup	130	1	0	404	31	4	4
Corn, Sweet, Yellow, Frozen, Kernels on Cob	1 ear	123	1	0	6	29	4	4
Corn, Sweet, Yellow, Frozen, Kernels on Cob, Cooked, w/Salt	1 ear	59	0	0	151	14	2	2
Cucumber	1 large	45	0	0	6	11	2	2
Cucumber, Peeled, Sliced	1 cup	14	0	0	2	3	1	1
Cucumber, w/Peel, Sliced	1/2 cup	8	0	0	1	2	0	0
Eggplant, Cooked, w/Salt, Cubed	1/2 cup	16	0	0	118	4	1	0
Eggplant, Cubed	1 cup	20	0	0	2	5	3	1
Endive, Chopped	1 cup	9	0	0	11	2	2	1
Fennel, Bulb, Sliced	1 cup	27	0	0	45	6	3	1
Fiddlehead Ferns	1 oz	10	0	0	0	2	0	1
Garlic	1 tsp	4	0	0	0	1	0	0
Grape Leaves	1 cup	13	0	0	1	2	2	1
Grape Leaves, canned	1 leaf	3	0	0	114	0	0	0
GREENS								
Beet	1 cup	8	0	0	86	2	1	1
Beet, Cooked, w/Salt	1/2 cup	19	0	0	343	4	2	2
Chard, Swiss	1 cup	7	0	0	77	1	1	1
Chard, Swiss, Cooked, w/Salt, Chopped	1/2 cup	18	0	0	363	4	2	2
Collards, Chopped	1 cup	11	0	0	7	2	1	1
Collards, Cooked, w/Salt, Chopped	1/2 cup	25	0	0	239	5	3	2
Collards, Frozen, Cooked, w/Salt, Chopped	1/2 cup	31	0	0	243	6	2	3
Dandelion, Chopped	1 cup	25	0	0	42	5	2	1
Dandelion, Cooked, w/Salt, Chopped	1/2 cup	17	0	0	147	3	2	1
Kale, Chopped	1 cup	34	0	0	29	7	1	2

	SERVING SIZE	CALORIES	TOTAL FAT (G)	SAT FAT (G)	SODIUM (MG)	CARBS (G)	FIBER (G)	PROTEIN (G)
Kale, Chopped, Cooked, w/Salt	1/2 cup	18	0	0	168	4	1	1
Kale, Frozen	10 ounces	80	1	0	43	14	6	8
Kale, Frozen, Chopped, Cooked, w/Salt	1/2 cup	20	0	0	163	3	1	2
Mustard, Chopped	1 cup	15	0	0	14	3	2	2
Mustard, Cooked, w/Salt, Chopped	1/2 cup	11	0	0	176	1	1	2
Mustard, Frozen, Cooked, w/Salt, Chopped	1/2 cup	14	0	0	196	2	2	2
Spinach	1 cup	7	0	0	24	1	1	1
Spinach, Canned	1 cup	49	1	0	689	7	5	6
Spinach, Cooked, w/Salt	1/2 cup	21	0	0	275	3	2	3
Spinach, Frozen, Chopped	1 cup	45	1	0	115	7	5	6
Spinach, Frozen, Cooked, w/Salt, Chopped	1/2 cup	32	1	0	306	5	4	4
Turnip, Canned	1/2 cup	16	0	0	324	3	2	2
Turnip, Canned, w/o Salt	1/2 cup	14	0	0	21	2	1	1
Turnip, Chopped	1 cup	18	0	0	22	4	2	1
Turnip, Chopped, Cooked, w/Salt	1/2 cup	14	0	0	191	3	3	1
Turnip, Frozen, Cooked, w/Salt	1/2 cup	24	0	0	206	4	3	3
Hearts of Palm, Canned	1 cup	41	1	0	622	7	4	4
Jerusalem Artichokes, Sliced	1 cup	110	0	0	6	26	2	3
Jicama, Sliced	1 cup	46	0	0	5	11	6	1
Kohlrabi	1 cup	36	0	0	27	8	5	2
Kohlrabi, Cooked, w/Salt, Sliced	1/2 cup	24	0	0	212	6	1	1
Leeks	1 cup	54	0	0	18	13	2	1
Leeks, Cooked, w/Salt, Chopped	1/4 cup	8	0	0	64	2	0	0
LETTUCE								
Butterhead/Boston/Bibb, Shredded or Chopped	1 cup	7	0	0	3	1	1	1
Green Leaf, Shredded	1 cup	5	0	0	10	1	0	0
Iceberg/Crisphead, Shredded	1 cup	10	0	0	7	2	1	1
Red Leaf, Shredded	1 cup	4	0	0	7	1	0	0
Romaine, Shredded	1 cup	8	0	0	4	2	1	1
MUSHROOMS								
Brown/Italian/Crimini, Whole	1 cup	19	0	0	5	4	1	2
Canned	1 cup	39	0	0	663	8	4	3
Chanterelle	1 cup	21	0	0	5	4	2	1
Enoki	1 large	2	0	0	0	0	0	0

common foods

	SERVING SIZE	CALORIES	TOTAL FAT (G)	SAT FAT (G)	SODIUM (MG)	CARBS (G)	FIBER (G)	PROTEIN (G)
Maitake, Diced	1 cup	22	0	0	1	5	2	1
Morel	1 cup	20	0	0	14	3	2	2
Oyster	1 large	49	1	0	27	9	3	5
Portabella, Diced	1 cup	19	0	0	8	3	1	2
Portabella, Grilled, Sliced	1 cup	35	1	0	13	5	3	4
Shiitake, Cooked, w/Salt	1 cup	81	0	0	348	21	3	2
Shiitake, Dried	1 mushroom	11	0	0	0	3	0	0
Shiitake, Whole	1 mushroom	6	0	0	2	1	0	0
Straw, Canned	1 cup	58	1	0	699	8	5	7
White, Cooked, w/Salt	1 cup	44	1	0	371	8	3	3
White, Pieces or Sliced	1 cup	15	0	0	4	2	1	2
Okra	1 cup	31	0	0	8	7	3	2
Okra, Cooked, w/Salt, Sliced	1/2 cup	18	0	0	193	4	2	1
Okra, Frozen, Cooked, w/Salt, Sliced	1/2 cup	31	0	0	220	6	2	2
Onions, Canned, Chopped or Diced	1/2 cup	21	0	0	416	5	1	1
Onions, Chopped	1 cup	64	0	0	6	15	3	2
Onions, Cooked, w/Salt	1/2 cup	44	0	0	251	10	1	1
Onions, Dehydrated	1 tbsp	17	0	0	1	4	0	0
Onions, Frozen, Chopped	10 ounces	82	0	0	34	19	5	2
Onions, Frozen, Cooked, w/Salt, Chopped	1/2 cup	31	0	0	37	1	0	0
Onions, Frozen, Cooked, w/Salt, Whole	1/2 cup	27	0	0	256	6	1	1
Onions, Spring or Scallions (Tops & Bulb), Chopped	1 cup	32	0	0	16	7	3	2
Onions, Sweet	1 onion	106	0	0	26	25	3	3
Onions, Yellow, Sautéed, Chopped	1 cup	115	9	1	10	7	1	1
Parsnips, Cooked, w/Salt, Sliced	1/2 cup	55	0	0	192	13	3	1
PEPPERS								
Ancho, Dried	1 pepper	48	1	0	7	9	4	2
Banana	1 small	9	0	0	4	2	1	1
Chili, Green, Canned	1/4 cup	7	0	0	138	2	1	0
Chili, Green, Hot	1 pepper	18	0	0	3	4	1	1
Chili, Green, Hot, Canned, Chopped or Diced	1/2 cup	14	0	0	798	3	1	1
Chili, Red, Hot	1 pepper	18	0	0	4	4	1	1
Chili, Red, Hot, Canned, Chopped or Diced	1/2 cup	14	0	0	798	3	1	1

	SERVING SIZE	CALORIES	TOTAL FAT (G)	SAT FAT (G)	SODIUM (MG)	CARBS (G)	FIBER (G)	PROTEIN (G)
Hungarian	1 pepper	8	0	0	0	2	0	0
Jalapeño, Sliced	1/4 cup	7	0	0	1	1	1	0
Jalapeño, Canned, Chopped	1/4 cup	37	1	0	2273	6	4	1
Pasilla, Dried	1 pepper	24	1	0	6	4	2	1
Serrano, Chopped	1/4 cup	8	0	0	3	2	1	0
Sweet, Green, Canned, Halved	1 cup	25	0	0	1917	5	2	1
Sweet, Green, Chopped	1 cup	30	0	0	4	7	3	1
Sweet, Green, Cooked, w/Salt	1/2 cup	3	0	0	28	1	0	0
Sweet, Green, Frozen, Cooked, w/Salt, Chopped or Strips	1/2 cup	11	0	0	162	2	1	1
Sweet, Red, Canned, Halves	1 cup	25	0	0	1917	5	2	1
Sweet, Red, Cooked, w/Salt	1 pepper	19	0	0	174	4	1	1
Sweet, Red, Frozen, Cooked, w/Salt, Chopped or Strips	1/2 cup	11	0	0	162	2	1	1
Sweet, Red, Sliced	1 cup	29	0	0	4	6	2	1
Sweet, Yellow	1 large	50	0	0	4	12	2	2
POTATOES								
Au Gratin, Homemade, w/Butter	1 cup	323	19	12	1061	28	4	12
Au Gratin, Homemade, w/Margarine	1 cup	323	19	9	1061	28	4	12
Baked, Peeled, w/Salt	1 medium	145	0	0	376	34	2	3
Baked, w/Salt	1 medium	161	0	0	17	37	4	4
Baked Skin, w/Salt	1 skin	115	0	0	149	27	5	2
Boiled in Skin, Peeled, w/Salt	1 medium	118	0	0	326	27	3	3
Boiled w/o Skin, Peeled, w/Salt	1 medium	144	0	0	402	33	3	3
Canned, Drained	1 cup	108	0	0	394	24	4	3
Hash Browns, Homemade	1 cup	413	20	3	534	55	5	5
Mashed, Instant, Flakes, w/Whole Milk & Butter	1 cup	204	11	7	344	23	2	4
Mashed, w/Whole Milk	1 cup	174	1	1	634	37	3	4
Mashed, w/Whole Milk & Butter	1 cup	237	9	5	666	35	3	4
Mashed, w/Whole Milk & Margarine	1 cup	237	9	2	699	36	3	4
Microwaved, w/Salt	1 medium	212	0	0	493	49	5	5
Red, Baked in Skin	1 medium	154	0	0	21	34	3	4
Russet, Baked in Skin	1 medium	168	0	0	24	37	4	5
Scalloped, Homemade, w/Butter	1 cup	216	9	6	821	26	5	7
Sweet Potato, Baked in Skin, w/Salt	1 medium	105	0	0	280	24	4	2
Sweet Potato, Boiled, Mashed	1 cup	249	0	0	863	58	8	4

common foods

	SERVING SIZE	CALORIES	TOTAL FAT (G)	SAT FAT (G)	SODIUM (MG)	CARBS (G)	FIBER (G)	PROTEIN (G)
Sweet Potato, Boiled w/o Skin, w/Salt	1 medium	115	0	0	397	27	4	2
Sweet Potato, Canned in Syrup	1 cup	212	1	0	76	50	6	3
Sweet Potato, Canned, Mashed	1 cup	258	1	0	191	59	4	5
Sweet Potato, Frozen, Cubed, Cooked, w/Salt	1 cup	176	0	0	429	41	3	3
White, Baked in Skin	1 medium	130	0	0	10	29	3	3
Pumpkin, Canned, w/Salt	1 cup	83	1	0	590	20	7	3
Pumpkin, Cooked, w/Salt, Mashed	1 cup	49	0	0	581	12	3	2
Pumpkin Flowers, Cooked, w/Salt	1/2 cup	10	0	0	162	2	1	1
Radicchio, Shredded	1 cup	9	0	0	9	2	0	1
Radishes	1 large	1	0	0	4	0	0	0
Radishes, Hawaiian-Style, Pickled	1 cup	42	0	0	1184	8	3	2
Radishes, Sliced	1 cup	19	0	0	45	4	2	1
Radishes, Daikon	1 radish	61	0	0	71	14	5	2
Radishes, Daikon, Cooked, w/Salt, Sliced	1 cup	25	0	0	366	5	2	1
Rhubarb, Diced	1 cup	26	0	0	5	6	2	1
Rhubarb, Frozen, Cooked w/Sugar	1 cup	278	0	0	2	75	5	1
Rutabagas, Cooked, w/Salt, Mashed	1/2 cup	47	0	0	305	10	0	2
Seaweed, Kelp	2 tbsp	4	0	0	23	1	0	0
Seaweed, Wakame	2 tbsp	5	0	0	87	1	0	0
Shallots, Chopped	1 tbsp	7	0	0	1	2	0	0
Spirulina, Dried	1 tbsp	20	1	0	73	2	0	4
SPROUTS								
Alfalfa	1/4 cup	2	0	0	0	0	0	0
Bean, Kidney	1/4 cup	13	0	0	3	2	0	2
Bean, Mung	1/4 cup	8	0	0	2	2	0	1
Bean, Mung, Canned, Drained	1/4 cup	4	0	0	44	1	0	0
Bean, Mung, Cooked, w/Salt	1/4 cup	6	0	0	76	1	0	1
Bean, Navy	1/4 cup	17	0	0	3	3	0	2
Lentil	1/4 cup	20	0	0	2	4	0	2
Pea	1/4 cup	37	0	0	6	8	0	3
Radish	1/4 cup	4	0	0	1	0	0	0
Soybean	1/4 cup	21	1	0	2	2	0	2
Soybean, Cooked	1/4 cup	19	1	0	2	2	0	2
SQUASH								
Acorn, Cooked, w/Salt, Cubed	1/2 cup	57	0	0	246	15	5	1
Acorn, Cooked, w/Salt, Mashed	1/2 cup	42	0	0	293	11	3	1

	SERVING SIZE	CALORIES	TOTAL FAT (G)	SAT FAT (G)	SODIUM (MG)	CARBS (G)	FIBER (G)	PROTEIN (G)
Butternut, Cooked, w/Salt, Cubed	1/2 cup	41	0	0	246	11	3	1
Butternut, Frozen, Cooked, w/Salt, Mashed	1/2 cup	47	0	0	286	12	0	1
Hubbard, Cooked, w/Salt, Cubed	1/2 cup	51	1	0	250	11	5	3
Hubbard, Cooked, w/Salt, Mashed	1/2 cup	35	0	0	284	8	3	2
Spaghetti, Cooked, w/Salt	1/2 cup	21	0	0	197	5	1	1
Yellow, Cooked, w/Salt, Sliced	1/2 cup	17	0	0	213	3	1	1
Yellow, Frozen, Cooked, w/Salt, Sliced	1/2 cup	24	0	0	232	5	1	1
Yellow, Frozen, Sliced	1 cup	26	0	0	6	6	2	1
Yellow, Sliced	1 cup	24	0	0	3	5	1	1
Tomatillos, Chopped or Diced	1 cup	42	1	0	1	8	3	1
TOMATOES								
Tomato Paste, Canned	1/2 cup	107	1	0	1035	25	5	6
Tomato Puree, Canned, w/Salt	1 cup	95	1	0	998	22	5	4
Tomato Sauce, Canned	1 cup	59	0	0	1284	13	4	3
Tomatoes, Canned, Stewed	1 cup	66	0	0	564	16	3	2
Tomatoes, Cherry	1 cup	27	0	0	7	6	2	1
Tomatoes, Green	1 large	42	0	0	24	9	2	2
Tomatoes, Orange, Chopped	1 cup	25	0	0	66	5	1	2
Tomatoes, Red, Canned, in Juice	1 cup	41	0	0	343	10	2	2
Tomatoes, Red, Chopped or Sliced	1 cup	32	0	0	9	7	2	2
Tomatoes, Red, Cooked	1/2 cup	22	0	0	13	5	1	1
Tomatoes, Red, Cooked, w/Salt	1/2 cup	22	0	0	296	5	1	1
Tomatoes, Red, Stewed	1/2 cup	40	1	0	230	7	1	1
Tomatoes, Sun-Dried	1/4 cup	35	0	0	33	8	2	2
Tomatoes, Sun-Dried, in Oil, Drained	1/4 cup	59	4	1	73	6	2	1
Tomatoes, Yellow, Chopped	1 cup	21	0	0	32	4	1	1
Turnips	1 large	51	0	0	123	12	3	2
Turnips, Cooked, w/Salt, Cubed	1/2 cup	25	0	0	329	6	2	1
Turnips, Cooked, w/Salt, Mashed	1/2 cup	25	0	0	329	6	2	1
Turnips, Cubed	1 cup	36	0	0	87	8	2	1
Turnips, Frozen, Cooked, w/Salt	1/2 cup	16	0	0	212	3	2	1
Turnips & Greens, Frozen, Cooked, w/Salt	1/2 cup	28	0	0	208	4	3	2
Vegetables, Mixed, Canned	1 cup	80	0	0	243	15	5	4
Vegetables, Mixed, Frozen, Cooked, w/Salt	1/2 cup	55	0	0	247	12	4	3
Water Chestnuts, Chinese, Canned, Sliced	1/4 cup	18	0	0	3	4	1	0

	SERVING SIZE	CALORIES	TOTAL FAT (G)	SAT FAT (G)	SODIUM (MG)	CARBS (G)	FIBER (G)	PROTEIN (G)
Water Chestnuts, Chinese (Matai), Sliced	1/4 cup	30	0	0	4	7	1	0
Watercress, Chopped	1 cup	4	0	0	14	0	0	1
Yam, Cubed, Cooked, w/Salt	1 cup	155	0	0	332	37	5	2
Zucchini, Baby	1 large	3	0	0	0	0	0	0
Zucchini, Chopped	1 cup	21	0	0	10	4	1	2
Zucchini, Cooked, w/Salt, Sliced	1/2 cup	14	0	0	215	2	1	1
Zucchini, Frozen, Cooked, w/Salt	1/2 cup	16	0	0	265	3	1	1
Zucchini, Italian Style, Canned	1/2 cup	66	0	0	849	16	0	2

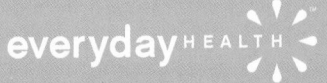

store brands

store brands

	SERVING SIZE	CALORIES	TOTAL FAT (G)	SAT FAT (G)	SODIUM (MG)	CARBS (G)	FIBER (G)	PROTEIN (G)
3 Musketeers								
Original	1 bar	260	8	5	110	46	1	2
7 UP								
Original	12 fl oz	153	0	n/a	45	39	n/a	0
A&W								
Cream Soda	12 fl oz	180	0	0	68	47	n/a	0
Root Beer	12 fl oz	180	0	0	83	48	n/a	0
A.1.								
Steak Sauce, Original	1 tbsp	15	0	0	280	3	0	0
Activia								
Raspberry, Light	1 container	70	0	0	75	13	2	4
Strawberry & Cereal	1 container	110	2	1	60	20	3	4
Vanilla, Light	1 container	70	0	0	70	14	3	5
Vanilla & Cereal	1 container	110	2	1	60	19	3	4
Alexia Foods								
APPETIZERS								
Beer Battered Onion Rings	6 rings	180	8	1	240	24	4	2
Cheddar Bites	3 bites	110	6	3	160	8	0	4
Mozzarella Stix, w/Italian Herbs & Olive Oil	2 sticks	120	6	2.5	230	10	1	5
Panko Breaded Onion Rings, w/Sea Salt	6 rings	240	13	2	150	27	2	4
Potato Bites	3 bites	220	12	3.5	630	19	2	7
OVEN BAKED FRENCH FRIES								
Classic Oven Crinkles	13 fries	120	4	0	170	19	3	2
Oven Fries, w/Olive Oil & Sea Salt	8 fries	110	2	0	210	22	3	2
Sweet Potato Puffs	2/3 cup	130	4	0	230	23	2	1
Waffle Fries, w/Seasoned Salt	1 cup	160	7	5	330	21	2	2
POTATOES								
Hashed Browns, w/Seasoned Salt	2/3 cup	60	0	0	300	13	2	2
Oven Reds, w/Olive Oil, Parmesan & Roasted Garlic	8 pieces	120	4	0.5	270	19	2	3
All-Bran								
Original	1/2 cup	80	1	0	80	23	10	4
Amy's Kitchen								
BOWLS								
Brown Rice & Vegetables	1 bowl	260	9	1	550	36	5	9
Pesto Tortellini	1 bowl	430	19	8	640	45	3	20

	SERVING SIZE	CALORIES	TOTAL FAT (G)	SAT FAT (G)	SODIUM (MG)	CARBS (G)	FIBER (G)	PROTEIN (G)
Stuffed Pasta Shells	1 bowl	310	13	7	740	30	5	19
BURRITOS								
Bean & Cheese	1 burrito	310	9	2.5	580	46	7	11
Black Bean Vegetable	1 burrito	280	8	1	580	44	4	9
Breakfast	1 burrito	270	8	1	540	38	5	11
ENTRÉES								
Cheese Enchilada	1 entrée	370	15	7	680	41	9	17
Lasagna, Vegetable	1 entrée	310	12	4.5	680	35	5	16
Macaroni & Cheese	1 entrée	410	16	10	590	47	3	16
Macaroni & Soy Cheeze	1 entrée	370	15	2	500	42	4	16
SOUPS								
Chunky Vegetable	1 cup	60	0	0	680	13	3	3
No Chicken Noodle	1 cup	100	3	0	540	13	2	5
Split Pea	1 cup	100	0	0	670	19	6	7
Vegetable Barley	1 cup	70	1	0	580	13	3	2

Annie Chun's
RICE EXPRESS, STICKY RICE

	SERVING SIZE	CALORIES	TOTAL FAT (G)	SAT FAT (G)	SODIUM (MG)	CARBS (G)	FIBER (G)	PROTEIN (G)
Black Pearl	1 tray	270	2	0	5	57	2	6
Sprouted Brown	1 tray	270	1	0	0	59	3	6
White	1 tray	300	0	0	0	67	0	6
SOUP, FROZEN, WONTON								
Chicken & Garlic	1 bowl	140	2	0	630	22	3	7
Spicy Vegetable	1 bowl	130	2	0	990	25	3	6

Applegate Farms
BACON

	SERVING SIZE	CALORIES	TOTAL FAT (G)	SAT FAT (G)	SODIUM (MG)	CARBS (G)	FIBER (G)	PROTEIN (G)
Natural Canadian Bacon	2 slices	90	4	1.5	500	1	0	12
Turkey Bacon, Natural or Organic	1 slice	35	2	0	200	0	0	6
HOT DOGS								
Chicken, Average of Natural & Organic	1 hot dog	65	4	1.5	405	0	0	7
Natural, Big Apple	1 hot dog	110	9	3.5	360	1	0	7
Turkey, Average of Natural & Organic	1 hot dog	60	4	1	320	1	0	7
SAUSAGES, ORGANIC								
Chicken & Apple	1 sausage	140	7	1.5	500	6	1	14
Spinach & Feta	1 sausage	120	7	2.5	470	2	0	13
Sweet Italian	1 sausage	130	6	2	500	2	1	15

AriZona Beverage Co.

	SERVING SIZE	CALORIES	TOTAL FAT (G)	SAT FAT (G)	SODIUM (MG)	CARBS (G)	FIBER (G)	PROTEIN (G)
Arnold Palmer, Half & Half, Lite	20 fl oz	125	0	0	63	35	0	0

store brands

	SERVING SIZE	CALORIES	TOTAL FAT (G)	SAT FAT (G)	SODIUM (MG)	CARBS (G)	FIBER (G)	PROTEIN (G)
Black Tea, w/Ginseng	20 fl oz	150	0	0	50	38	0	0
Coconut Water	14-1/2 fl oz	70	0	0	220	18	0	0
Green Tea, w/Ginseng & Honey	20 fl oz	175	0	0	50	45	0	0
Lemonade	20 fl oz	275	0	0	25	68	0	0
Sweet Tea	20 fl oz	225	0	0	50	58	0	0
Aunt Jemima **SYRUP**								
Lite	1/4 cup	100	0	0	190	26	1	0
Original	1/4 cup	210	0	0	120	52	0	0
Banquet **BROWN 'N SERVE SAUSAGES**								
Link, Maple	3 links	190	17	5	480	2	0	8
Link, Maple, Lite	3 links	120	9	2.5	520	2	0	9
Link, Original	2 links	150	13	4.5	350	1	0	6
Patty, Original	2 patties	170	15	5	410	2	0	6
CHICKEN								
Boneless Breast Nuggets, Average of Bag & Box	6 nuggets	210	11	2	365	18	3	11
Boneless Breast Tenders	5 tenders	210	10	1.5	330	19	3	11
Country Fried Chicken	1 piece	350	24	5	1180	11	1	24
Hot & Spicy Wings, Bag	3 oz	270	18	4.5	470	11	1	15
ENTRÉES								
Dinner, Macaroni & Cheese	1 entrée	260	6	3	760	39	3	10
Dinner, Salisbury Steak	1 entrée	250	12	4.5	1020	25	3	11
Select Recipes, Fried Chicken, Original	1 entrée	350	17	4	930	35	5	12
Select Recipes, Homestyle Pot Roast	1 entrée	170	5	2	860	19	5	13
Barber Foods Chicken, w/Broccoli, Cheese & Ham	1 piece	280	15	4.5	540	15	1	22
Chicken Cordon Bleu	1 piece	280	14	4	550	14	<1	24
Chicken Parmesan	1 piece	290	14	3.5	530	19	1	22
Barq's Root Beer Original	12 fl oz	160	0	0	70	45	0	0
Bear Naked **GRANOLA, 100% PURE & NATURAL**								
Fruit & Nut	1/4 cup	140	7	1.5	0	18	2	3
Heavenly Chocolate	1/4 cup	130	4	1	10	21	2	3

	SERVING SIZE	CALORIES	TOTAL FAT (G)	SAT FAT (G)	SODIUM (MG)	CARBS (G)	FIBER (G)	PROTEIN (G)
TRAIL MIX, 100% PURE & NATURAL								
Chocolate Cherry	1/4 cup	120	5	0.5	5	20	2	2
Cranberry Protein	1/4 cup	140	7	0.5	10	17	2	4
Ben & Jerry's								
ICE CREAM								
Cherry Garcia	1/2 cup	240	13	9	35	28	< 1	4
Chocolate Chip Cookie Dough	1/2 cup	270	14	8	60	33	0	4
Chubby Hubby	1/2 cup	340	20	10	140	33	1	7
Chunky Monkey	1/2 cup	290	18	10	35	29	1	4
Everything But The...	1/2 cup	290	17	11	70	31	1	5
Half Baked	1/2 cup	270	13	7	70	35	1	4
Phish Food	1/2 cup	280	13	8	80	39	2	4
ICE CREAM BARS								
Cherry Garcia	1 bar	260	16	11	40	23	1	8
Fudgy Brownies	1 bar	350	20	12	75	38	2	4
Half Baked	1 bar	360	22	13	100	37	1	4
Bertolli								
FROZEN ENTRÉES								
Chicken Alfredo & Penne	1/2 package	530	28	16	1040	35	3	25
Chicken Florentine & Farfalle	1/2 package	570	31	17	1070	40	4	25
Chicken Parmigiana & Penne	1/2 package	480	21	6	1460	49	4	23
Garlic Shrimp, Penne & Cherry Tomatoes	1/2 package	340	11	1.5	750	42	5	13
Grilled Chicken & Roasted Vegetables	1/2 package	360	16	2.5	880	35	4	20
Italian Sausage & Rigatoni	1/2 package	500	26	8	1120	46	4	18
Shrimp Scampi & Linguine	1/2 package	540	24	11	850	55	2	18
Steak, Rigatoni & Portabella Mushrooms	1/2 package	390	17	5	890	38	4	19
Tuscan-Style Braised Beef, w/Gold Potatoes	1/2 package	310	11	2.5	920	35	3	16
Betty Crocker								
FROSTING								
Butter Cream, Whipped	2 tbsp	100	5	1.5	25	15	0	0
Chocolate, Rich & Creamy	2 tbsp	130	5	1.5	95	21	< 1	0
Fluffy White, Whipped	2 tbsp	100	5	1.5	25	15	n/a	0
Vanilla, Rich & Creamy	2 tbsp	140	5	1	70	23	0	0
POTATOES, PREPARED								
Au Gratin	1/2 cup	150	5	1.5	640	23	1	2

store brands

	SERVING SIZE	CALORIES	TOTAL FAT (G)	SAT FAT (G)	SODIUM (MG)	CARBS (G)	FIBER (G)	PROTEIN (G)
Mashed, Butter & Herb	2/3 cup	140	7	4	480	18	1	2
Mashed, Home-Style, Reds	2/3 cup	80	1	0.5	410	18	1	1
Mashed, Loaded	2/3 cup	160	0	0	460	17	1	2
SUPER MOIST CAKE MIX, PREPARED								
Butter Recipe, Yellow	1/10 cake	240	9	5	370	36	<1	3
Chocolate Fudge	1/10 cake	280	14	2.5	390	35	1	4
Party Rainbow Chip	1/10 cake	280	14	2.5	340	35	<1	3
Birds Eye								
FRESHLIKE SAUCED & SEASONED								
Classic Cheddar Pasta	2 cups	126	5	1	313	15	1	4
Garlic Herb Pasta	2 cups	144	6	2	186	19	1	4
SAUCED & SEASONED								
California Blend & Cheddar Cheese Sauce	1/2 cup	71	4	2	347	7	1	2
Green Beans & Spaetzle in Bavarian Sauce	1 cup	96	4	2	249	10	2	3
Pasta & Vegetables in Creamy Cheese Sauce	1 cup	125	3	1	453	20	1	4
Roasted Potatoes & Broccoli	1/3 cup	86	3	1	433	13	1	2
Rotelle & Vegetables, w/Herbed Garlic Sauce	1 cup	85	1	0.5	350	15	1	3
STEAMFRESH CHEF'S FAVORITES								
Lightly Sauced Rigatoni & Vegetables, w/Tomato Parmesan Sauce	2 cups	121	3	1	222	19	1	4
Lightly Sauced Rotini & Broccoli, w/Smooth Creamy Cheese Sauce	2 cups	115	2	1	334	20	1	4
Lightly Sauced Rotini & Vegetables, w/Oven-Roasted Garlic Butter Sauce	2 cups	127	4	2	188	19	2	3
VOILA REGULAR SIZE								
Alfredo Chicken	1-1/2 cups	136	6	3.5	294	13	1	7
Beef Lo Mein	2-1/4 cups	108	1	0.5	530	18	1	6
Chicken Stir-Fry	2 cups	94	1	0	482	15	1	5
Garlic Shrimp	2 cups	128	5	1	228	15	1	6
Shrimp Scampi	1-3/4 cups	86	1	0.5	242	14	1	5
Teriyaki Chicken	1-2/3 cups	82	1	0	366	14	1	5
Blue Bunny								
ICE CREAM								
Birthday Party Cake	1/2 cup	150	6	4	45	21	0	2

	SERVING SIZE	CALORIES	TOTAL FAT (G)	SAT FAT (G)	SODIUM (MG)	CARBS (G)	FIBER (G)	PROTEIN (G)
Bunny Tracks, Premium	1/2 cup	190	11	6	95	21	< 1	4
Orange Dream	1/2 cup	120	5	3	40	19	0	1
Peanut Butter Brownie Sensation	1/2 cup	170	10	4.5	80	17	< 1	3
Strawberry Cheesecake	1/2 cup	130	5	3.5	40	19	0	2
ICE CREAM BARS								
Big Alaska	1 bar	260	20	15	55	25	< 1	3
Chocolate Raspberry	1 bar	270	18	12	45	25	1	3
Naturally Strawberry	1 bar	140	8	6	35	14	0	2
Orange Dream	1 bar	70	1	0.5	25	15	0	< 1
Root Beer Float	1 bar	90	3	1.5	25	15	0	< 1
Bob's Red Mill								
Granola, Natural, No Fat Added	1/2 cup	160	3	0	10	35	4	5
Grits, Corn, Polenta, Organic	1/4 cup	130	0	0	0	27	2	3
Muesli, Old Country-Style	1/4 cup	110	3	0	0	21	4	4
Boca								
CHIK'N								
Nuggets, Original	1/4 package	180	7	1	500	17	3	14
Patties, Original	1 patty	160	6	1	430	15	2	11
MEATLESS BREAKFAST LINKS & CRUMBLES								
Breakfast Links	1/5 package	70	3	1	330	5	2	8
Ground Crumbles	1/6 package	60	1	0	270	6	3	13
MEATLESS BURGERS								
Cheeseburger	1 burger	100	5	1.5	320	6	4	13
Grilled Vegetable	1 burger	80	1	0	300	7	4	12
Original Vegan	1 burger	70	1	0	280	6	4	13
Bolthouse Farms								
BEVERAGES								
Juice, 100% Carrot	8 fl oz	70	0	0	150	14	1	2
Juice, 100% Pomegranate	8 fl oz	150	0	0	20	38	0	0
Perfectly Protein, Vanilla Chai Tea	8 fl oz	170	4	0.5	70	27	1	9
Protein Plus, Chocolate	8 fl oz	190	3	1.5	150	28	1	16
Smoothie, Strawberry Banana	8 fl oz	120	0	0	10	29	1	1
SALAD DRESSINGS								
Chunky Blue Cheese	2 tbsp	35	3	1	135	1	0	2
Classic Ranch	2 tbsp	45	3	0.5	270	3	0	1
Honey Mustard	2 tbsp	45	2	0.5	115	6	0	1

store brands

	SERVING SIZE	CALORIES	TOTAL FAT (G)	SAT FAT (G)	SODIUM (MG)	CARBS (G)	FIBER (G)	PROTEIN (G)
Breyers								
ICE CREAM								
Cherry Vanilla	1/2 cup	130	6	4	55	18	0	2
Chocolate Chip Cookie Dough	1/2 cup	160	8	5	60	20	0	2
Cookies & Cream	1/2 cup	150	7	4.5	90	19	0	2
Vanilla, Lactose-Free	1/2 cup	130	7	4.5	35	14	0	2
PURE FRUIT BARS								
Berry Swirls	1 bar	40	0	0	0	10	0	0
Pomegranate Blends	1 bar	40	0	0	0	10	0	0
Strawberry, Tropical, or Raspberry, No Sugar Added	1 bar	25	0	0	0	5	0	0
Buitoni								
ENTRÉES								
Butternut Squash Ravioli, w/Brown Butter Sage Sauce	1/2 package	490	14	7	620	76	5	16
Chicken & Mushroom Ravioli, w/Marsala Wine Sauce	1/2 package	530	20	11	1140	59	5	29
Chicken & Mushroom Risotto	1/2 package	350	13	7	690	37	3	22
Chicken Fiorentina, w/Asiago Cream Sauce	1/2 package	400	14	8	870	40	3	29
Five Cheese Cannelloni, w/Tomato Basil Sauce	1/2 package	560	27	15	1560	52	5	27
Shrimp & Lobster Ravioli, w/Garlic Butter Sauce	1/2 package	500	16	9	1170	68	0	21
PASTAS								
Ravioli, Chicken & Four Cheese	1 cup	290	10	5	660	32	2	17
Ravioli, Four Cheese	1- 1/4 cup	340	12	4	630	42	3	15
Ravioli, Spicy Beef & Sausage	1 cup	260	8	3.8	830	33	3	13
Tortellini, Spinach Cheese	1 cup	320	7	3.5	510	49	3	15
Tortellini, Three Cheese	1 cup	330	9	3	460	46	4	16
Bush's Best								
Baked Beans, Bold & Spicy	1/2 cup	110	1	0	560	24	5	6
Baked Beans, Honey	1/2 cup	160	1	0	540	32	6	6
Baked Beans, Original	1/2 cup	140	1	0	550	29	5	6
Butterfinger								
Crisp	1 bar	270	11	6	135	43	1	4
Original	1 bar	270	11	6	135	43	1	4

	SERVING SIZE	CALORIES	TOTAL FAT (G)	SAT FAT (G)	SODIUM (MG)	CARBS (G)	FIBER (G)	PROTEIN (G)
Campbell's								
CHUNKY SOUP								
Creamy Chicken & Dumplings	1 cup	160	8	2	890	16	3	7
Hearty Beef Barley	1 cup	140	2	0.5	790	24	4	8
Hearty Chicken, w/Vegetables	1 cup	110	2	0.5	710	17	3	6
Hearty Italian Style Wedding	1 cup	140	3	1	650	21	4	8
Hearty Tomato, w/Pasta	1 cup	140	1	0.5	650	30	3	4
Manhattan Clam Chowder	1 cup	130	4	1	800	19	3	5
New England Clam Chowder	1 cup	210	10	1.5	890	23	3	6
Old-Fashioned Vegetable Beef	1 cup	120	3	1	890	17	3	7
Split Pea 'N Ham	1 cup	170	3	1	790	25	5	11
CONDENSED SOUP								
Broccoli Cheese	1/2 cup	100	5	2	820	12	0	2
Chicken Gumbo, Light	1/2 cup	60	1	0.5	480	11	1	2
Chicken Noodle	1/2 cup	60	2	0.5	890	8	1	3
Chicken, w/Rice	1/2 cup	70	2	0.5	610	13	1	2
Cream of Mushroom	1/2 cup	100	6	1	870	9	2	1
Green Pea	1/2 cup	180	3	1	870	28	4	9
Italian-Style Wedding, Light	1/2 cup	80	2	1	480	12	2	3
Lentil	1/2 cup	140	1	0.5	800	24	5	8
Minestrone	1/2 cup	90	1	0.5	650	17	3	4
Tomato	1/2 cup	90	0	0	480	20	1	2
Vegetable	1/2 cup	100	1	0	890	20	2	3
Canada Dry								
Ginger Ale	12 fl oz	135	0	0	53	38	0	0
Carr's								
Poppy Sesame Crackers	4 crackers	80	5	2.5	135	9	<1	2
Rosemary Crackers	4 crackers	70	3	0	140	11	<1	2
Table Water Crackers	5 crackers	70	2	0.5	100	13	<1	2
Cascadian Farm								
CEREALS								
Hearty Morning	3/4 cup	200	3	1	360	43	8	5
Multi Grain Squares	3/4 cup	110	1	0	115	25	2	3
Purely O's	1 cup	110	1	0	200	24	3	3
GRANOLA BARS								
Chewy, Dark Chocolate, Almond	1 bar	130	4	1	100	25	5	2
Chewy, Fruit & Nut	1 bar	140	4	1	100	24	1	2

store brands	SERVING SIZE	CALORIES	TOTAL FAT (G)	SAT FAT (G)	SODIUM (MG)	CARBS (G)	FIBER (G)	PROTEIN (G)
Chewy, Oatmeal Raisin	1 bar	70	2	0	65	17	3	1
Sweet & Salty Mixed Nut	1 bar	160	8	3	125	20	1	3
Cedarlane Natural								
BURRITO								
Low-Fat Beans, Rice & Cheese Style	1 burrito	260	1	0	490	48	7	13
Roasted Vegetable & Cheese	1 burrito	330	8	1	590	48	3	14
ENTRÉE								
Eggplant Parmesan	1 entrée	240	13	5	680	21	5	13
Enchiladas, Low-Fat Garden Vegetable	1 enchilada	140	3	1.5	310	20	3	9
Manicotti, Spinach & Three-Cheese Stuffed	1 entrée	380	13	7	660	45	5	21
Stuffed Focaccia, Roma Tomato & Basil	1 focaccia	275	9	4	528	33	2	14
Veggie Wrap, Low-Fat Couscous & Vegetable	1 wrap	220	3	0	580	36	3	17
Cheerios								
Honey Nut	3/4 cup	110	2	0	160	22	2	2
Multi Grain	1 cup	110	1	0	120	24	3	2
Original	1 cup	100	2	0	160	20	3	3
Cheetos								
Puffs	1 oz	160	10	2	350	13	0	2
Cheez Whiz								
Original	2 tbsp	90	7	1.5	440	4	0	3
Chef Boyardee								
Beefaroni, Original	1 cup	250	9	4	730	32	3	9
PASTA								
Cheesy Burger Macaroni	1 cup	200	6	2.5	700	28	3	9
Mini O's	1 cup	170	1	0	650	34	3	5
Spaghetti & Meatballs	1 cup	260	12	4.5	750	28	3	9
RAVIOLI								
Beef	1 cup	230	7	2.5	750	34	3	7
Cheese	1 cup	230	6	3	750	34	4	9
Chex								
CEREAL								
Corn	1 cup	120	1	0	240	26	2	2
Multi-Bran	3/4 cup	160	2	0	270	39	6	4
Rice	1 cup	100	0	0	240	23	1	2
Wheat	3/4 cup	160	1	0	270	39	6	5

	SERVING SIZE	CALORIES	TOTAL FAT (G)	SAT FAT (G)	SODIUM (MG)	CARBS (G)	FIBER (G)	PROTEIN (G)
MIX								
Bold Party Blend	1/2 cup	120	4	1	190	20	1	2
Cheddar	1/2 cup	130	4	0.5	220	21	1	2
Sweet 'N Salty, Trail Mix	1/2 cup	150	5	1.5	95	24	1	3
Traditional	1/2 cup	120	4	1	210	20	1	2
Chips Ahoy								
Original	3 cookies	160	8	2.5	110	22	1	2
Reduced-Fat	3 cookies	140	5	2	150	23	1	2
Ciao Bella								
GELATO								
Chocolate Jalapeño	1/2 cup	230	14	8	65	23	1	4
Chocolate S'mores	1/2 cup	310	18	7	105	35	1	4
Dulce de Leche	1/2 cup	230	12	7	85	27	0	4
Strawberry	1/2 cup	190	10	5	50	27	1	3
SORBET								
Blackberry Cabernet	1/2 cup	110	0	0	0	27	2	1
Coconut	1/2 cup	190	10	9	40	22	0	1
Dark Chocolate	1/2 cup	160	6	4	0	25	2	2
Raspberry	1/2 cup	120	0	0	0	28	2	1
Classico								
Basil Pesto Sauce	1/4 cup	240	23	4	580	5	1	3
Creamy Alfredo Sauce	1/4 cup	100	9	5	410	3	0	2
Light Creamy Alfredo Sauce	1/4 cup	60	5	3	330	3	0	1
Tomato Basil Sauce	1/2 cup	50	1	0	380	9	1	2
Traditional Sweet Basil Sauce	1/2 cup	70	1	0	470	13	3	2
Vodka Sauce	1/2 cup	100	5	2	420	11	3	3
Club								
Multi Grain Cracker	4 crackers	70	3	0	120	9	<1	1
Original Cracker	4 crackers	70	3	0.5	125	9	<1	<1
Coca-Cola								
Classic	12 fl oz	140	0	0	45	39	0	0
Vanilla or Cherry	12 fl oz	150	0	0	35	42	0	0
Coffee-Mate								
French Vanilla	1 tbsp	35	2	0	30	5	0	0
French Vanilla, Sugar-Free	1 tbsp	15	1	0	0	2	0	0
Hazelnut	1 tbsp	35	2	0	0	5	0	0
Original	1 tbsp	20	1	0	0	2	0	0

store brands

	SERVING SIZE	CALORIES	TOTAL FAT (G)	SAT FAT (G)	SODIUM (MG)	CARBS (G)	FIBER (G)	PROTEIN (G)
Original, Fat-Free	1 tbsp	10	0	0	0	1	0	0
Combos								
Cheddar Cheese Cracker	1/3 cup	140	6	3	290	18	0	2
Cheddar Cheese Pretzel	1/2 cup	130	5	3	300	19	1	2
Pepperoni Pizza Cracker	1/3 cup	140	7	3	290	18	1	2
Corn Flakes								
Original	1 cup	100	0	0	200	24	1	2
Country Time								
Lemonade Iced Tea	23 grams	90	0	0	10	22	0	0
Original Lemonade	17 grams	60	0	0	25	16	0	0
Crunchmania								
Cinnamon Bun Graham Snacks	1 package	220	7	2	230	37	2	4
French Toast Graham Snacks	1 package	210	7	2	220	37	2	4
Dannon								
ALL NATURAL YOGURT								
Plain	8 oz	160	8	5	120	12	0	9
Plain, Nonfat	6 oz	80	0	0	120	12	0	9
Vanilla	6 oz	150	3	1.5	100	25	0	7
FRUIT ON THE BOTTOM YOGURT								
Apple Cinnamon	1 container	150	2	1	130	28	1	6
Banana Crème Pie	1 container	150	2	1	110	30	0	6
Blueberry	1 container	140	2	1	130	26	1	6
Strawberry Banana	1 container	150	2	1	95	26	1	6
GREEK YOGURT								
Honey	1 container	130	0	0	50	21	0	12
Plain	1 container	80	0	0	50	6	0	15
Strawberry	1 container	120	0	0	50	19	0	12
Vanilla	1 container	120	0	0	45	19	0	12
LIGHT & FIT YOGURT								
Blueberry	1 container	80	0	0	75	16	0	5
Cherry Vanilla	1 container	80	0	0	80	16	0	5
Strawberry	1 container	80	0	0	80	16	0	5
Digiorno								
Classic Thin Crust, Four Cheese	1/5 pizza	330	14	7	670	33	3	19
Rising Crust, Four Cheese	1/6 pizza	310	11	5	850	40	2	15
Rising Crust, Supreme	1/6 pizza	360	15	6	990	41	3	16
Stuffed Crust, Pepperoni	1/5 pizza	380	16	8	1040	40	3	19

	SERVING SIZE	CALORIES	TOTAL FAT (G)	SAT FAT (G)	SODIUM (MG)	CARBS (G)	FIBER (G)	PROTEIN (G)
Stuffed Crust, Supreme	1/6 pizza	350	16	7	950	34	3	17
Ultimate Toppings, Pepperoni	1/5 pizza	370	19	9	1080	34	2	17
Dole								
JUICE								
Orange, Peach, or Mango	8 fl oz	120	0	0	25	29	0	1
Orange, w/Pulp	8 fl oz	120	0	0	10	27	0	1
Pineapple	8 fl oz	130	0	0	10	30	0	1
Strawberry or Kiwi	8 fl oz	120	0	0	25	31	0	0
Doritos								
Baked Nacho Cheese	1 oz	120	4	0.5	230	21	2	2
Cool Ranch	1 oz	150	8	1	180	18	2	2
Nacho Cheese	1 oz	150	8	1.5	210	17	1	2
Dove								
CHOCOLATES								
Bar, Silky Smooth, Milk & Peanut Butter	1 bar	180	12	7	75	17	1	3
Promises, Silky Smooth, Dark Chocolate	5 pieces	210	13	8	0	24	3	2
Promises, Silky Smooth, Milk Chocolate & Caramel	5 pieces	200	11	7	30	23	1	2
ICE CREAM								
Bar, Milk Chocolate, w/Almonds	1 bar	340	23	13	135	28	1	6
Beyond Vanilla	1/2 cup	240	15	10	60	23	2	4
Irresistibly Raspberry	1/2 cup	240	12	8	40	30	1	3
Dr Pepper								
Cherry	12 fl oz	165	0	0	60	44	0	0
Original	12 fl oz	150	0	0	53	41	0	0
Drumstick								
Chocolate	1 Item	310	17	9	115	34	2	5
Vanilla	1 Item	290	16	9	100	33	2	4
Vanilla Fudge	1 Item	310	16	9	10	37	2	5
DRYER'S, See Edy's								
Duncan Hines								
BROWNIE MIX, PREPARED								
Chewy Fudge	1 item	170	8	1.5	105	24	1	2
Dark Chocolate	1 item	190	9	2	135	25	<1	2
Milk Chocolate	1 item	170	9	2	75	22	1	2
FROSTINGS								
Creamy Home-Style, Butter Cream	2 tbsp	140	6	1.5	70	23	0	0

store brands

	SERVING SIZE	CALORIES	TOTAL FAT (G)	SAT FAT (G)	SODIUM (MG)	CARBS (G)	FIBER (G)	PROTEIN (G)
Chocolate, Whipped	3 tbsp	140	7	2	70	20	< 1	1
Fluffy White, Whipped	3 tbsp	150	7	2	60	22	0	0
Vanilla, Whipped	3 tbsp	150	7	2	60	22	0	0
MOIST DELUXE CAKE MIX, PREPARED								
Angel Food	1 piece	140	0	0	280	31	0	3
Classic Yellow	1 piece	270	12	2.5	310	36	0	3
Confetti	1 piece	100	3	0.5	140	17	0	1
Devil's Food	1 piece	290	15	3.5	380	35	1	4
Red Velvet	1 piece	270	13	3	280	35	1	4
Edy's								
FRUIT BARS								
Peach	1 bar	100	0	0	0	24	0	0
Pomegranate	1 bar	70	0	0	0	17	0	0
Raspberry, No Sugar Added	1 bar	30	0	0	0	8	1	0
Strawberry	1 bar	80	0	0	0	21	1	0
ICE CREAM								
Chocolate Peanut Butter Cup	1/2 cup	170	8	4	85	21	1	3
Coffee, Rich & Creamy	1/2 cup	100	4	2	35	15	0	2
Cookies 'N Cream	1/2 cup	130	5	2.5	80	20	0	1
Fudge Tracks, Rich & Creamy	1/2 cup	120	4	2.5	35	19	0	3
Mint Chocolate Chip	1/2 cup	150	8	6	35	18	0	2
Nestlé Drumstick Sundae Cone	1/2 cup	160	7	4	60	21	0	2
Nestlé Toll House Cookie Dough	1/2 cup	150	6	3	65	23	0	1
Rocky Road	1/2 cup	160	8	4	35	19	1	3
Egg Beaters								
Egg Whites	3 tbsp	25	0	0	75	1	0	5
Original	3 tbsp	25	0	0	90	1	0	5
El Monterey								
BURRITOS								
Beef & Bean	1 burrito	300	14	5	410	34	2	9
Butcher-Wrapped Chicken & Cheese	1 burrito	480	17	5	1010	58	3	23
Chicken, Rice & Beans	1 burrito	240	7	1.5	570	34	1	10
Supreme, Shredded Steak & Cheese	1 burrito	290	9	3	590	41	1	12
XX Large, Spicy Red Hot Beef & Bean	1 burrito	790	43	13	790	80	7	22
CHIMICHANGAS								
Jalapeño Bean & Cheese	1 chimichanga	240	8	1.5	340	34	2	8

	SERVING SIZE	CALORIES	TOTAL FAT (G)	SAT FAT (G)	SODIUM (MG)	CARBS (G)	FIBER (G)	PROTEIN (G)
Supreme, Chicken & Monterey Jack Cheese	1 chimichanga	280	10	3	640	37	2	12
TAQUITOS								
Egg, Bacon & Cheese Breakfast	2 taquitos	210	11	1	290	22	1	6
Shredded Steak & Cheese	2 taquitos	230	12	1.5	340	24	1	8
Enjoy Life								
Beach Bash Trail Mix	1/4 cup	130	7	1	45	13	2	4
Boom Choco Boom Rice Milk Bar	1 bar	230	17	11	25	21	1	1
Chocolate Chip Chewy Soft-Baked Cookies	2 cookies	130	5	1	105	21	2	1
Double Chocolate Brownie Soft-Baked Cookies	2 cookies	120	5	1	105	20	2	1
Very Berry Crunch Granola	1/2 cup	170	2	0	10	35	2	3
Entenmann's								
CAKES								
Chocolate Fudge	1/8 cake	240	10	3.5	190	37	2	2
Coffee Crumb	1/10 cake	260	13	4	210	34	1	3
Coffee Crumb, Cheese Filled	1/9 cake	200	10	4	190	25	1	4
Golden Thick Fudge, Iced	1/8 cake	260	11	3.5	150	37	1	2
Sour Cream Loaf	1/8 cake	210	12	3.5	150	24	0	2
DANISHES								
Cheese Twist	1/8 danish	230	12	5	210	29	1	3
Cherry Cheese	1/8 danish	180	6	2.5	120	28	1	3
DONUTS, 12 PACK								
Frosted Mini	1 doughnut	160	11	7	90	15	< 1	1
Glazed	1 doughnut	210	11	3	190	25	< 1	3
Softee, Plain	1 doughnut	190	11	5	210	21	< 1	2
LITTLE BITES								
Blueberry Muffins	1 packet	180	8	1.5	190	25	0	2
Brownies	1 packet	270	14	4	200	35	2	3
Chocolate Chip Muffin	1 packet	190	9	2.5	135	26	< 1	2
Famous Amos								
Chocolate Chip Cookies	4 cookies	150	7	3	105	20	1	1
Vanilla Sandwich Cookies	3 cookies	170	7	3	100	25	1	2
Fanta								
Grape	12 fl oz	180	0	0	35	48	0	0
Orange	12 fl oz	160	0	0	55	44	0	0

store brands

	SERVING SIZE	CALORIES	TOTAL FAT (G)	SAT FAT (G)	SODIUM (MG)	CARBS (G)	FIBER (G)	PROTEIN (G)
Farm Rich								
Cheese Sticks	2 sticks	180	10	4	410	14	1	8
Mini Bacon Cheeseburgers	2 pieces	150	7	3.5	470	14	1	7
Mini Philly Cheese Steaks	2 pieces	210	11	6	640	16	1	11
Mini Pizza Slices	4 pieces	250	12	5	470	23	1	12
Flatout								
FLATBREAD								
Harvest Wheat	1 flatbread	120	3	0	310	23	6	7
Garden Spinach	1 flatbread	130	2	0	340	25	3	7
Original, Light	1 flatbread	90	3	0	320	16	9	9
The Original	1 flatbread	130	2	0	310	24	3	7
FLATBREAD CRISPS, BAKED								
Four Cheese	15 chips	130	5	0.5	290	15	5	6
Sea Salt	15 chips	120	4	0	150	17	1	6
Florida's Natural								
Home-Squeezed Style Lemonade	8 fl oz	110	0	n/a	20	28	n/a	0
Orange Pineapple Juice	8 fl oz	130	0	n/a	0	31	n/a	1
Original Orange Juice	8 fl oz	110	0	n/a	0	26	n/a	2
Ruby Red Grapefruit Juice	8 fl oz	90	0	n/a	0	22	n/a	1
Food Should Taste Good								
Average of All Flavors	1 oz	141	7	0.6	110	18	3	2
Fritos								
Original	1 oz	160	10	1.5	170	15	1	2
Scoops	1 oz	160	10	1.5	110	16	1	2
Froot Loops								
Original	1 cup	110	1	0.5	135	25	3	1
Full Throttle Energy Drinks								
Citrus	16 fl oz	220	0	0	160	58	0	0
Mocha	16 fl oz	270	7	4.5	390	50	2	4
Gardenburger								
Black Bean Chipotle	1 burger	100	3	0	390	16	5	5
Original Veggie Burger	1 burger	100	3	1	400	18	5	5
Veggie Medley	1 burger	100	3	0	380	17	5	3
Gatorade								
01 Prime, Pre-Game Fuel	1 pouch	100	0	0	110	25	0	0

	SERVING SIZE	CALORIES	TOTAL FAT (G)	SAT FAT (G)	SODIUM (MG)	CARBS (G)	FIBER (G)	PROTEIN (G)
02 Perform, Original G, Thirst Quencher, All Flavors	8 fl oz	50	0	0	110	14	0	0
03 Recover, Post-Game Protein	8 fl oz	60	0	0	120	7	0	8

Glutenfreeda
BURRITOS & PIZZA WRAPS

Beef & Potato Burrito	1 burrito	260	14	6	320	23	1	11
Pesto Chicken Pizza Wrap	1 wrap	240	10	2	450	27	4	15
Three Cheese Pizza Wrap	1 wrap	220	6	2	500	29	4	14
Vegetarian & Dairy Free Burrito	1 burrito	177	3	0	261	33	4	5

GRANOLA & OATMEAL

Banana Maple, w/Flax Oatmeal	1 packet	180	3	0.5	110	35	4	6
Raisin Almond Honey Granola	1/4 cup	120	4	0	0	19	2	3

Good Humor
ICE CREAM BARS

Chocolate Éclair	1 bar	210	9	4	40	30	1	3
Oreo	1 bar	240	13	6	150	31	1	3
The Original	1 bar	250	15	10	60	27	< 1	3

ICE CREAM SANDWICHES

Chocolate Chip Cookie	1 sandwich	270	10	6	200	44	1	3
Giant Neapolitan	1 sandwich	220	5	3	190	40	1	4
Vanilla	1 sandwich	140	3	1.5	135	26	< 1	2

Gorton's
FILLETS

Beer Battered	2 fillets	250	18	4.5	550	16	1	7
Breaded, Lemon Herb	2 fillets	240	13	2.5	720	21	n/a	9
Grilled, Italian Herb	1 fillet	90	3	0.4	310	2	1	14
Salmon, Grilled	1 fillet	100	3	0.5	270	2	n/a	15
Tilapia, Grilled, w/Roasted Garlic & Butter	1 fillet	80	3	0.5	150	< 1	n/a	14

Green Giant
FROZEN VEGETABLES, W/SAUCE

Baby Sweet Peas in Butter Sauce	3/4 cup	80	2	1	350	14	4	5
Carrots, Honey Glazed	1 cup	90	3	2	190	15	2	< 1
Cauliflower & Cheese Sauce	1/2 cup	50	3	1	380	6	1	2
Corn Niblets & Butter Sauce	2/3 cup	90	2	1	310	15	3	2
Cut Leaf Spinach in Butter Sauce	1/2 cup	30	1	0	340	4	2	2
Green Bean Casserole	2/3 cup	110	8	3	630	9	2	2

store brands

	SERVING SIZE	CALORIES	TOTAL FAT (G)	SAT FAT (G)	SODIUM (MG)	CARBS (G)	FIBER (G)	PROTEIN (G)
VALLEY FRESH STEAMERS, PREPARED								
Basil Vegetable Medley	3/4 cup	45	1	0	270	10	2	2
Broccoli & Cheese Sauce	2/3 cup	60	3	1	430	7	1	2
Buttery Rice & Vegetables	1 cup	180	2	1	410	37	2	4
Roasted Red Potatoes, Green Beans & Rosemary Butter Sauce	3/4 cup	100	1	0.5	330	21	3	3
Häagen-Dazs								
BARS								
Chocolate & Dark Chocolate	1 bar	290	20	12	30	24	2	4
Vanilla & Almonds	1 bar	310	22	13	40	22	< 1	5
Vanilla & Milk Chocolate	1 bar	280	20	13	40	21	0	4
Five Ice Cream, Average of All Flavors	1/2 cup	240	11	7	59	26	0	5
ICE CREAM								
Butter Pecan	1/2 cup	310	23	11	110	21	< 1	5
Chocolate Chip Cookie Dough	1/2 cup	310	20	12	125	29	0	4
Chocolate Peanut Butter	1/2 cup	360	24	11	100	27	2	8
Coffee	1/2 cup	270	18	11	70	21	0	5
Cookies & Cream	1/2 cup	270	17	10	95	23	0	5
Dulce de Leche	1/2 cup	290	17	10	95	28	0	5
Rocky Road	1/2 cup	300	18	9	75	29	1	5
Hamburger Helper								
CLASSIC, PREPARED, W/HAMBURGER								
Beef Pasta	1 cup	280	11	4.5	770	24	< 1	21
Cheddar Cheese Melt	1 cup	300	13	5	700	24	< 1	22
Cheeseburger Macaroni	1 cup	320	13	5	860	28	< 1	23
Stroganoff	1 cup	320	13	6	860	27	< 1	23
ITALIAN, PREPARED, W/HAMBURGER								
Cheesy Italian Shells	1 cup	310	13	5	820	28	1	22
Lasagna	1 cup	290	11	4.5	730	28	< 1	20
Tomato Basil Penne	1 cup	300	11	4	650	31	1	20
MEXICAN, PREPARED								
Cheesy Nacho	1 cup	330	12	5	660	35	< 1	21
Chili Macaroni	1 cup	270	12	4	590	22	< 1	20
Hawaiian Snacks								
POTATO CHIPS								
Original	13 chips	140	9	2.5	120	15	1	1
Wasabi	13 chips	140	9	1.5	200	18	3	2

	SERVING SIZE	CALORIES	TOTAL FAT (G)	SAT FAT (G)	SODIUM (MG)	CARBS (G)	FIBER (G)	PROTEIN (G)
SNACK RINGS								
Luau Barbecue	27 rings	130	6	1	300	19	< 1	2
Sweet Maui Onion	27 rings	130	6	1	370	19	< 1	2
Health Valley Organic								
CEREAL								
Amaranth Flakes	1-1/4 cup	210	2	0.5	190	43	5	6
Fiber 7	1 cup	160	1	0	100	37	7	6
Golden Flax	1 cup	190	4	0.5	65	37	6	6
Heart Wise	1 cup	200	3	0	140	37	5	11
Oat Bran Flakes, w/Raisins	1 cup	200	2	0	160	43	4	5
Cereal Bars, Average of All Varieties	1 bar	130	3	0.5	89	26	3	2
CHILI, VEGETARIAN								
Regular Varieties, Average of All Flavors	1 cup	200	3	0	468	38	8	10
Tame Tomato, No Salt Added	1 cup	210	3	0	70	41	8	10
Crackers, Average of All Varieties	4 crackers	70	3	0	185	10	1	1
Granola, Low-Fat, Average of All Flavors	2/3 cup	190	2	0	90	42	5	5
Granola Bars, Chewy, Average of All Varieties	1 bar	110	2	1	25	23	3	1
Toaster Tarts, Average of All Varieties	1 tart	148	3	0	93	29	3	2
Healthy Choice								
100% NATURAL								
Asian Potstickers	1 entrée	340	5	1	560	66	5	8
Portabella Spinach Parmesan Pasta	1 entrée	270	7	2	550	39	5	11
Pumpkin Squash Ravioli	1 entrée	310	6	2	600	52	5	9
Tortellini Primavera Parmesan	1 entrée	230	5	2	490	37	5	10
CAFÉ STEAMERS								
Barbeque Seasoned Steak, w/Red Potatoes	1 entrée	330	6	2	550	47	4	20
Beef Teriyaki	1 entrée	300	6	2	570	44	3	16
Cajun Style Chicken & Shrimp	1 entrée	230	2	0.5	570	36	3	15
Grilled Vegetables Mediterranean, w/Rice	1 entrée	230	3	0.5	600	44	7	6
Roasted Beef Merlot	1 entrée	210	6	2	600	23	5	15
Sweet Sesame Chicken	1 entrée	340	5	1	330	55	4	17
SOUPS, CANNED								
Chicken, w/Rice	1 cup	110	2	1	390	17	2	5
Garden Vegetable	1 cup	130	1	0	450	25	5	5
Old-Fashioned Chicken Noodle	1 cup	90	1	0	390	12	1	8
Tomato Basil	1 cup	100	0	0	450	22	3	2

store brands

	SERVING SIZE	CALORIES	TOTAL FAT (G)	SAT FAT (G)	SODIUM (MG)	CARBS (G)	FIBER (G)	PROTEIN (G)
Vegetable Beef	1 cup	130	2	0	420	21	4	9
STEAMING ENTRÉES								
Garlic Herb Shrimp	1 entrée	260	7	2	570	37	5	11
Honey Balsamic Chicken	1 entrée	220	4	1	540	34	5	12
Portabella Parmesan Risotto	1 entrée	220	4	2	590	35	4	9
Sundried Tomato Chicken	1 entrée	320	3	0.5	290	53	5	18
Hebrew National								
BEEF FRANKS								
Franks	1 frank	150	14	6	460	1	1	6
Jumbo	1 frank	270	25	10	810	2	0	10
Reduced-Fat	1 frank	110	9	3.5	490	2	0	5
BEEF KNOCKWURST & POLISH SAUSAGE								
Knockwurst	1 item	270	25	10	810	2	0	10
Polish Sausage	1 item	250	23	9	870	< 1	0	10
Heinz								
Gravy, Classic Chicken	1/4 cup	30	2	0.5	250	3	0	0
Gravy, Roasted Turkey	1/4 cup	25	1	0	290	3	0	1
Gravy, Sausage	1/4 cup	45	2	0.5	250	6	0	2
Tomato Ketchup	1 tbsp	20	0	0	160	4	0	0
Hershey's								
CHOCOLATE BARS								
Milk Chocolate	1 bar	210	13	8	35	26	1	3
Milk Chocolate, w/Almonds	1 bar	210	14	6	25	21	2	4
Special Dark	1 bar	180	12	8	15	25	3	2
Chocolate Syrup	2 tbsp	100	0	0	15	24	1	1
KISSES								
Milk Chocolate	9 pieces	200	12	7	35	25	1	3
Special Dark Chocolate	9 pieces	180	12	8	15	25	3	2
Hi-C								
Fruit Punch	1 box	90	0	0	15	25	0	0
Honest Tea								
OTHER BEVERAGES								
Cacao Mint Cocoa Nova	10.1 fl oz	50	0	0	5	13	0	0
Cranberry Lemonade Ade	16.9 fl oz	100	0	0	10	25	0	0
Super Fruit Punch Ade	16.9 fl oz	100	0	0	5	25	0	0
TEA								
Black Forest Berry	16.9 fl oz	60	0	n/a	5	8	n/a	0

	SERVING SIZE	CALORIES	TOTAL FAT (G)	SAT FAT (G)	SODIUM (MG)	CARBS (G)	FIBER (G)	PROTEIN (G)
Green Honey	16.9 fl oz	70	0	n/a	10	18	n/a	0
Half & Half	16.9 fl oz	100	0	n/a	10	24	n/a	0
White Mango Acai	8 fl oz	35	0	n/a	5	9	n/a	0

Hormel
CHILI, 15-OZ CAN

Chili, w/o Beans	1 cup	220	9	4	970	18	3	16
Chunky, w/Beans	1 cup	260	7	3	1080	33	7	16
Turkey, w/o Beans	1 cup	190	3	1	1230	16	3	23
Vegetarian, w/Beans	1 cup	190	1	0	780	35	10	11

COMPLEATS

Café Creations Cheese Manicotti	1 entrée	290	9	4.5	990	42	4	10
Café Creations Teriyaki Chicken, w/Rice	1 entrée	250	2	0.5	940	50	2	10
Home-Style Beef Pot Roast	1 entrée	230	6	3	1470	22	2	21
Home-Style Chicken & Rice	1 entrée	280	11	3.5	990	34	1	11
Home-Style Salisbury Steak	1 entrée	280	11	5	950	30	2	16
Home-Style Swedish Meatballs	1 entrée	350	18	8	960	32	2	16
Home-Style Turkey & Dressing	1 entrée	290	9	3	960	31	2	20

Hot Pockets
BREAKFAST SANDWICHES

Ham, Egg & Low-Fat Cheese	1 sandwich	300	12	5	590	38	1	11
Sausage, Egg & Low-Fat Cheese	1 sandwich	320	15	7	470	34	1	11

CRISPY CRUST PIZZERIA

Pepperoni	1 sandwich	370	21	10	680	34	2	10

SANDWICHES

Cheeseburger	1 sandwich	310	12	5	600	39	1	10
Meatballs & Mozzarella	1 sandwich	340	15	7	560	39	2	10
Philly Steak & Cheese	1 sandwich	310	13	7	590	37	1	10

Husman's
POTATO CHIPS

Bar-B-Q	13 chips	150	10	2	280	14	1	2
Honey Bar-B-Q	17 chips	150	9	1.5	230	16	< 1	1
Kettle Cooked, Average of All Flavors	13 chips	148	9	2	278	15	1	2
Original	18 chips	150	10	2	125	14	1	2
Vlasic Dill Pickle	17 chips	150	10	1.5	280	14	1	1
Wavy Cheddar & Sour Cream	16 chips	150	10	2	260	14	1	2

OTHER SNACKS

Baked Cheese Curls	1-1/3 cups	170	13	2	230	12	0	2

store brands	SERVING SIZE	CALORIES	TOTAL FAT (G)	SAT FAT (G)	SODIUM (MG)	CARBS (G)	FIBER (G)	PROTEIN (G)
Bar-B-Q Pork Skins	1/2 oz	80	5	1.5	210	0	0	8
Ian's								
BREAKFAST								
Cinnamon French Toast Sticks	4 pieces	170	6	0	95	27	0	2
Maple Cheddar & Egg Wafflewich	1 sandwich	350	15	4	580	46	1	7
Maple Sausage & Egg Wafflewich	1 sandwich	370	18	4	710	42	1	9
CHICKEN								
Organic Nuggets	5 pieces	210	10	1	250	12	0	12
Patties	1 patty	210	10	0.5	370	15	< 1	15
Tenders	3 oz	160	6	0.5	210	7	< 1	20
COOKIES								
Chocolate Chip Buttons	23 cookies	130	5	1.5	130	21	1	2
Chocolate-Covered Wafer Bites	5 cookies	160	9	4	30	19	0	< 1
Crunchy Cinnamon, Buttons	23 cookies	120	5	0.4	80	22	1	1
Fish Sticks	5 pieces	220	11	1	200	21	< 1	10
PIZZA								
French Bread Pizza, Pepperoni	1 slice	180	6	0.5	500	30	3	2
French Bread Pizza, Soy Cheesy	1 slice	180	6	0.5	500	30	3	2
International Delight								
Amaretto	1 tbsp	35	2	1	0	6	0	0
Caramel Macchiato	1 tbsp	35	2	1	0	6	0	0
Hazelnut	1 tbsp	35	2	1	0	6	0	0
Skinny Caramel Macchiato	1 tbsp	30	0	0	5	7	0	0
Vanilla Caramel Cream	1 tbsp	35	2	1	0	6	0	0
Jack Link's								
BEEF JERKY								
Beef Steak, Original	1 oz	60	1	0.5	640	2	0	12
Beef Stick, Original	1 oz	110	9	4	460	1	0	6
Jerky Chew, Original	1/3 oz	30	0	0	450	0	0	9
Original Jerky	1 oz	80	1	0	590	3	0	15
Teriyaki Jerky	1 oz	80	1	0	600	5	0	14
Jell-O								
COOK & SERVE PUDDING, UNPREPARED								
Chocolate	1/4 box	90	0	0	110	22	1	1
Chocolate, Sugar-Free	1/4 box	30	0	0	110	7	1	1
Lemon	1/6 box	50	0	0	70	12	0	0

	SERVING SIZE	CALORIES	TOTAL FAT (G)	SAT FAT (G)	SODIUM (MG)	CARBS (G)	FIBER (G)	PROTEIN (G)
GELATIN DESSERT								
Cherry	1/4 box	80	0	0	100	19	0	2
Cherry, Sugar-Free, Low-Calorie	1/4 box	10	0	0	70	0	0	1
GELATIN SNACKS								
Strawberry, Sugar-Free, Low-Calorie	1 container	10	0	0	45	0	0	1
Strawberry & Raspberry	1 container	70	0	0	40	17	0	1
INSTANT PUDDING, UNPREPARED								
Butterscotch	1/4 box	90	0	0	400	23	0	0
Chocolate	1/4 box	100	0	0	420	25	1	0
Vanilla	1/4 box	90	0	0	350	23	0	0
Vanilla, Sugar-Free, Fat-Free	1/4 box	25	0	0	300	6	0	0
NO-BAKE DESSERT MIX, DRY								
Double Chocolate Silk	1/6 box	190	2	2.5	430	33	2	2
Home Style Cheesecake	1/6 box	230	5	3	380	44	1	2
Real Cheesecake	1/8 box	290	15	7	330	39	2	4
PUDDING SNACK CUPS								
Chocolate, Original	1 container	120	2	1.5	190	25	1	2
Chocolate, Sugar-Free, Reduced-Calorie	1 container	60	2	1	180	13	1	2
Tapioca, Original	1 container	110	2	1.5	200	25	0	1
Vanilla, Original	1 container	110	2	1.5	190	23	0	1
Jiffy Mix								
CAKE MIX, UNPREPARED								
Devil's Food	1/5 box	210	5	1.5	450	39	1	3
Golden Yellow	1/5 box	210	5	1	340	40	0	2
White	1/5 box	210	5	1	340	40	0	2
MUFFIN MIX, UNPREPARED								
Banana	1/6 box	150	5	2	310	25	< 1	2
Blueberry	1/5 box	160	5	2	320	26	0	2
Corn	1/6 box	150	5	2	340	27	< 1	2
OTHER MIXES								
Baking Mix, All Purpose	1/7 box	130	5	1	310	21	< 1	2
Biscuit Mix, Buttermilk	1/6 box	160	5	2	420	27	< 1	3
Pancake & Waffle Mix, Complete, Buttermilk	1/26 box	170	5	2	380	30	< 1	3
Jiffy Pop								
Butter Popcorn, Popped	4 cups	140	7	1.5	220	19	3	3

store brands

	SERVING SIZE	CALORIES	TOTAL FAT (G)	SAT FAT (G)	SODIUM (MG)	CARBS (G)	FIBER (G)	PROTEIN (G)
Jimmy Dean								
BREAKFAST SANDWICHES								
Bacon, Egg & Cheese Biscuit	1 sandwich	320	18	7	800	27	1	12
Delights Canadian Bacon Honey Wheat Muffin	1 sandwich	230	5	3	760	30	2	15
Ham & Cheese Croissant	1 sandwich	280	13	4	760	29	1	12
Sausage, Egg & Cheese Biscuits	1 sandwich	440	31	11	850	27	1	13
SAUSAGE, FULLY COOKED								
Links, Maple	3 links	170	14	5	400	2	0	7
Links, Original	3 links	240	22	8	450	1	0	9
Patties, Maple	2 patties	250	22	8	510	3	0	8
Patties, Original	2 patties	240	23	8	610	1	0	9
Kashi								
BARS								
GOLEAN Crunchy! Chocolate Peanut	1 bar	180	5	2	250	30	6	9
GOLEAN Oatmeal Raisin	1 bar	190	5	2.5	105	33	5	10
GOLEAN Peanut Butter & Chocolate	1 bar	200	5	3.5	180	32	5	10
TLC Chewy Granola, Peanut Peanut Butter	1 bar	140	5	0.5	85	19	4	7
TLC Crunchy Granola, Roasted Almond Crunch	2 bars	170	6	0.5	150	26	4	6
TLC Layered Granola, Dark Chocolate Coconut	1 bar	120	4	1.5	50	21	4	4
CEREAL								
7 Whole Grain Flakes	1 cup	180	1	0	150	41	6	6
GOLEAN Crunch!	1 cup	190	3	0	100	37	8	9
GOLEAN Original	1 cup	140	1	0	85	30	10	13
Good Friends, Original	1 cup	160	2	0	110	42	12	5
Heart to Heart, Honey Toasted Oat	3/4 cup	120	2	0	85	26	5	3
TLC CRACKERS								
Fire-Roasted Veggie	15 crackers	120	4	0	200	19	3	4
Original 7-Grain	15 crackers	120	4	0	160	19	3	4
Keebler Fudge Shoppe								
Deluxe Grahams	3 cookies	140	7	4.5	70	18	< 1	1
Fudge Sticks, Jumbo	1 cookie	160	8	5	35	21	< 1	< 1
Fudge Sticks, Original	3 cookies	150	8	5	40	20	< 1	< 1
Grasshopper, Fudge Mint	4 cookies	140	7	5	75	20	< 1	1

	SERVING SIZE	CALORIES	TOTAL FAT (G)	SAT FAT (G)	SODIUM (MG)	CARBS (G)	FIBER (G)	PROTEIN (G)
Kit Kat								
Bar, Milk Chocolate	4 wafers	210	11	7	30	28	1	3
Klondike Bars								
Heath	1 bar	230	15	11	80	25	<1	2
Krunch	1 bar	250	14	11	55	30	1	3
Original	1 bar	250	14	11	55	29	1	3
Kraft								
EASY MAC								
Original Cheesy	1 package	220	4	2.5	670	40	<1	6
Triple Cheese Cheesy	1 package	220	5	2.5	660	39	1	7
MACARONI & CHEESE								
Original, prepared	1 cup	400	19	4.6	720	48	1	7
Three Cheese, prepared	1 cup	400	17	4	740	54	2	9
SALAD DRESSING								
Balsamic Vinaigrette	2 tbsp	90	8	1	310	4	0	0
Catalina	2 tbsp	130	11	1.5	380	7	0	0
Creamy French	2 tbsp	150	14	2	260	5	0	1
Italian, Fat-Free	2 tbsp	20	0	0	380	4	0	0
Zesty Italian	2 tbsp	70	6	0	370	3	0	0
Krusteaz								
Muffin, Banana Nut, prepared	1 muffin	250	13	2.6	240	29	1	2
Muffin, Chocolate Chunk, prepared	1 muffin	260	13	4	230	32	1	2
Muffin, Wild Blueberry, prepared	1 muffin	220	14	2.6	210	28	<1	1
Quick Bread, Banana, prepared	1/10 loaf	250	11	2	288	35	<1	2
Lay's								
POTATO CHIPS								
Baked Original	15 crisps	120	2	0	135	23	2	2
Cheddar & Sour Cream	15 chips	160	10	1	170	15	1	2
Classic	15 chips	160	10	1	170	15	1	2
Kettle Cooked, Original	16 chips	160	9	1	90	16	1	2
Light, Original	15 chips	75	0	0	200	17	1	2
Stax, Original	12 crisps	150	9	2.5	140	16	1	1
Wavy	11 chips	160	10	1	140	15	1	2
Lean Pockets								
Breakfast, Applewood Bacon, Egg & Cheese	1 pocket	260	9	3.5	510	37	3	11
Culinary Creations, Chicken Bacon Dijon	1 pocket	270	8	4	540	38	3	12
Italian Meatballs & Mozzarella	1 pocket	300	9	4	540	40	3	12

store brands	SERVING SIZE	CALORIES	TOTAL FAT (G)	SAT FAT (G)	SODIUM (MG)	CARBS (G)	FIBER (G)	PROTEIN (G)
Philly Steak & Cheese	1 pocket	270	8	3.5	560	40	2	10
Pizza, Sausage & Pepperoni	1 pocket	280	8	3.5	550	40	2	11
Pizza, Whole Grain Supreme	1 pocket	220	6	3	550	33	4	10
Quesadilla, Stuffed Grilled Chicken Fajita	1 pocket	170	4	1.5	340	24	1	8

Lender's
FRESH BAGELS

Average of All Varieties	1 bagel	240	2	0	440	48	3	9

FROZEN BAGELS

Blueberry	1 bagel	150	1	0	240	32	1	5
Cinnamon	1 bagel	150	2	0	260	32	2	5
Egg	1 bagel	150	1	0	300	30	1	6
Onion	1 bagel	140	1	0	290	30	1	5
Plain	1 bagel	140	1	0	300	29	1	5
Soft	1 bagel	200	3	0.5	340	38	2	6

Lightlife
CHICK'N & MORE

Smart Strips, Chick'n	3 oz	80	0	0	520	6	4	14
Smart Strips, Steak	3 oz	80	0	0	570	6	5	14
Smart Tenders, Lemon Pepper	3 tenders	110	1	0	600	9	3	18
Smart Wings, Buffalo	4 wings	110	3	0	680	6	4	13

DELI, HOT DOGS & SAUSAGE

Smart Deli, Baked Ham	4 slices	70	1	0	390	3	0	12
Smart Deli, Pepperoni	13 slices	50	1	0	240	2	1	9
Smart Deli, Roast Turkey	4 slices	100	4	0.5	300	5	2	13
Smart Dogs	1 link	45	0	0	310	2	1	8
Smart Sausages, Italian	1 link	140	7	1	500	7	1	13
Tofu Pups	1 link	60	3	0.5	300	2	1	8

GROUNDS & BURGERS

Light Burgers, Mushroom	1 burger	160	5	1	480	13	3	15
Light Burgers, Original	1 burger	120	2	0	500	12	3	16
Smart Ground, Original	1/3 cup	70	0	0	310	6	3	12

Lean Cuisine
CULINARY COLLECTION

Beef Pot Roast	1 entrée	210	6	2	550	26	3	14
Chicken Club Panini	1 entrée	360	9	4	675	45	4	24
Chicken Parmesan	1 entrée	300	8	2	660	39	3	18

	SERVING SIZE	CALORIES	TOTAL FAT (G)	SAT FAT (G)	SODIUM (MG)	CARBS (G)	FIBER (G)	PROTEIN (G)
Herb Roasted Chicken	1 entrée	170	3	1	540	19	3	16
Meatloaf & Whipped Potatoes	1 entrée	250	8	2	590	25	3	20
Roasted Turkey & Vegetables	1 entrée	200	7	1	580	18	4	16
Roasted Vegetable Deep Dish Pizza	1 entrée	320	5	2	480	52	3	16
Steak Tips Portobello	1 entrée	150	4	2	430	14	3	15
Three-Meat Deep Dish Pizza	1 entrée	390	9	3	610	55	3	22
MARKET COLLECTION								
Asiago Cheese Tortelloni	1 entrée	270	7	4	670	39	5	14
Chicken Fettuccini, w/Broccoli	1 entrée	330	6	3	770	42	4	26
Chicken Margherita	1 entrée	300	8	2	660	38	5	21
Jumbo Rigatoni, w/Meatballs	1 entrée	420	9	3	860	62	7	22
Salisbury Steak, w/Honey-Glazed Carrots	1 entrée	270	8	3	690	32	5	19
Shrimp Scampi	1 entrée	250	7	4	690	32	4	15
SIMPLE FAVORITES								
Cheese Ravioli	1 entrée	220	5	3	620	33	3	11
Fettuccini Alfredo	1 entrée	330	7	3	600	54	3	12
Lasagna, w/Meat Sauce	1 entrée	320	8	4	630	45	4	17
Macaroni & Cheese	1 entrée	280	6	3	570	43	1	14
Spaghetti, w/Meatballs	1 entrée	270	6	2	580	38	3	16
SPA COLLECTION								
Butternut Squash Ravioli	1 entrée	260	7	2	550	40	5	9
Chicken Mediterranean	1 entrée	240	4	1	620	34	5	16
Tuscan Style Vegetable Lasagna	1 entrée	320	5	2	650	50	4	18
Salmon, w/Basil	1 entrée	210	6	2	590	25	5	15
Mama Rosie's								
Gnocchi, Potato	3/4 cup	270	5	0	190	57	2	8
Manicotti, Cheese & Spinach, w/Sauce	1 piece	250	10	5	810	29	1	12
Manicotti, w/Sauce	1 piece	170	6	4	480	23	0	7
Ravioli, Cheese & Spinach	9 pieces	260	3	1	240	45	2	12
Ravioli, Cheese, Low-Fat, Made w/Whole Grains	9 pieces	210	3	0.5	160	35	5	10
Shells, Stuffed, Jumbo	1 pieces	140	7	3.5	390	13	0	6
Shells, Stuffed, Jumbo, Four Cheese, w/Sauce	1 pieces	190	10	5	480	16	< 1	8
Tortellini, Cheese	2/3 cup	290	6	2	360	47	2	13
Tortellini, Cheese, Tri-Color	2/3 cup	290	6	2	360	47	2	13

store brands

	SERVING SIZE	CALORIES	TOTAL FAT (G)	SAT FAT (G)	SODIUM (MG)	CARBS (G)	FIBER (G)	PROTEIN (G)
Manwich								
Bold	1/4 cup	60	0	0	610	13	2	1
Original	1/4 cup	35	0	0	430	7	2	< 1
Thick & Chunky	1/4 cup	45	0	0	430	10	0	< 1
Marie Callender's								
ENTRÉES								
Beef & Broccoli	1 entrée	400	14	4.5	1200	52	3	22
Cheesy Chicken & Rice	1 entrée	430	16	9	1330	38	4	33
Chicken Parmesan	1 entrée	620	30	7	830	57	9	29
Fettuccine Alfredo, w/Garlic Bread	1 entrée	650	34	17	1220	61	5	24
Herb-Roasted Chicken	1 entrée	460	21	6	940	32	5	30
Lasagna, Meat	1 cup	260	10	5	960	32	4	10
Meat Loaf, w/Gravy	1 entrée	450	18	7	1090	41	6	29
Pot Pie, Turkey	1 entrée	630	36	13	1180	58	4	19
Pot Roast, Old-Fashioned Beef	1 entrée	260	6	2.5	1130	31	7	20
Salisbury Steak Dinner	1 entrée	370	15	5	1040	35	5	24
Spaghetti, w/Meat Sauce	1 entrée	490	14	4	1030	67	7	23
Turkey, w/Stuffing	1 entrée	350	10	2.5	1200	43	9	23
Marie's								
DIPS								
Buttermilk Ranch	2 tbsp	100	9	3	230	2	0	1
Buttermilk Ranch, Lite	2 tbsp	60	5	1.5	230	3	0	1
Roasted French Onion	2 tbsp	100	10	3	220	2	0	1
Spinach Parmesan	2 tbsp	90	9	3	200	2	0	2
DRESSINGS								
Blue Cheese, Chunky	2 tbsp	160	17	3.5	160	0	0	1
Blue Cheese, Chunky, Lite	2 tbsp	70	7	1	290	1	0	1
Caesar	2 tbsp	170	19	3.5	150	1	0	1
Italian, Creamy Garlic	2 tbsp	180	19	3	135	1	0	1
Ranch, Creamy	2 tbsp	170	19	3	150	1	0	1
Ranch, Creamy, Lite	2 tbsp	60	6	1	200	2	0	1
Sesame Ginger	2 tbsp	100	8	1.5	250	7	0	0
McCain								
FRENCH FRIES								
Classic Cut	3 oz	120	3	0	220	21	1	2
Premium Golden Crisp, Crinkle Cut	3 oz	150	4	0.5	200	26	1	2
Steak Cut	3 oz	100	3	0	280	16	1	1

	SERVING SIZE	CALORIES	TOTAL FAT (G)	SAT FAT (G)	SODIUM (MG)	CARBS (G)	FIBER (G)	PROTEIN (G)
Sweet Potato	3 oz	160	7	1	190	25	3	1
Tasti Taters	9 pieces	160	8	1	340	23	1	1

Milky Way
Regular	1 bar	260	10	7	95	41	1	2

Minute Maid
Grape Punch	8 fl oz	120	0	0	15	32	0	0
Lemonade	8 fl oz	100	0	0	35	28	0	0
Lemonade Iced Tea	8 fl oz	110	0	0	20	29	0	0
Orangeade	8 fl oz	110	0	0	15	31	0	0
Tropical Punch	8 fl oz	110	0	0	15	30	0	0

Minute Rice
Brown & Wild	1 container	230	5	0.5	135	42	5	5
Chicken, Mix	1 container	230	5	0.5	1020	41	2	6
Multi-Grain Medley	1 cup	220	4	0.5	230	41	6	6
Pilaf, Mix	1 container	220	4	0	1350	41	2	5
Steamers, Broccoli & Cheese	1 cup	200	4	1.5	720	37	1	6
Steamers, Spanish	1 cup	280	6	1.5	990	51	2	5

Miss Vickie's
POTATO CHIPS
Crinkle Cut, Original	31 chips	250	14	1	210	31	1	3
Lime & Black Pepper	28 chips	260	15	1.5	460	29	2	4
Original Recipe	31 chips	270	16	1.5	210	29	2	4
Sweet Chili & Sour Cream	28 chips	260	15	1.5	400	29	2	3
Unsalted	31 chips	270	16	1.5	0	29	2	4

Mission Tortillas
96% Fat-Free, Burrito, Large	1 tortilla	180	3	1	430	36	3	5
96% Fat-Free, Fajita, Small	1 tortilla	90	1	0	210	17	1	2
96% Fat-Free, Whole Wheat, Taco, Soft, Medium	1 tortilla	130	2	0.5	300	24	4	3
Flour, Multi Grain, Fajita, Small	1 tortilla	110	3	1	230	17	3	3
Flour, Multi Grain, Taco, Soft, Medium	1 tortilla	150	4	1.5	310	23	5	4
Whole Wheat, Taco, Soft, Medium	1 tortilla	130	3	1	280	22	3	4

Monster
ENERGY SUPPLEMENTS
Energy	8 fl oz	100	n/a	n/a	180	27	n/a	n/a
Energy, Import	8 fl oz	90	n/a	n/a	200	22	n/a	n/a
Energy, M 80	8 fl oz	90	n/a	n/a	15	23	n/a	n/a

store brands

	SERVING SIZE	CALORIES	TOTAL FAT (G)	SAT FAT (G)	SODIUM (MG)	CARBS (G)	FIBER (G)	PROTEIN (G)
Java Monster, Average of All Flavors	8 fl oz	92	2	1	307	15	n/a	5
Nitrous, Anti Gravity	12 fl oz	160	n/a	n/a	300	39	n/a	n/a
X-Presso, Hammer	9-2/3 fl oz	130	3	2	400	20	n/a	6
Morningstar Farms								
Chik'n Buffalo Wings	5 wings	200	8	1	640	20	3	12
Chik'n Nuggets	4 nuggets	190	9	1.5	600	19	4	12
Chik'n Patties, Original	1 patty	140	5	0.5	590	16	2	8
Chipotle Black Bean Burger	1 burger	210	7	1	700	24	7	17
Garden Veggie Patties	1 burger	110	4	0.5	350	9	3	10
Grillers, 1/4 Pounder Burger	1 burger	250	12	2	490	10	3	26
Grillers, Chik'n Patties	1 patty	80	3	0	350	7	5	9
Grillers, Original Burger	1 burger	130	6	1	260	5	2	15
Hickory BBQ Riblets	1 riblet	210	4	0	620	35	6	16
Veggie Bacon Strips	2 strips	60	5	0.5	230	2	1	2
Veggie Corn Dogs	1 corn dog	150	3	0.5	470	26	3	8
Veggie Sausage, Breakfast Links	2 links	80	3	0.5	300	3	2	9
Mountain Dew								
Original	12 fl oz	170	0	0	65	46	0	0
Mrs. Paul's								
Deviled Crab Cakes	1 cake	220	12	2	320	12	< 1	20
Fish Fillets, Beer-Battered	1 fillet	210	10	3	680	21	1	10
Fish Fillets, Crunchy Fish	1 fillet	280	14	3.5	510	25	< 1	13
Fish Fillets, Sandwich	1 fillet	190	10	2.5	360	18	3	6
Fish Sticks, Crunchy	6 sticks	230	10	2.5	480	22	< 1	11
Fish Tenders, Crispy	1 tender	230	11	2.5	800	21	< 1	11
Fried Clams	18 pieces	270	12	3	600	31	1	8
Parchment Bake, Tilapia, Classic Grilled	1 fillet	80	1	0	360	4	2	15
Parchment Bake, Tilapia, Lemon Pepper	1 fillet	70	0	0	220	5	0	13
Popcorn Fish, Crunchy	1/5 box	270	13	3	510	25	< 1	14
Mrs. Smith's								
PIES, PRE-BAKED								
Apple	1/8 pie	340	16	7	440	46	2	3
Blueberry	1/8 pie	330	16	7	430	45	2	3
Cherry	1/8 pie	350	16	7	360	48	1	3
Chocolate Creme	1/8 pie	390	24	17	190	40	1	2
Lemon Meringue	1/8 pie	310	12	6	170	46	1	2
Pumpkin	1/8 pie	320	12	5	380	49	2	5

	SERVING SIZE	CALORIES	TOTAL FAT (G)	SAT FAT (G)	SODIUM (MG)	CARBS (G)	FIBER (G)	PROTEIN (G)
Mrs. T's								
PIEROGIES								
Potato & Four Cheese, Blend	3 pierogies	220	7	1.5	540	34	1	6
Potato, Sour Cream & Chive	3 pierogies	190	5	2	480	32	1	5
Sauerkraut	3 pierogies	140	2	0	670	28	3	4
Nature's Path								
CEREAL								
Corn Flakes, Fruit-Juice Sweetened	3/4 cup	110	0	0	150	24	2	2
Crispy Rice	3/4 cup	110	2	0	160	24	2	2
Crunchy Maple Sunrise	2/3 cup	110	1	0	130	25	3	2
Flax Plus, Maple Pecan Crunch	3/4 cup	220	7	1	190	38	5	6
Flax Plus, Organic, Raisin, Bran	3/4 cup	190	3	0	190	41	8	6
Whole O's	2/3 cup	120	2	0	115	25	3	2
Granola, Average of All Flavors	3/4 cup	253	9	2	70	37	5	6
OATMEAL, INSTANT								
Apple Cinnamon	1 packet	210	3	0	100	40	4	5
Maple Nut	1 packet	210	4	0.5	100	38	4	5
WAFFLES, FROZEN								
Buckwheat, Wildberry	2 waffles	190	7	1	330	33	1	2
Home-Style, Gluten-Free	2 waffles	270	10	1.5	420	44	2	2
Nesquik								
Chocolate Syrup	1 tbsp	50	0	0	30	13	0	0
Strawberry Syrup	1 tbsp	50	0	0	0	13	0	0
Nestea								
Green, Sweetened	8 fl oz	80	0	0	0	20	0	0
Iced, Sweetened	8 fl oz	80	0	0	15	21	0	0
Nestlé Toll House								
MORSELS								
Butterscotch	1 tbsp	70	4	3.5	10	9	0	0
Milk Chocolate	1 tbsp	70	4	2.5	5	9	0	0
Peanut Butter, Swirled	1 tbsp	75	5	2.5	20	8	0	0
Semi-Sweet, Chocolate	1 tbsp	70	4	2.5	0	9	0	0
REFRIGERATED COOKIE DOUGH, PREPARED								
Chocolate Chip	1 cookie	130	6	2.5	90	17	0	1
Sugar	1 cookie	160	7	2.5	120	23	0	2
Ultimates, Peanut Butter Lovers	1 cookie	170	8	4	190	23	1	2
Ultimates, White Chocolate, Macadamia Nut	1 cookie	190	10	5	160	22	0	2

store brands

	SERVING SIZE	CALORIES	TOTAL FAT (G)	SAT FAT (G)	SODIUM (MG)	CARBS (G)	FIBER (G)	PROTEIN (G)
Newman's Own								
BEVERAGES								
Old-Fashioned Roadside Virgin Lemonade	8 fl oz	110	0	0	40	27	0	0
Virgin Lemon-Aided Iced Tea	8 fl oz	110	0	0	40	27	0	0
Virgin Limeade	8 fl oz	140	0	0	35	34	0	0
PASTA SAUCE								
Alfredo	1/4 cup	90	8	4.5	410	3	0	1
Five Cheese	1/2 cup	80	3	1.5	610	10	2	3
Marinara, Average of All Flavors	1/2 cup	70	2	0	530	12	3	2
Vodka Sauce	1/2 cup	110	5	1.5	440	11	2	5
PIZZA, THIN & CRISPY								
Four Cheese	1/3 pizza	300	13	6	610	31	2	16
Margherita	1/3 pizza	280	12	4.5	650	31	1	12
Roasted Vegetable	1/3 pizza	240	7	2.5	550	33	3	11
Supreme	1/3 pizza	320	15	5	750	33	2	14
POPCORN, MICROWAVE								
Average of All Flavors	3-1/2 cups	123	4	2	209	18	3	2
SALAD DRESSING								
Balsamic Vinaigrette	2 tbsp	90	9	1	290	3	0	0
Caesar	2 tbsp	150	16	2.5	420	1	0	1
Italian, Family Recipe	2 tbsp	130	13	2	360	1	0	1
Ranch	2 tbsp	150	16	2.5	310	2	0	0
Newtons								
COOKIES								
Fig	2 cookies	110	2	0	130	22	1	1
Fig, Fat-Free	2 cookies	90	0	0	125	22	1	1
Nilla Wafers								
Original	8 wafers	140	6	1.5	115	21	0	1
Reduced-Fat	8 wafers	120	2	0	110	24	0	1
Northland								
JUICE								
Blueberry Acai	8 fl oz	130	0	0	15	32	0	0
Cranberry Pomegranate	8 fl oz	140	0	0	25	34	0	0
Nutri-Grain								
Apple Cinnamon	1 bar	120	3	0.5	110	24	3	2
Raspberry	1 bar	120	3	0.5	110	24	3	2
Strawberry Yogurt	1 bar	130	4	0.5	110	25	3	2

	SERVING SIZE	CALORIES	TOTAL FAT (G)	SAT FAT (G)	SODIUM (MG)	CARBS (G)	FIBER (G)	PROTEIN (G)
Ocean Spray								
Craisins, Original	1/3 cup	130	0	0	0	33	0	0
Cranberry Sauce, Jellied	1/4 cup	110	0	0	10	25	0	0
JUICE & JUICE DRINKS								
Cran-Apple Juice Drink	8 fl oz	130	0	0	80	32	0	0
Cran-Raspberry Juice Drink	8 fl oz	110	0	0	70	28	0	0
Cranberry & Concord Grape Juice Drink, Light	8 fl oz	50	0	0	35	13	0	0
Cranberry Juice, Diet	8 fl oz	5	0	0	50	2	0	0
Odwalla								
BARS								
Banana Nut	1 bar	220	5	0.5	105	39	5	4
Choco Walla	1 bar	210	5	1.5	75	39	5	4
Chocolate Chip Peanut	1 bar	230	8	1.5	170	33	4	7
Super Protein	1 bar	210	5	1	150	30	4	14
DRINKS								
C Monster, Citrus	12 fl oz	230	0	0	20	50	2	3
Protein Monster, Chocolate Shake	12 fl oz	320	6	1	360	40	3	25
Smoothie, Strawberry Banana	12 fl oz	190	1	0	5	45	2	2
Superfood, Berries Go Mega	12 fl oz	240	3	0	20	50	5	3
On Cor								
Char-Broiled Jumbo Beef Patties, w/ 1/2 cup Gravy	1 patty	240	14	6	1240	12	4	16
Chicken Parmagiana, w/ 1/3 Cup Tomato Sauce	1 patty	220	13	4	650	16	2	9
Lasagna, w/Meat Sauce	1 cup	220	9	4	800	26	1	9
Macaroni & Cheese	1 cup	170	3	2	1000	29	1	8
Salisbury Steak, w/ 1/3 Cup Gravy	1 patty	160	11	2.5	690	8	1	8
Sliced White Turkey, w/ 1/3 Cup Gravy	1 patty	70	3	0.5	620	7	1	4
Ore Ida								
Crispers!	3 oz	230	14	2.5	390	23	2	2
Golden Crinkles, Extra-Crispy	3 oz	170	6	1.5	370	25	2	3
Seasoned Crinkles	3 oz	150	6	1	450	22	2	2
Tater Tots, Extra-Crispy	3 oz	170	9	1.5	480	21	2	2
Tater Tots, Original	3 oz	160	8	1.5	420	20	2	2
Oreo								
Double Stuf	2 cookies	140	7	2	105	21	1	1

store brands	SERVING SIZE	CALORIES	TOTAL FAT (G)	SAT FAT (G)	SODIUM (MG)	CARBS (G)	FIBER (G)	PROTEIN (G)
Mini, Bite-Size	9 cookies	130	6	2	160	21	1	1
Original	3 cookies	160	7	2	160	25	1	1
Reduced-Fat	3 cookies	150	5	1	160	27	1	1

Oscar Mayer
BACON

Original	14 grams	70	6	2	290	0	0	4
Original, Turkey	15 grams	35	3	1	180	0	0	2

HOT DOGS

Beef & Cheddar Franks	1 frank	170	15	7	600	2	0	7
Beef Franks	1 frank	130	12	5	470	1	0	5
Turkey Franks	1 frank	100	8	2.5	510	2	0	5

Pacific Natural Foods
NON-DAIRY BEVERAGES

Almond Milk, Original, Low-Fat, Organic	8 fl oz	60	3	0	140	8	0	1
Almond Milk, Vanilla, Low-Fat, Organic	8 fl oz	70	3	0	140	11	0	1

SOUPS

Minestrone, w/Chicken Meatballs, Organic	8 fl oz	130	4	1	700	19	3	6
Savory White Bean, w/Smoked Bacon, Organic	8 fl oz	220	7	2	780	27	8	13
Vegetable, Lentil & Roasted Red Pepper	8 fl oz	150	1	0	760	27	7	8

Pasta Roni, Prepared

Chicken & Broccoli	1 cup	360	15	4	870	49	3	10
Fettuccine Alfredo	1 cup	450	24	7	1050	44	2	11
White Cheddar & Broccoli	1 cup	300	13	4	710	39	2	9

Pepperidge Farm
COOKIES

Milano, Original	3 cookies	180	10	5	80	21	< 1	2
Pirouette, Rolled Wafers, Chocolate Fudge	2 wafers	120	5	2.5	40	18	< 1	1
Soft Baked, Nantucket, Dark Chocolate	1 cookie	140	6	3	75	22	0	1
Verona, Apricot Raspberry	3 cookies	140	5	2.5	55	22	< 1	2

GOLDFISH CRACKERS

Cheddar	55 pieces	140	5	1	250	20	< 1	4
Grahams, Honey	37 pieces	140	5	1	150	23	1	2

Pepsi

Regular	12 fl oz	150	0	0	30	41	0	0

	SERVING SIZE	CALORIES	TOTAL FAT (G)	SAT FAT (G)	SODIUM (MG)	CARBS (G)	FIBER (G)	PROTEIN (G)
Pillsbury								
BISCUITS, ROLLS, CRUSTS & BREADSTICKS								
Biscuits, Country-Style	3 biscuits	150	2	0	540	30	1	4
Biscuits, Grands, Home-Style, Original	1 biscuit	170	6	1.5	580	25	< 1	3
Crescent Rolls, Big & Buttery	1 roll	150	7	3	330	19	< 1	2
Crescent Rolls, Original	1 roll	100	6	2.5	220	11	0	1
Garlic Breadsticks	2 sticks	180	9	3.5	540	23	< 1	3
CINNAMON ROLLS								
Cinnamon, w/Icing	1 roll	140	5	1.5	340	23	< 1	2
Grands, Cinnamon, w/Icing	1 roll	290	11	4	480	43	1	5
COOKIES, READY-TO-BAKE								
Chocolate Chip	2 cookies	170	8	2.5	125	23	< 1	2
Oatmeal Chocolate Chip	2 cookies	160	7	3.5	95	24	< 1	1
TOASTER STRUDELS								
Average of All Flavors	1 pastry	173	7	3	176	25	< 1	3
Pirate's Booty								
Original	1 oz	130	5	1	140	19	0	2
Planters								
Almonds, Cocoa & Cinnamon, Flavor Grove Blend	24 almonds	160	12	1	40	9	3	5
NUT-RITION MIXES								
Antioxidant	1/4 cup	160	11	3	0	15	2	4
Digestive Health	1/4 cup	150	8	1	40	18	5	4
Heart Healthy	30 whole nuts	170	15	1.5	50	5	3	6
Omega-3	1/4 cup	160	10	1.5	0	16	2	3
Pistachios, Harvest Grove Blend	28 pieces	160	13	1.5	100	7	2	6
Trail Mix, Nuts & Chocolate	24 pieces	160	12	1	40	9	3	5
POM Wonderful								
100% Juice, Pomegranate, Average of All Flavors	8 fl oz	144	0	0	5	35	0	< 1
Juice Cocktail, Pomegranate, Lite, Average of All Flavors	8 fl oz	79	0	0	0	20	0	0
Pop Secret								
94% Fat-Free Butter	5 cups	110	2	0.5	270	19	4	3
Butter	4-1/2 cups	180	12	2.5	310	15	3	2
Kettle Corn	4 cups	180	13	3	110	15	3	2

store brands

	SERVING SIZE	CALORIES	TOTAL FAT (G)	SAT FAT (G)	SODIUM (MG)	CARBS (G)	FIBER (G)	PROTEIN (G)
Popsicle								
Creamsicle, Low-Fat	1 bar	70	1	0	20	13	0	< 1
Fudgsicle, Low-Fat	1 bar	60	2	0	55	12	0	1
Orange, Cherry, or Grape	1 bar	45	0	0	0	11	0	0
Pop Tarts								
Brown Sugar Cinnamon, Frosted	1 pastry	210	7	2	170	34	1	2
Frosted S'mores	1 pastry	200	5	1.5	210	36	<1	3
Strawberry, Frosted, Low-Fat	1 pastry	180	3	1	180	37	3	2
Strawberry, Unfrosted	1 pastry	200	5	2	180	37	1	2
Post								
Grape-Nuts	1/2 cup	200	1	0	290	48	7	6
Honey Bunches of Oats, w/Almonds	3/4 cup	130	3	0	135	26	2	2
Honeycomb	1-1/2 cups	130	1	0	180	28	1	2
Raisin Bran	1 cup	190	1	0	250	46	8	5
Shredded Wheat	2 biscuits	160	1	0	0	37	6	5
Powerade								
All Flavors	8 fl oz	50	0	0	100	14	0	0
Prego								
Classic, Flavored, w/Meat	1/2 cup	80	3	0.5	480	13	3	2
Classic, Italian Sausage & Garlic	1/2 cup	90	3	1	480	13	3	3
Classic, Marinara	1/2 cup	80	3	0.5	480	10	3	2
Pringles								
BBQ	16 chips	150	9	3	150	15	1	1
Light, Average of All Flavors	15 chips	70	0	0	167	15	1	1
Original	16 chips	150	9	2.5	150	15	1	1
Salt & Vinegar	16 chips	150	9	2.5	220	15	1	1
Sour Cream & Onion	16 chips	150	9	2.5	150	15	1	1
Progresso Soup								
Chicken Noodle	8 fl oz	100	3	0.5	690	12	1	7
Chicken Noodle, Light	8 fl oz	70	2	0.5	690	10	1	5
Chicken Rice, w/Vegetables	8 fl oz	100	2	0.5	640	16	1	5
Hearty Tomato	8 fl oz	110	1	0	690	24	3	3
Italian-Style Wedding	8 fl oz	120	4	1.5	690	11	2	7
Minestrone	8 fl oz	100	2	0.5	690	20	4	4
New England Clam Chowder	8 fl oz	180	9	2	890	20	1	6
Potato, Broccoli & Cheese Chowder	8 fl oz	210	12	3.5	860	20	2	5
Vegetable	8 fl oz	80	0	0	660	15	3	5

	SERVING SIZE	CALORIES	TOTAL FAT (G)	SAT FAT (G)	SODIUM (MG)	CARBS (G)	FIBER (G)	PROTEIN (G)
Quaker								
CHEWY GRANOLA BARS								
Chocolate Chip	1 bar	100	3	1	75	17	1	1
Chocolate Chip & Peanut Butter	1 bar	100	3	1	95	17	1	2
GRANOLA								
Natural, Low-Fat	2/3 cup	210	3	0.5	130	44	5	5
Natural Oats & Honey	1/2 cup	200	6	0.5	25	35	5	5
INSTANT OATMEAL								
Apples & Cinnamon	1 packet	130	2	0	160	27	3	3
Maple & Brown Sugar	1 packet	160	3	0.5	260	32	3	4
Original	1 packet	100	2	0	75	19	3	4
LIFE CEREAL								
Average of All Flavors	3/4 cup	120	2	0	150	25	3	3
RICE CAKES								
Buttered Popcorn	1 cake	35	0	0	45	8	0	1
Caramel Corn	1 cake	50	0	0	30	11	0	1
Lightly Salted	1 cake	35	0	0	15	7	0	1
Mini, Caramel Corn	13 cakes	110	1	0	310	26	1	1
Mini, Cheddar Cheese	18 cakes	140	5	0.5	410	21	1	2
Quorn								
BURGER								
Cheese Burger	1 burger	100	4	1	370	8	3	11
Classic	1 burger	90	3	0.5	290	7	3	11
CHIK'N								
Cranberry & Goat Cheese Cutlets	1 cutlet	280	17	5	600	25	5	12
Garlic & Herb	1 cutlet	200	9	1	570	22	3	12
Gruyere Cutlets	1 cutlet	260	15	4	510	23	3	11
Naked Cutlets	1 cutlet	80	3	0.5	420	5	2	11
Nuggets	4 nuggets	180	8	1	460	21	2	10
Patties	1 patty	150	6	0.5	400	17	2	9
Tenders	1 cup	80	2	0.5	390	9	4	10
TURK'Y								
Burgers	1 burger	90	4	0.5	200	6	2	10
Roast	1/5 roast	90	2	0.5	470	9	5	14
Ragu								
Alfredo, Cheesy Classic	1/4 cup	90	8	2.5	330	2	0	1
Chunky, Tomato, Garlic & Onion	1/2 cup	90	2	0	460	14	2	2

	SERVING SIZE	CALORIES	TOTAL FAT (G)	SAT FAT (G)	SODIUM (MG)	CARBS (G)	FIBER (G)	PROTEIN (G)
OLD-WORLD-STYLE SAUCE								
Marinara	1/2 cup	80	3	0	470	10	3	2
Meat	1/2 cup	70	3	0.5	470	9	2	2
Reese's								
Peanut Butter Cups	1 cup	210	13	4.5	150	27	1	5
Pieces Candy	51 pieces	200	9	8	55	25	2	5
Rice-A-Roni								
Chicken Fajita, Prepared	1 cup	260	9	1.5	1090	41	2	5
Country Cheddar, Prepared	1 cup	370	16	5	990	50	2	8
Creamy Four Cheese, Prepared	1 cup	270	12	3.5	740	37	1	6
Garden Vegetable, Prepared	1 cup	270	10	2.5	830	40	2	7
Parmesan Chicken, Prepared	1 cup	370	15	4	1240	52	3	8
Spanish Rice	2 oz	260	8	1.5	1250	44	3	6
Rice Krispies								
Cereal	1-1/4 cup	130	0	0	190	29	< 1	2
Treats, Original	1 bar	90	2	0.5	105	17	0	< 1
Rold Gold								
PRETZELS								
Hard Sourdough	1 pretzel	90	1	0	500	19	2	2
Honey Mustard, Tiny Twists	1 oz	110	1	0	430	23	1	3
Honey Wheat, Braided	1 oz	110	1	0	200	24	1	3
Rods	1 oz	110	1	0	450	22	1	3
Tiny Twists	1 oz	110	1	0	450	23	1	2
Rolo								
Original	1 package	220	10	7	80	33	0	2
Ruffles								
BAKED CRISPS								
Original	1 oz	120	3	0	135	22	2	2
POTATO CHIPS								
Authentic Barbeque	11 chips	160	10	1	170	16	1	2
Natural Sea Salted, Reduced-Fat	15 chips	140	7	0.5	160	17	1	2
Original	12 chips	160	10	1	160	15	1	2
Original, Reduced-Fat	13 chips	140	7	1	180	18	1	2
Sour Cream & Onion	11 chips	160	10	1	150	15	1	2
Sandies								
Pecan Shortbread	2 cookies	170	10	3	110	18	< 1	2
Simply Shortbread	2 cookies	160	9	4	90	19	0	2

	SERVING SIZE	CALORIES	TOTAL FAT (G)	SAT FAT (G)	SODIUM (MG)	CARBS (G)	FIBER (G)	PROTEIN (G)
Santa Cruz Organic								
FRUIT SPREAD								
Blackberry Pomegranate	1 fl oz	45	0	0	5	11	0	0
Red Raspberry, Seedless	1 fl oz	40	0	0	5	10	0	0
Strawberry	1 fl oz	40	0	0	5	10	0	0
JUICE BOX								
Grape	8 fl oz	100	0	0	10	23	0	0
Orange Drink	8 fl oz	100	0	0	10	25	0	1
Tropical Punch	8 fl oz	110	0	0	5	27	0	0
Shake 'N Bake								
Chicken, Original	1/8 packet	40	1	0	220	7	0	1
Pork, Original	1/8 packet	40	0	0	240	8	0	1
Snackwell								
Cereal Bars, Peanut Butter	35 grams	140	5	2	115	17	3	8
Cookie Cakes, Devil's Food	16 grams	50	0	0	25	12	0	1
Cookies, Crème Sandwich	25 grams	110	3	1	90	20	0	1
Popcorn, Caramel, Fudge Drizzled	30 grams	130	3	2.5	200	24	1	1
Sierra Mist								
Regular	12 fl oz	100	0	0	20	27	0	0
Siggi's Yogurt								
NON-FAT SKYR								
Average of All Flavors	1 container	100	0	0	60	11	0	14
Plain	1 container	80	0	0	60	5	0	15
Silk								
PURE								
Almond, Original	1 cup	60	3	0	150	8	1	1
Coconut, Original	1 cup	80	5	5	30	7	0	1
Vanilla Almond	1 cup	90	3	0	150	16	1	1
SOYMILK								
Original	1 cup	90	4	0.5	120	8	1	6
Original, Light	1 cup	60	2	0	125	6	1	6
Vanilla	1 cup	100	4	0.5	95	11	1	6
Vanilla, Light	1 cup	70	2	0	100	7	1	6
Simply Orange								
Simply Apple	8 fl oz	120	0	0	5	30	n/a	2
Simply Grapefruit	8 fl oz	90	0	0	10	21	n/a	1
Simply Lemonade	8 fl oz	120	0	0	15	30	n/a	0

	SERVING SIZE	CALORIES	TOTAL FAT (G)	SAT FAT (G)	SODIUM (MG)	CARBS (G)	FIBER (G)	PROTEIN (G)
Simply Orange, Average of All Flavors	8 fl oz	115	0	0	0	28	n/a	2
Simply Potatoes								
Hash Browns, Shredded	1/2 cup	70	0	0	55	16	2	1
Mashed Potatoes, Traditional	1/2 cup	130	6	4	420	16	2	3
Red Potato Wedges	1/2 cup	50	0	0	250	10	2	2
Skinny Cow								
Fudge Bars	1 bar	100	1	0.5	45	22	4	4
ICE CREAM CUPS								
Chocolate Fudge Brownie	1 container	150	2	1	70	29	4	5
Cookies & Cream	1 container	150	2	1	100	30	4	5
Dulce de Leche	1 container	150	1	0	85	32	4	4
Strawberry Cheesecake	1 container	150	1	0.5	65	33	4	4
Ice Cream Sandwiches, Average of All Flavors	1 sandwich	147	2	1	132	30	3	4
TRUFFLE BARS								
Caramel	1 bar	160	3	2	85	33	4	4
Chocolate	1 bar	100	3	2	50	19	3	3
Cookies & Cream	1 bar	110	3	2	55	20	3	3
French Vanilla	1 bar	100	2	2	45	18	3	3
Slim Jim								
Giant Stick, Original	1 stick	150	13	5	430	2	< 1	6
Snapple								
JUICE DRINK								
Kiwi Strawberry	8 fl oz	100	0	0	10	23	0	0
Lemonade	8 fl oz	90	0	0	45	24	0	0
Mango Madness	8 fl oz	100	0	0	10	23	0	0
Raspberry Peach	8 fl oz	110	0	0	5	27	0	0
TEA								
Green	8 fl oz	60	0	0	5	16	0	0
Peach	8 fl oz	80	0	0	5	20	0	0
Sweet	8 fl oz	90	0	0	5	24	0	0
Snickers								
Candy Bar, Original	1 bar	280	14	5	140	35	1	4
Ice Cream Bar	1 bar	180	11	6	60	18	1	3
Snyder of Berlin								
CORN SNACKS								
Baked Cheese Crunch	1 cup	140	8	1	330	17	< 1	2

	SERVING SIZE	CALORIES	TOTAL FAT (G)	SAT FAT (G)	SODIUM (MG)	CARBS (G)	FIBER (G)	PROTEIN (G)
Puff 'N Corn Cheese	2 cups	180	14	3	250	12	0	1
POTATO CHIPS								
Honey Bar-B-Q	17 chips	150	9	1.5	230	16	< 1	1
Kettle Cooked, Buffalo Wing	13 chips	150	9	1	190	15	< 1	1
Kettle Cooked, Sea Salt & Cracked Pepper	13 chips	140	9	2.5	390	15	1	2
Red Hot	17 chips	150	10	2	180	14	1	2
Rippled	17 chips	150	10	2	150	14	1	2
Wavy Cheddar & Sour Cream	16 chips	150	10	2	260	14	1	2
PRETZELS								
Hard Sourdough	1 pretzel	100	1	0	470	21	< 1	3
Pittsburgh Pretzel Rods	3 pieces	110	1	0	340	22	< 1	3
Snyder's of Hanover								
Pretzels, Nibblers, Honey Mustard & Onion	30 grams	130	3	1.5	95	23	< 1	3
PRETZELS, STICKS								
Gluten-Free	30 sticks	120	2	0.5	260	25	< 1	0
Multi-Grain	7 sticks	120	2	0	160	23	3	3
PRETZEL TWISTS, BRAIDED								
Honey Wheat	8 twists	120	2	0	230	24	2	3
Multi-Grain	9 twists	120	2	0	160	23	3	3
Sprite								
Original	12 fl oz	100	0	0	45	26	0	0
Stouffer's								
EASY EXPRESS SKILLETS								
Cheesy Meatball Rigatoni	1/2 package	470	21	9	1190	48	5	21
Chicken Alfredo	1/2 package	410	10	4	980	48	6	31
Grilled Chicken & Vegetables	1/2 package	360	9	2.5	860	43	4	26
MACARONI & CHEESE								
Broccoli, Signature Classics	12 oz	480	20	8	1000	52	5	22
Macaroni & Cheese	10 oz	350	17	7	920	34	2	15
PIZZA								
Cheese	1 pizza	360	15	6	530	43	4	14
Deluxe	1 pizza	430	21	7	820	44	4	15
Grilled Vegetables	1 pizza	340	12	4.5	570	44	5	13
Three Meat	1 pizza	470	25	9	990	43	4	19
SIGNATURE CLASSICS								
Chicken Broccoli & Cheddar Stromboli	1 entrée	360	11	4.5	750	45	4	20
Pepperoni & Provolone Stromboli	1 entrée	430	17	7	1110	45	5	24

store brands

	SERVING SIZE	CALORIES	TOTAL FAT (G)	SAT FAT (G)	SODIUM (MG)	CARBS (G)	FIBER (G)	PROTEIN (G)
Smoked Turkey Club Panini	1 entrée	380	15	6	870	37	4	24
Three Cheese & Ham Panini	1 entrée	420	18	8	940	42	4	22

Special K
CEREAL

Fruit & Yogurt	3/4 cup	120	1	0	140	27	3	2
Low-Fat Granola, Touch of Honey	1/2 cup	190	3	0.5	115	39	5	7
Original	1 cup	120	1	0	220	23	0	6
Protein Plus	3/4 cup	100	3	0.5	110	14	5	10
Vanilla Almond	3/4 cup	110	2	0	170	25	3	2
Cereal Bars, Average of All Flavors	1 bar	90	2	1	93	17	3	1

PROTEIN BARS & SHAKES

Meal Bar, Chocolate Peanut Butter	1 bar	180	6	3.5	250	25	5	10
Meal Bar, Chocolatey Chip	1 bar	170	5	3.5	180	26	5	10
Meal Bar, Strawberry	1 bar	170	5	4	160	25	5	10
Protein Shakes, Average of All Flavors	1 bottle	185	5	0.5	223	29	5	10
Snack Bars, Average of All Flavors	1 bar	110	3	2	78	16	1	4

Sun Chips

Multigrain Snacks, Average of All Flavors	15 chips	140	6	1	160	19	3	2

Talenti
GELATO

Cappuccino	1/2 cup	200	11	6	45	23	0	5
Double Dark Chocolate	1/2 cup	210	10	6	35	28	2	4
Sea Salt Caramel	1/2 cup	240	11	5	190	38	2	4
Sicilian Pistachio	1/2 cup	210	10	6	55	27	0	4
Toasted Almond	1/2 cup	230	12	5	50	28	1	5
Sorbetto, Average of All Flavors	1/2 cup	120	0	0	0	30	1	0

Tastee Choice

Chicken Parmigiana & Penne Pasta	1/2 package	380	8	4	760	60	29	17
Dijon Cilantro Tilapia, w/Basmati Rice	1 package	436	12	7	766	54	26	28
Lemon Herb Tilapia, w/Basmati Rice	1 package	446	18	13	809	52	26	19
Orange Chicken	1/2 package	370	9	1.5	670	56	6	15
Shrimp, Basmati Rice & Vegetables	1/2 package	320	2	0.5	1470	58	4	16
Shrimp Scampi, w/Linguine	1 package	368	10	7.3	577	48	8	22

Terra
POTATO CHIPS

Red Bliss, Made w/Olive Oil	1 oz	140	7	1	190	18	2	1
Yukon Gold, Salt & Pepper	1 oz	130	5	0.5	120	19	1	2

	SERVING SIZE	CALORIES	TOTAL FAT (G)	SAT FAT (G)	SODIUM (MG)	CARBS (G)	FIBER (G)	PROTEIN (G)
POTATO CHIPS, KETTLES								
Au Natural, Unsalted	1 oz	150	9	0.5	0	15	2	2
Hickory BBQ, Unsalted	1 oz	150	9	0.5	5	15	1	2
Lemon Pepper, Unsalted	1 oz	150	10	0.5	5	15	1	2
VEGETABLE CHIPS								
Crinkles, Classic Cut, Sweets & Carrots	1 oz	150	9	1	20	15	5	2
Crinkles, Sweet Potato, Sea Salt	1 oz	160	11	1	90	15	3	1
Exotic Harvest, Sea Salt	1 oz	130	6	0.5	160	16	3	2
Tim's Cascade Snacks								
ERIN'S ALL NATURAL POPCORN								
Low-Fat, Low-Salt	4 cups	130	6	0.5	135	18	1	3
White Cheddar	2 cups	150	8	1.5	240	15	3	4
POTATO CHIPS								
Cheddar & Sour Cream	13 chips	140	9	1.5	200	18	1	2
Johnny's Seasoned	13 chips	130	9	1	220	15	1	2
Mesquite BBQ, Natural	13 chips	130	6	1.5	170	18	1	2
Original	13 chips	140	9	1.5	110	15	1	2
Sea Salt, Natural	15 chips	130	6	1.5	110	18	1	2
Tofurky								
Franks	1-3/5 oz	80	2	0	370	5	2	10
Italian Deli Slices	5 slices	110	4	1	360	7	4	11
Jerky, Original	4 pieces	100	2	0	260	9	1	12
Links, Breakfast	1-3/5 oz	120	6	0	320	6	2	10
Oven-Roasted Deli Slices	5 slices	100	3	0	300	6	3	13
Pepperoni Deli Slices	8 slices	60	1	0	170	6	4	7
Total Cereal								
Plus Omega-3, Honey Almond Flax	1 cup	200	4	0.5	90	40	4	5
Raisin Bran	1 cup	160	1	0	230	40	5	3
Whole Grain	3/4 cup	100	1	0	190	23	3	2
Totino's								
FAMILY SIZE, FROZEN								
Cheese	1/3 pizza	330	16	5	610	35	2	10
Sausage	1/2 pizza	390	21	6	770	39	2	13
Party Pizza, Frozen, Average of All Varieties	1/2 pizza	356	18	6	731	35	2	12
Pizza Roll Snacks, Average of All Varieties	6 rolls	206	9	3	384	24	1	7

	SERVING SIZE	CALORIES	TOTAL FAT (G)	SAT FAT (G)	SODIUM (MG)	CARBS (G)	FIBER (G)	PROTEIN (G)
Town House								
CRACKERS								
Original	5 crackers	80	5	1	130	10	< 1	< 1
Reduced-Fat	6 crackers	60	2	0	130	12	< 1	1
Wheat	5 crackers	80	4	0.5	140	10	< 1	1
Flatbread Crisps, Average of Flavors	6 crackers	70	2	0	140	12	1	1
Toppers, Original Crackers	3 crackers	70	3	0.5	135	9	0	1
Tribe								
HUMMUS								
Average of All Flavors	2 tbsp	61	4	0	129	4	1	2
Roasted Eggplant	2 tbsp	45	3	0	150	3	1	2
Triscuit								
Original	6 crackers	120	5	1	180	19	3	3
Reduced-Fat	7 crackers	120	3	0.5	160	21	3	3
True North Crunch								
Almond Pecan	1 oz	170	12	1	90	9	3	5
Cashew	1 oz	120	7	1.5	150	12	1	4
Chocolate	1 oz	160	11	2	75	11	3	4
Peanut	1 oz	170	13	2	75	9	3	5
Turkey Hill								
FROZEN YOGURT								
Chocolate Chip Cookie Dough	1/2 cup	120	3	1.5	80	22	1	3
Fudge Ripple	1/2 cup	100	0	0	65	21	0	3
Peanut Butter Pie	1/2 cup	160	7	2.5	95	22	1	4
Vanilla Bean	1/2 cup	90	0	0	60	19	0	3
ICE CREAM								
Black Raspberry	1/2 cup	130	7	4.5	40	16	0	2
Chocolate	1/2 cup	150	7	4.5	45	19	1	2
Fudge Ripple	1/2 cup	140	6	4	45	20	0	2
Neapolitan	1/2 cup	140	7	4.5	40	17	0	2
Peanut Butter Ripple	1/2 cup	170	11	4.5	75	15	0	3
Rocky Road	1/2 cup	170	8	3.5	125	23	1	3
ICE CREAM, LIGHT								
Cookies 'N Cream	1/2 cup	120	3	1.5	80	20	1	2
Moose Tracks	1/2 cup	140	6	2.5	65	20	1	3
Skinny Minty	1/2 cup	140	5	2	80	21	1	2
Vanilla Bean	1/2 cup	100	2	1.5	55	17	1	2

	SERVING SIZE	CALORIES	TOTAL FAT (G)	SAT FAT (G)	SODIUM (MG)	CARBS (G)	FIBER (G)	PROTEIN (G)
Sherbet, Average of All Flavors	1/2 cup	120	1	0.5	18	27	0	1
Twizzlers								
Bites, Cherry	17 pieces	140	1	0	95	32	0	1
Pull 'n Peel, Sugar-Free	6 pieces	130	1	0	110	34	0	1
Twists, Black Licorice	4 pieces	150	1	0	210	35	0	1
Twists, Strawberry	4 pieces	160	1	0	95	36	0	1
Tyson								
ANYTIZERS								
Buffalo-Style Boneless Chicken Bites	3 pieces	150	7	1.5	680	8	0	12
Honey BBQ Flavored Wings	3 oz	190	12	3	390	8	0	13
Popcorn Chicken	7 pieces	180	9	1.5	560	11	0	13
Quesa Dippers, Chicken Fajita, w/o Salsa	2 pieces	190	9	4	540	17	1	10
Quesa Dippers, Chicken Taco Seasoned, w/o Salsa	2 pieces	200	11	4.5	470	16	0	9
CHICKEN BREAST								
Nuggets	5 pieces	220	13	3	470	15	1	12
Patties	1 piece	200	13	3	400	10	0	9
Patties, Spicy	1 piece	180	11	2.5	420	10	1	9
CHICKEN STRIPS								
Buffalo Chicken	3 oz	190	9	1.5	1040	17	1	12
Home-Style, Breaded	4 oz	220	10	2	570	14	2	19
Udi's Gluten-Free								
BAGELS								
Cinnamon Raisin	1 bagel	280	8	1	450	45	3	6
Plain	1 bagel	310	10	1	530	47	3	7
Whole Grain	1 bagel	280	9	1	470	43	3	7
BREAD								
Cinnamon Raisin	2 slices	160	4	0	220	29	1	3
Millet Chia	2 slices	170	5	0.5	300	28	6	5
White, Sandwich	2 slices	140	4	0	270	22	1	3
Whole Grain	2 slices	140	4	0	270	22	1	3
COOKIES								
Chocolate Chip	2 cookies	150	7	4.5	85	22	1	1
Oatmeal Raisin	2 cookies	170	7	4	110	26	2	3
Snickerdoodle	2 cookies	150	6	3.5	110	23	0	1
GRANOLA								
Average of All Flavors	1/4 cup	123	5	0	0	18	3	3

store brands

	SERVING SIZE	CALORIES	TOTAL FAT (G)	SAT FAT (G)	SODIUM (MG)	CARBS (G)	FIBER (G)	PROTEIN (G)
Uncle Ben's Rice								
COUNTRY INN								
Broccoli Rice Au Gratin	1 cup	210	3	1.5	840	41	1	6
Chicken & Wild Rice	1 cup	200	1	0	910	45	1	4
Mexican Fiesta Rice	1 cup	190	1	0	710	42	1	5
Rice Pilaf	1 cup	200	1	0	650	44	1	5
READY RICE								
Butter & Garlic	1 cup	220	4	0.5	750	41	2	4
Garden Vegetable	1 cup	200	3	0	830	41	1	4
Spanish Style	1 cup	200	3	0	620	40	2	4
WHOLE GRAIN MEDLEY								
Brown & Wild	1 cup	220	4	0	730	42	3	6
Chicken Medley	1 cup	210	4	0	730	41	4	5
Vegetable Harvest	1 cup	220	3	0	780	44	5	5
Uncle Sam								
Cereal, w/Mixed Berries	1 cup	190	5	0.5	130	39	10	7
Toasted Whole Wheat Flakes & Flaxseed	3/4 cup	190	5	0.5	135	38	10	7
UTZ								
Baked Crisps, Original	1 oz	110	2	0	170	23	2	2
KETTLE CLASSIC POTATO CHIPS								
Regular	1 oz	140	8	1.5	120	15	1	2
Salt & Malt Vinegar	1 oz	150	9	1.5	260	15	1	2
POPCORN								
Butter	2 cups	170	12	3	250	13	2	2
Cheese	2 cups	160	11	1.5	300	14	3	2
White Cheddar	2 cups	150	9	1.5	240	15	3	3
Pork Rinds, Regular	1/2 oz	80	5	1.5	230	10	0	8
POTATO CHIPS								
Reduced-Fat	1 oz	140	7	1.5	120	18	1	2
Regular	1 oz	150	9	2	95	14	1	2
V8								
SPLASH								
Berry Blend	8 fl oz	70	0	0	50	18	0	0
Tropical Blend	8 fl oz	70	0	0	50	18	0	0
Vegetable Juice, Original	8 fl oz	50	0	0	420	10	2	2
V-FUSION								
Cranberry Blackberry	8 fl oz	100	0	0	90	26	0	0

	SERVING SIZE	CALORIES	TOTAL FAT (G)	SAT FAT (G)	SODIUM (MG)	CARBS (G)	FIBER (G)	PROTEIN (G)
Strawberry Banana	8 fl oz	120	0	0	70	28	0	1
Strawberry Banana, Light	8 fl oz	50	0	0	60	12	0	0
Van Camp's								
Baked Beans, Hickory & Bacon	1/2 cup	170	1	0	470	32	5	7
Baked Beans, Original	1/2 cup	160	1	0	510	30	5	7
Beanee Weenees, Baked	1 can	290	8	2.5	1160	42	6	13
Beanee Weenees, Original	1 can	240	8	3	990	29	8	14
Chili, w/Beans	1 cup	350	18	8	900	31	7	17
Chili, w/o Beans	1 cup	390	26	11	1080	20	6	20
VAN DE KAMP'S, See Mrs. Paul's								
Van's Natural Foods								
8 Whole Grains Multigrain Waffles	2 waffles	160	6	0	230	28	6	3
Belgian Waffles, Home-Style	2 waffles	210	9	0.5	430	29	1	3
Buttermilk Pancakes	2 pancakes	170	2	0	300	34	1	4
Cinnamon French Toast, Wheat-Free	2 slices	190	4	0	310	39	1	2
Vanilla Sticks Waffles	1 stick	70	1	0	130	14	1	2
Velveeta								
CHEESE PRODUCTS								
2% Milk	1/4 inch slice	60	3	1.5	410	4	0	5
Regular	1/4 inch slice	80	6	3.5	410	3	0	5
PASTAS								
Rotini & Cheese, Whole Grain	1 cup	310	12	3	830	40	3	11
Shells & Cheese, Original	1 cup	360	12	3.5	840	49	2	13
Vienna Fingers								
Creme-Filled	2 cookies	150	6	2	95	23	< 1	1
Creme-Filled, Reduced-Fat	2 cookies	140	5	1.5	115	24	< 1	1
Vitamin Water								
Average of All Flavors	12 fl oz	120	0	0	0	33	0	0
Vitasoy								
Organic Original	8 fl oz	90	4	0.5	150	9	1	7
Organic Original Lite Plus	8 fl oz	60	2	0.4	130	6	0	4
Wanchai Ferry								
ENTRÉES, PREPARED								
Beef & Broccoli	1/2 entrée	360	6	1	1300	61	3	18
General Tso's Spicy Garlic Chicken	1-3/4 cups	570	22	3	1270	79	3	15
Orange Chicken	1-3/4 cups	610	22	3	1180	90	3	15
Shrimp Lo Mein	2 cups	600	16	3	1600	92	6	20

	SERVING SIZE	CALORIES	TOTAL FAT (G)	SAT FAT (G)	SODIUM (MG)	CARBS (G)	FIBER (G)	PROTEIN (G)
Weight Watchers Smart Ones								
ANYTIME SELECTIONS								
Cheeseburger, Mini	1 burger	200	9	4	360	20	3	10
Pizza, Cheese, Mini	2 pizzas	270	8	3.5	490	37	6	13
Pizza, Pepperoni, Mini	2 pizzas	280	7	2.5	460	42	6	12
Quesadilla, Fiesta	1 quesadilla	230	5	2.5	490	35	9	10
BREAKFAST, MORNING EXPRESS								
Cheesy, Scramble, w/Hashbrowns	1 entrée	210	9	4	510	18	3	15
French Toast, w/Turkey Sausage	1 entrée	280	8	2	570	39	2	14
Smart Morning Wrap, Egg, Sausage & Cheese	2 wraps	240	8	2.5	560	32	7	11
DESSERTS								
Brownie, à la Mode	1 brownie	130	4	2.5	120	120	2	3
Pie, Key Lime	1 pie	150	3	1	55	28	< 1	2
Strawberry Shortcake	1 cake	120	4	2	210	19	< 1	2
Sundae, Brownie, Chocolate Fudge	1 sundae	140	3	1.5	65	24	1	2
ENTRÉES								
Beef, Pot Roast, Home-Style	1 entrée	180	5	2	670	18	4	17
Broccoli & Cheddar Roasted Potatoes	1 entrée	240	7	3.5	520	35	4	10
Chicken Parmesan	1 entrée	290	5	1.5	630	35	4	26
Chicken Teriyaki Stir-Fry	1 entrée	340	6	1	600	49	5	25
Lasagna Bake, w/Meat Sauce	1 entrée	270	4	1.5	560	46	4	13
Macaroni & Cheese	1 entrée	270	2	1	790	52	2	11
Pasta Primavera	1 entrée	250	4	2	610	41	4	11
Roast Beef, Mashed Potatoes & Gravy	1 entrée	230	11	3.5	530	18	2	16
Sesame Chicken	1 entrée	360	7	1.5	490	49	6	25
Spaghetti, w/Meat Sauce	1 entrée	290	6	1.5	520	44	5	16
Turkey Breast, w/Stuffing, Home-Style	1 entrée	260	5	1.5	700	39	4	14
Ziti, w/Meatballs & Cheese	1 entrée	390	9	4	730	52	6	25
Welch's								
JAM, JELLY & SPREAD								
Concord Grape Jam or Jelly	1 tbsp	50	0	0	10	13	0	0
Strawberry Spread	1 tbsp	50	0	0	10	13	0	0
Wheatables								
Original Golden	17 crackers	140	6	1.5	210	20	1	2
Toasted Honey	17 crackers	140	6	1.5	200	20	1	2

	SERVING SIZE	CALORIES	TOTAL FAT (G)	SAT FAT (G)	SODIUM (MG)	CARBS (G)	FIBER (G)	PROTEIN (G)
Wheat Thins								
Fiber Selects, 5-Grain	13 crackers	120	5	0.5	260	22	5	2
Multigrain	15 crackers	140	5	0.5	230	22	2	2
Original	16 crackers	140	5	1	230	22	2	2
Reduced-Fat	16 crackers	130	4	0.5	230	22	2	2
Whoppers								
Original	18 pieces	190	7	7	115	31	0	1
Wise								
CHEEZ DOODLES								
Cheese Balls	43 pieces	150	8	2	320	17	0	2
Crunchy	1/2 cup	150	9	2.5	230	17	0	1
Puffed	23 pieces	150	8	2	320	17	0	2
POTATO CHIPS								
All Natural	16 chips	150	10	3	160	14	1	2
Kettle Cooked, New York Deli	13 chips	150	9	2.5	170	15	1	2
Lightly Salted	15 chips	150	10	3	80	14	1	2
Wonder Bread								
100% Whole Wheat, Soft	2 slices	110	2	0	220	20	3	5
Wheat, Light	1 slice	40	0	0	120	9	3	3
White, Classic	1 slice	70	1	0	150	14	0	2
Yoplait Yogurt								
Fiber One, All Flavors	1 container	50	0	0	55	13	5	3
Greek, Honey Vanilla	1 container	150	0	0	120	25	n/a	12
Greek, Plain	1 container	120	0	0	115	13	n/a	15
Greek, Strawberry	1 container	160	0	0	100	26	n/a	12
Lactose Free, All Flavors	1 container	170	2	1	85	33	n/a	5
Light, All Flavors	1 container	100	0	0	85	19	n/a	5
Light, Thick & Creamy, All Flavors	1 container	100	0	0	90	21	n/a	5
Light, w/Granola, All Flavors	1 container	190	3	0	105	1	n/a	5
Original, All Flavors	1 container	170	2	1	85	33	n/a	5
Thick & Creamy, All Flavors	1 container	180	3	1.5	110	31	n/a	7
York Peppermint Pattie								
Original	1 pattie	140	3	1.5	10	31	1	1
Yumnuts								
Chocolate Cashews	1/4 cup	150	10	2	0	11	2	5
Dark Chocolate Almonds	28 grams	150	11	1	0	10	3	5

	SERVING SIZE	CALORIES	TOTAL FAT (G)	SAT FAT (G)	SODIUM (MG)	CARBS (G)	FIBER (G)	PROTEIN (G)
Sea Salt Cashews	1/4 cup	160	11	2	105	9	2	6
Zatarain's								
Dirty Rice, Original, prepared	1 cup	130	0	0	620	29	< 1	3
Red Beans & Rice, Spicy, prepared	1 cup	200	0	0	890	40	5	7
Yellow Rice, prepared	1 cup	190	0	0	930	43	< 1	4

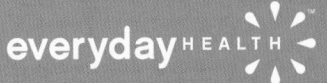

restaurants

	SERVING SIZE	CALORIES	TOTAL FAT (G)	SAT FAT (G)	SODIUM (MG)	CARBS (G)	FIBER (G)	PROTEIN (G)
A&W								
BURGERS & CHICKEN								
Bacon Double Cheeseburger	1 burger	760	45	17	1570	45	4	44
Cheeseburger	1 burger	420	21	7	1040	37	4	23
Chicken Strips	3 pieces	500	29	5	1050	32	2	28
Double Cheeseburger	1 burger	680	38	14	1330	44	4	40
Grilled Chicken Sandwich	1 sandwich	400	15	3	820	31	4	35
Hamburger	1 burger	380	19	6	860	33	3	21
Papa Burger	1 burger	690	39	14	1350	44	4	40
HOT DOGS								
Cheese	1 hot dog	350	22	9	940	26	1	12
Coney Chili Cheese	1 hot dog	380	23	9	1100	28	2	14
Plain	1 hot dog	310	19	8	740	23	1	11
SIDES								
Breaded Onion Rings, Regular	as served	350	16	3.5	710	45	2	5
Cheese Curds, Regular	as served	570	40	21	1220	27	2	27
Cheese Fries	as served	390	18	4.5	870	50	4	4
Chili	1 bowl	190	6	2	640	22	5	12
Chili Fries	as served	370	15	4	790	49	5	8
Corn Dog Nuggets, Regular	8 pieces	280	13	3	830	32	2	9
French Fries, Regular	as served	310	12	3	460	45	4	3
SWEETS & TREATS								
Cherry Limeades, Medium	16 fl oz	300	0	0	45	79	0	0
Hot Fudge Sundae	1 sundae	350	11	6	140	54	1	8
Reese's Peanut Butter Fudge Blendrrr, Medium	20 fl oz	710	41	30	180	108	3	7
Reese's Polar Swirl	12 fl oz	740	31	14	380	97	3	18
Root Beer Float, Medium	20 fl oz	350	5	3	105	77	0	2
Root Beer Freeze, Medium	20 fl oz	480	10	6	230	89	1	9
Strawberry Banana Smoothee, Medium	20 fl oz	420	6	4.5	100	86	0	3
Vanilla Shake, Medium	20 fl oz	900	39	24	260	121	0	15
Vanilla Soft Serve Cone, Regular	1 item	200	5	3	115	32	0	6
Watermelon Slushee, Medium	16 fl oz	360	0	0	65	99	0	0
Applebee's								
APPETIZERS								
Appetizer Sampler	as served	2530	167	48	6230	184	15	92
Boneless Wings, Classic Buffalo	as served	1170	69	16	3780	66	8	70

	SERVING SIZE	CALORIES	TOTAL FAT (G)	SAT FAT (G)	SODIUM (MG)	CARBS (G)	FIBER (G)	PROTEIN (G)
Cheeseburger Sliders, w/Applewood-Smoked Bacon	as served	1340	87	27	2550	82	4	56
Chili Cheese Nachos	as served	1680	107	40	4270	134	17	48
ENTRÉES								
Bruschetta Chicken	1 entrée	850	43	14	2760	56	9	61
Cajun Shrimp Pasta	1 entrée	1210	72	28	3250	96	8	44
Chicken Broccoli Pasta Alfredo	1 entrée	1350	71	35	2760	111	9	68
Chicken Parmesan Stack	1 entrée	1690	95	42	4110	130	10	82
Double Crunch Shrimp	1 entrée	1280	69	13	3270	133	10	33
Garlic Herb Salmon	1 entrée	680	29	8	1450	62	5	46
Grilled Dijon Chicken & Portobellos	1 entrée	470	16	7	1820	30	5	55
New England Fish & Chips	1 entrée	1930	138	24	3180	121	12	51
Provolone-Stuffed Meatballs, w/Fettuccine	1 entrée	1510	89	42	4000	117	8	62
Shrimp Fettuccine Alfredo	1 entrée	1420	81	40	3610	113	9	64
Sizzling Chili Lime Chicken	1 entrée	470	10	3	1970	56	8	52
Sizzling Skillet Fajitas, Chicken	1 entrée	1370	52	24	4870	149	11	78
Sizzling Steak & Cheese	1 entrée	1000	64	23	3260	39	6	67
REALBURGERS & SANDWICHES, W/O FRIES								
Cheeseburger	1 burger	940	58	22	1700	51	3	54
Chicken Fajita Rollup	1 sandwich	1060	59	27	3360	62	6	119
Cowboy Burger	1 burger	1180	70	25	2720	77	5	61
Hamburger	1 burger	790	46	15	1220	50	3	46
Honey BBQ Chicken Sandwich	1 sandwich	1000	41	16	2650	88	4	70
Quesadilla Burger	1 burger	1420	103	43	3630	46	6	79
SALADS, SIDES & SOUPS								
Chicken Tortilla Soup	1 bowl	160	8	2.5	1110	14	1	8
Chili	1 bowl	410	27	13	1010	14	6	27
Chili Cheese Fries	as served	590	32	11	1510	60	7	17
Crunchy Onion Rings	as served	530	28	5	1320	63	4	7
Fries	as served	390	18	3.5	720	53	4	5
Grilled Chicken Caesar, w/Dressing	1 salad	820	57	11	1740	25	6	54
Oriental Chicken, w/Dressing	1 salad	1380	99	15	1430	91	11	40
STEAKS & TOPPERS								
Asiago Peppercorn Steak, w/Sides	1 entrée	380	14	6	1520	25	5	44
Chicken Fried Steak, w/Mashed Potatoes, Gravy & Vegetables	1 entrée	1200	59	16	3920	112	10	57
Roasted Garlic Sirloin, w/o Sides	as served	450	18	7	1910	33	5	42

restaurants

	SERVING SIZE	CALORIES	TOTAL FAT (G)	SAT FAT (G)	SODIUM (MG)	CARBS (G)	FIBER (G)	PROTEIN (G)
Steak & Grilled Shrimp Combo, w/o Sides	as served	540	36	9	1960	2	< 1	51
Steak & Honey BBQ Chicken Combo, w/o Sides	as served	600	15	6	2160	37	< 1	78

Arby's
CHICKEN

Chicken Bacon & Swiss, Crispy	1 sandwich	610	30	7	1400	51	3	33
Chicken Bacon & Swiss, Roast	1 sandwich	480	20	6	1280	43	2	31
Cravin' Chicken Sandwich, Crispy	1 sandwich	510	22	4	1110	51	4	26
Cravin' Chicken Sandwich, Roast	1 sandwich	380	12	2.5	1000	42	3	24
Prime-Cut Chicken Tenders	5 pieces	590	28	4	1610	42	4	42

SALADS

Chopped Farmhouse Chicken, Crispy	1 salad	430	24	9	1000	26	4	29
Chopped Farmhouse Chicken, Roast	1 salad	250	14	7	670	11	3	23

SANDWICHES

Angus Philly	1 sandwich	590	29	9	1760	48	3	34
Angus Three Cheese & Bacon	1 sandwich	640	33	12	1820	45	2	41
Market Fresh Reuben	1 sandwich	640	30	8	1610	62	4	32
Market Fresh Roast Turkey, Ranch & Bacon	1 sandwich	800	36	9	2200	78	5	45
Roast Beef 'n Cheddar, Classic	1 sandwich	440	18	5	1290	47	2	23
Roast Beef 'n Cheddar, Mid	1 sandwich	530	23	7	1720	48	2	34
Roast Beef, Classic	1 sandwich	350	12	4	950	39	2	25
Roast Beef, Mid	1 sandwich	440	17	6	1380	40	2	33
Signature Bacon Beef 'n Cheddar	1 sandwich	510	23	7	1510	48	2	28
Signature French Dip & Swiss, w/Au Jus	1 sandwich	430	14	6	2120	52	2	26

SIDES

Curly Fries, Medium	as served	540	29	4	1200	62	7	6
Potato Cakes	4 pieces	460	27	4.5	930	50	5	3
Steakhouse Onion Rings	5 pieces	410	20	3	1690	51	3	6

Atlanta Bread
BAGELS

Asiago	1 bagel	390	11	7	820	53	2	17
Cinnamon Raisin	1 bagel	270	1	0	420	55	3	10
Everything	1 bagel	350	4	0.5	1660	66	4	13
Plain	1 bagel	300	2	0	500	60	3	11
Whole Grain	1 bagel	260	2	0	450	52	4	10

	SERVING SIZE	CALORIES	TOTAL FAT (G)	SAT FAT (G)	SODIUM (MG)	CARBS (G)	FIBER (G)	PROTEIN (G)
BAKERY								
Bear Claw	1 pastry	540	24	10	320	71	3	9
Cheese Croissant	1 croissant	360	19	10	320	41	1	6
Chocolate Croissant	1 croissant	560	28	16	330	68	4	9
Ciabatta	1 roll	270	2	1	500	55	2	10
French Roll	1 roll	160	1	0	370	34	1	6
Gooey Butter Danish	1 danish	560	26	15	380	74	2	8
Sticky Bun	1 pastry	560	30	17	320	66	1	6
BREAD								
Cinnamon Raisin	1 slice	270	5	2	330	50	2	6
French Baguette	1 slice	90	0	0	210	19	1	4
Honey Wheat	1 slice	140	2	0.5	290	28	2	5
Nine Grain	1 slice	120	2	0.5	240	22	2	5
Pumpernickel Loaf	1 slice	110	1	0	230	22	2	5
Rye Loaf	1 slice	90	1	0	170	18	2	4
Sourdough	1 slice	140	0	0	300	28	1	5
MUFFIN								
Apple, Low-Fat	1 muffin	230	3	0.5	290	48	1	5
Banana Nut	1 muffin	610	36	5	330	63	2	11
Blueberry	1 muffin	320	15	2.5	250	41	1	5
MUFFIN TOP								
Banana Nut	1 muffin top	420	26	3.5	200	39	2	7
Blueberry	1 muffin top	250	12	2	190	31	1	4
Chocolate Chip	1 muffin top	390	19	6	220	51	2	6
Pumpkin, Low-Fat	1 muffin top	200	2	0	220	43	2	4
SANDWICHES								
ABC Special	1 sandwich	750	38	10	1980	57	3	45
California Avocado	1 sandwich	930	50	11	1120	98	14	25
Honey Maple Ham on Honey Wheat	1 sandwich	410	5	2	1370	64	5	27
Turkey Bacon Rustica	1 sandwich	960	56	19	2480	62	3	53
Turkey on Nine Grain	1 sandwich	370	6	2	1240	50	4	29
Veggie on Nine Grain	1 sandwich	500	25	8	820	52	5	18
SOUP & SALADS								
Baja Chicken Enchilada Soup	1-1/4 cups	330	19	9	1560	23	4	16
Chicken Peppercorn Soup	1-1/4 cups	430	34	18	1530	13	0	15
Chopstix Chicken Salad, w/o Dressing	1 salad	240	10	1.5	530	22	4	18
Salsa Fresca Salmon Salad, w/o Dressing	1 salad	560	29	4.5	590	40	6	38

restaurants

	SERVING SIZE	CALORIES	TOTAL FAT (G)	SAT FAT (G)	SODIUM (MG)	CARBS (G)	FIBER (G)	PROTEIN (G)
Au Bon Pain								
BAKERY								
Bagel, Cinnamon Raisin	1 bagel	320	1	0	450	68	3	11
Bagel, Plain	1 bagel	280	1	0	440	57	2	11
Breadstick, Sesame	1 breadstick	170	3	0	220	30	2	6
Brownie, Chocolate Cheesecake	1 brownie	420	21	7	250	57	1	5
Classic Chicken Salad Sandwich	1 sandwich	450	11	1.5	1000	60	3	27
Croissant, Ham & Cheese	1 croissant	390	21	11	580	35	1	15
Croissant, Plain	1 croissant	240	12	8	320	26	1	5
Danish, Sweet Cheese	1 danish	470	24	12	410	54	2	9
Muffin, Blueberry	1 muffin	490	17	2	510	74	2	9
Pecan Roll	1 roll	810	41	14	430	99	3	12
Roll, Farm House	1 roll	360	7	1	670	63	3	12
Scone, Cinnamon	1 scone	530	28	17	400	60	2	9
SALADS								
Caesar Asiago	1 salad	220	12	6	470	18	3	11
Chicken Cobb, w/Avocado	1 salad	410	24	10	920	12	5	38
Mandarin Sesame Chicken	1 salad	310	11	2	440	31	4	20
Mediterranean Chicken	1 salad	290	16	6	1150	12	3	25
Thai Peanut Chicken	1 salad	200	5	1	300	18	4	22
SANDWICHES & WRAPS								
Angus Steak Teriyaki Hot Wrap	1 wrap	630	15	3	1420	100	5	26
Caprese on a Baguette	1 sandwich	680	32	15	1200	65	4	30
Grilled Chicken on Ciabatta	1 sandwich	470	4	1	1660	67	4	39
Ham & Swiss on a Baguette	1 sandwich	650	19	10	2040	82	4	41
Mediterranean Wrap	1 wrap	630	34	9	1350	61	10	21
Toasted Southwestern Black Bean Burger on Country White	1 sandwich	670	32	11	1500	66	8	33
Turkey Cranberry Brie on Multigrain	1 sandwich	590	20	10	1680	66	9	42
SOUP, CHILI & STEW, MEDIUM								
12 Veggie	12 fl oz	180	6	1	1290	25	4	5
Butternut Squash & Apple	12 fl oz	240	8	3	860	40	4	4
Chicken Florentine	12 fl oz	270	14	6	1140	27	1	9
Chili, Turkey	12 fl oz	380	14	3	1100	43	16	23
Clam Chowder	12 fl oz	340	19	8	1090	29	2	10
Lobster Bisque	12 fl oz	410	30	18	1400	25	0	8
Macaroni & Cheese	12 fl oz	560	35	22	1300	37	2	21

	SERVING SIZE	CALORIES	TOTAL FAT (G)	SAT FAT (G)	SODIUM (MG)	CARBS (G)	FIBER (G)	PROTEIN (G)
Auntie Anne's								
BEVERAGES								
Lemonade Mixers, Average of All Flavors	42 fl oz	645	0	0	46	163	0	0
Mocha Dutch Ice	20 fl oz	390	12	11	125	73	0	2
Strawberry Dutch Ice	20 fl oz	230	0	0	50	58	0	0
DIPPING SAUCES								
Caramel Dip	1-1/2 oz	130	3	1.5	95	23	0	1
Melted Cheese Dip	2 oz	150	12	3	850	6	0	5
Sweet Dip	1-1/2 oz	130	0	0	0	32	0	0
Sweet Mustard	1-1/4 oz	60	2	1	0	10	0	2
PRETZELS								
Pretzel, Cinnamon Sugar	1 pretzel	470	12	7	400	84	2	8
Pretzel, Garlic	1 pretzel	350	5	3	990	65	2	8
Pretzel, Jalapeño	1 pretzel	330	5	3	1060	63	2	8
Pretzel, Original	1 pretzel	340	5	3	990	65	2	8
Pretzel, Original, No Butter or Salt	1 pretzel	310	1	0	400	65	2	8
Pretzel, Pepperoni	1 pretzel	480	16	8	860	65	2	15
Pretzel, Raisin	1 pretzel	360	5	3	390	69	2	8
Pretzel Dog	1 item	360	20	9	740	33	1	11
Pretzel Dog, Jumbo	1 item	610	29	13	1150	67	2	19
Pretzel Pocket, Bacon, Egg & Cheese	1 item	580	23	10	790	71	2	23
Pretzel Pocket, Pepperoni	1 pretzel	650	27	12	1120	75	2	11
Pretzel Pocket, Turkey & Cheddar	1 item	470	10	5	1050	73	2	20
Pretzel Stix, Cinnamon Sugar	6 sticks	470	12	7	400	84	2	8
Pretzel Stix, Original	6 sticks	340	5	3	990	65	2	8
Back Yard Burgers								
BURGERS & CHICKEN SANDWICHES								
American Cheeseburger, 1/3 lb	1 burger	730	44	16	1300	47	3	39
Bacon Cheddar Burger	1 burger	850	54	22	1420	48	3	46
Black Jack Cheeseburger	1 burger	780	49	17	1340	48	4	40
Blackened Chicken	1 sandwich	540	24	4	1810	53	4	32
Burger, 2/3 lb	1 burger	1070	70	26	1130	47	3	64
Crispy Chicken	1 sandwich	590	26	5	1360	65	4	25
Grilled Chicken	1 sandwich	350	5	0.5	1280	47	3	31
Pepper Jack Cheeseburger, 1/3 lb	1 burger	740	45	17	1370	47	3	39
SIDES								
Chili	1 serving	150	9	3	690	8	1	8

restaurants

	SERVING SIZE	CALORIES	TOTAL FAT (G)	SAT FAT (G)	SODIUM (MG)	CARBS (G)	FIBER (G)	PROTEIN (G)
Seasoned Fries, Regular	as served	640	45	7	1160	58	6	6

Baja Fresh
BAJA FAVORITES

Carnitas Fajita, w/Flour Tortillas	as served	1190	43	14	3450	150	26	58
Charbroiled Steak Nachos	as served	2120	118	44	2990	163	31	96
Cheese Nachos	as served	1890	108	40	2530	163	31	63
Chicken Fajita, w/Flour Tortillas	as served	1140	33	10	3240	147	27	69
Chicken Taquitos, w/Beans	as served	780	40	12	1810	68	17	39
Mahi Mahi Fajita, w/Flour Tortillas	as served	1120	32	10	2800	147	25	64
Quesadillas, Average of All Flavors	as served	1318	82	38.4	2474	87	9	63
Steak Fajita, w/Flour Tortillas	as served	1240	45	15	3440	149	25	65
Torta, w/Chips	as served	880	35	9	1580	96	9	54

BURRITOS

Baja Chicken	as served	790	38	15	2140	65	8	52
Baja Shrimp	as served	760	37	15	2230	66	7	47
Baja Steak	as served	850	46	18	2260	67	7	49
Bare Veggie & Cheese	as served	580	10	4	1950	101	20	19
Bean & Cheese	as served	840	33	17	1790	96	20	39
Diablo Shrimp Burrito	as served	1000	34	12	2930	130	19	56
Grilled Veggie	as served	800	33	17	1880	94	16	32
Mexicano Chicken	as served	790	13	3.5	2270	117	20	50
Mexicano Steak	as served	860	21	7.0	2400	118	18	47
Nacho Burrito	as served	1250	42	17	3200	145	23	75
Salad Burritos, Average of All Flavors	as served	960	51	20	1850	78	10	49
Ultimo Chicken	as served	880	36	18	2190	84	9	54
Ultimo Shrimp	as served	860	36	18	2280	85	8	48

SALADS, W/O DRESSING

Baja Ensalada, w/Charbroiled Chicken	1 salad	310	7	2	1210	18	7	46
Mango Chipotle Chicken Salad	1 salad	930	52	33	1960	67	10	42
Tostada Salad, w/Charbroiled Chicken	1 salad	1140	55	14	2370	98	27	60

SIDES

Chips & Guacamole	as served	1340	83	8	950	141	20	21
Chips & Salsa Baja	as served	810	37	4	1140	98	14	13

TACOS

Americano Soft Tacos, Average of All Flavors	as served	243	11	5	628	21	2	15
Baja Breaded Fish, Fried	as served	250	13	2	420	27	2	8

	SERVING SIZE	CALORIES	TOTAL FAT (G)	SAT FAT (G)	SODIUM (MG)	CARBS (G)	FIBER (G)	PROTEIN (G)
Baja Tacos, Average of All Flavors	as served	215	6	1.5	263	28	2	11
Grilled Mahi Mahi	as served	230	9	1.5	300	26	4	12

Baskin Robbins
FLOATS, FREEZES & SHAKES, MEDIUM

	SERVING SIZE	CALORIES	TOTAL FAT (G)	SAT FAT (G)	SODIUM (MG)	CARBS (G)	FIBER (G)	PROTEIN (G)
Chocolate Shake w/Vanilla Ice Cream	24 fl oz	990	44	28	270	131	0	19
Freeze, w/Orange Sherbet	1 item	510	5	3.5	160	112	1	3
Ice Cream Float, w/Vanilla Ice Cream & Root Beer	1 item	680	30	19	190	99	0	8
Ice Cream Soda, w/Vanilla Ice Cream	1 item	720	30	19	190	103	0	8
Strawberry Shake, w/Very Berry Strawberry Ice Cream	24 fl oz	770	31	20	290	105	1	17
Vanilla Shake	24 fl oz	980	45	28	640	125	0	19
FRUIT BLASTS & SMOOTHIES, MEDIUM								
Fruit Blast, Peach Passion	24 fl oz	370	1	0	10	94	3	2
Fruit Blast, Wild Mango	24 fl oz	470	2	0	15	116	2	1
Smoothie, Mango	24 fl oz	620	2	0	120	148	3	7
Smoothie, Strawberry Banana	24 fl oz	560	1	0	110	135	5	8
ICE CREAM, BRIGHT CHOICES								
Chocolate Covered Bananas Ice Cream, Reduced-Fat, No Sugar Added	4 oz scoop	170	6	3.5	95	33	4	5
Chocolate Éclair Frozen Yogurt	4 oz scoop	240	8	4.5	105	40	1	5
Key Lime Pie Ice Cream, Reduced-Fat, No Sugar Added	4 oz scoop	210	8	4	110	37	3	5
Thin Mint Ice Cream, Reduced-Fat, No Sugar Added	4 oz scoop	180	9	6	80	31	4	6
Tin Roof Sundae, Reduced-Fat, No Sugar Added	4 oz scoop	190	7	4.5	100	34	4	5
Vanilla Frozen Yogurt, Fat-Free	4 oz scoop	150	0	0	105	32	0	6
ICE CREAM, CLASSIC FLAVORS								
Chocolate Chip Cookie Dough	4 oz scoop	300	15	10	135	36	0	5
Mint Chocolate Chip	4 oz scoop	260	16	10	90	28	1	5
Reese's Peanut Butter Cup	4 oz scoop	300	17	9	140	32	1	6
Vanilla	4 oz scoop	260	16	10	70	27	0	4
Very Berry Strawberry	4 oz scoop	220	11	7	70	27	0	4
World Class Chocolate	4 oz scoop	280	16	11	95	31	1	5
ICE CREAM, SOFT SERVE								
Oreo 31° Below Mix-In, Medium	16 oz	750	28	15	580	110	3	19

	SERVING SIZE	CALORIES	TOTAL FAT (G)	SAT FAT (G)	SODIUM (MG)	CARBS (G)	FIBER (G)	PROTEIN (G)
Reese's Peanut Butter Cup 31° Below, Medium	16 oz	880	40	20	560	115	4	25
Soft Serve Parfaits, Average of All Flavors	15 oz	786	35	17	454	105	4	19
Vanilla Soft Serve, Regular	6 oz	250	9	6	150	37	1	8
SUNDAES								
Classic Banana Split	1 dish	1010	34	20	240	173	8	12
Two-Scoop Sundae	1 dish	530	29	19	200	61	0	8

Bertucci's
BRICK OVEN PIZZA, INDIVIDUAL

	SERVING SIZE	CALORIES	TOTAL FAT (G)	SAT FAT (G)	SODIUM (MG)	CARBS (G)	FIBER (G)	PROTEIN (G)
Margherita	1 pizza	980	43	16	1040	115	6	35
Nolio	1 pizza	900	34	14	1590	119	5	28
Pucillo	1 pizza	1210	58	18	2080	131	8	42
Sofia	1 pizza	1160	61	19	1680	112	6	40
The Bertucci	1 pizza	1160	57	20	2230	119	6	42
Ultimate	1 pizza	1300	64	21	3140	123	7	60
BRICK OVEN PIZZA, LARGE								
Nolio	1 slice	250	8	3.5	390	36	1	8
Pizza Verde	1 slice	340	17	6	270	34	1	11
Plain Cheese	1 slice	290	11	4	440	36	2	10
Pucillo	1 slice	360	16	5	570	40	2	13
Silano	1 slice	350	15	5	730	40	3	16
Stella	1 slice	290	11	3.5	420	38	2	10
The Bertucci	1 slice	330	15	5	560	36	2	12
Ultimate	1 slice	380	18	6	840	37	2	17
ENTRÉE SALADS								
Chopped, w/Grilled Steak, w/o Dressing	1 salad	640	37	16	550	19	6	59
Giardino, Full, w/Grilled Chicken	1 salad	320	12	6	370	22	6	32
Tomato Mozzarella Caprese	1 salad	280	20	13	80	10	4	19
Tomato Mozzarella Caprese, w/Grilled Chicken	1 salad	450	28	17	180	11	4	44
Venetian Spinach, w/Grilled Salmon	1 salad	650	37	13	300	29	8	51
ENTRÉES								
Cheese Calzone	1 calzone	680	28	13	1040	80	4	27
Chicken Marsala, w/Mushrooms	1 entrée	670	33	14	1290	43	6	53
Chicken Parma	1 entrée	1180	47	18	1850	110	8	83
Chicken Piccata	1 entrée	1100	47	16	1700	106	6	65

	SERVING SIZE	CALORIES	TOTAL FAT (G)	SAT FAT (G)	SODIUM (MG)	CARBS (G)	FIBER (G)	PROTEIN (G)
Eggplant Parma, w/Pasta	1 entrée	1000	50	14	2000	110	15	36
Fettucine Alfredo, w/Chicken & Asparagus	1 entrée	1200	51	27	1580	140	8	58
Filet Mignon, w/Chianti Sauce	1 entrée	770	47	27	860	35	1	54
Four Cheese Ravioli	1 entrée	950	29	16	2110	117	7	54
Grilled Salmon Fillet	1 entrée	910	60	27	640	40	4	52
Grilled Steak & Chicken Combo	1 entrée	1200	78	41	1080	38	3	87
Lasagna Rustica	1 entrée	1310	65	29	2960	120	7	64
Lobster Ravioli	1 entrée	640	29	14	1730	64	3	28
Merluzzo di Mare	1 entrée	670	25	3.5	1350	25	3	80
Rigatoni Broccoli & Shrimp, w/Cream Sauce	1 entrée	970	31	16	1290	117	10	59
Salmon Florentine	1 entrée	560	35	8	890	11	2	49
Spaghetti Bolognese	1 entrée	1320	51	20	1900	178	7	50
Spaghetti, w/Meatballs & Bolognese Sauce	1 entrée	1880	91	36	3740	198	11	86
Taste of Bertucci's	1 entrée	1740	85	32	2790	188	13	70
Tuscan Vegetable Torta	1 entrée	730	34	6	740	90	9	16
SOUPS								
Sausage	1 bowl	230	12	4.5	1220	20	1	9
Shrimp & Corn Chowder	1 bowl	360	23	12	890	31	2	9
Tuscan Minestrone	1 bowl	220	6	3	1330	28	3	12

Big Apple Bagels & My Favorite Muffins

BAGELS

	SERVING SIZE	CALORIES	TOTAL FAT (G)	SAT FAT (G)	SODIUM (MG)	CARBS (G)	FIBER (G)	PROTEIN (G)
Blueberry	1/2 bagel	165	1	0	241	34	2	6
Cheddar Herb	1/2 bagel	176	3	2	302	30	1	7
Chocolate Chip	1/2 bagel	174	1	1	236	34	2	6
Cinnamon Raisin	1/2 bagel	168	1	0	232	35	2	6
Egg	1/2 bagel	164	1	0	246	33	1	6
Everything	1/2 bagel	168	1	0	389	34	2	6
French Toast	1/2 bagel	186	2	0	232	37	1	6
Plain	1/2 bagel	167	1	0	251	34	2	6
Wheat	1/2 bagel	165	1	0	238	34	2	6
BREAKFAST SANDWICHES								
Lox & Cream Cheese	1 sandwich	602	21	14	1456	78	4	29
Morning Classic	1 sandwich	486	11	5	861	73	3	23

restaurants	SERVING SIZE	CALORIES	TOTAL FAT (G)	SAT FAT (G)	SODIUM (MG)	CARBS (G)	FIBER (G)	PROTEIN (G)
Southern Tradition, w/Ham	1 sandwich	547	15	6	1362	73	3	29
MUFFINS, JUMBO								
Banana Nut	1/3 muffin	195	11	2	121	21	1	4
Blueberry, Fat-Free	1/3 muffin	108	0	0	192	26	1	2
Chocolate Chip	1/3 muffin	211	11	3	142	27	1	3
Cinnamon Crumb Cake	1/3 muffin	212	13	5	135	21	0	3
Lemon Poppyseed	1/3 muffin	201	10	3	161	25	0	3
Pumpkin Spice	1/3 muffin	181	8	3	128	26	0	2
SANDWICHES								
Gourmet, Classic Turkey	1 sandwich	552	14	2	1450	74	4	41
Overstuffed, Classic Rueben	1 sandwich	962	43	17	3017	57	4	60
Overstuffed, Ham & Cheese	1 sandwich	889	36	16	2893	79	4	40
Specialty, Big Apple Club	1 sandwich	797	37	13	2438	75	4	32
Specialty, Roma Italian	1 sandwich	764	34	14	2393	76	4	51
Toasted, Cafe Chicken Melt	1 sandwich	815	32	14	1767	80	4	60
Toasted, Tuna Melt	1 sandwich	641	23	8	1310	75	4	32

Biggby Coffee
DRINKS, W/2% MILK & WHIPPED CREAM

	SERVING SIZE	CALORIES	TOTAL FAT (G)	SAT FAT (G)	SODIUM (MG)	CARBS (G)	FIBER (G)	PROTEIN (G)
Butter Bear	16 fl oz	395	14	8.8	217	57	0	11
Café Au Lait	16 fl oz	180	10	6.5	91	13	0	8
Caramel Marvel	16 fl oz	388	14	9.1	236	55	0	50
Chai Creme Freeze	16 fl oz	550	17	11.6	102	93	0	5
Chai Latte	16 fl oz	396	14	8.5	176	55	0	14
Double Chocolate Creme Freeze	16 fl oz	565	18	11.6	144	93	2	5
Frozen Caramel Marvel	16 fl oz	480	16	11	125	80	0	3
Frozen Hot Chocolate	16 fl oz	565	18	11.6	144	93	2	5
Frozen Latte	16 fl oz	440	14	10	75	76	0	3
Frozen Mocha Mocha	16 fl oz	470	16	10.5	85	78	1	2
Frozen White Lightning	16 fl oz	480	15	10.5	130	81	0	3
Frozen Wild Zebra	16 fl oz	475	15	10.5	108	79	1	3
Iced Chai Latte	16 fl oz	423	16	10.4	155	55	0	12
Iced Hazelnut Mocha	16 fl oz	415	16	9.6	159	55	1	9
Iced Vanilla Bean	16 fl oz	347	16	10.1	131	38	0	11
Mint Mocha	16 fl oz	381	13	7.5	174	54	1	11
Mocha Mocha	16 fl oz	373	14	7.6	184	52	2	11
Nutty Buddy	16 fl oz	314	13	8.1	151	36	0	12

	SERVING SIZE	CALORIES	TOTAL FAT (G)	SAT FAT (G)	SODIUM (MG)	CARBS (G)	FIBER (G)	PROTEIN (G)
Orange Creme Freeze	16 fl oz	502	15	10.5	54	86	0	2
Vanilla Bean	16 fl oz	320	13	8.1	151	38	0	12
Vanilla Creme Freeze	16 fl oz	565	17	11.6	91	96	0	5
REDUCED-CALORIE DRINKS, W/O WHIPPED CREAM								
Banana Berry Creme Freeze	16 fl oz	285	3	2.2	31	67	3	2
Banana Creme Freeze	16 fl oz	274	3	2.2	30	64	3	2
Cocoa Carmella	16 fl oz	206	1	0.4	263	38	1	13
Dark Hot Chocolate	16 fl oz	217	0	0	319	39	2	14
Iced Chai Latte	16 fl oz	173	1	0	150	33	0	12
Iced Mocha Mocha	16 fl oz	190	1	0	282	36	2	11
Iced Vanilla Bean	16 fl oz	95	1	0	131	16	0	11

Blimpie
BURGERS & SANDWICHES

	SERVING SIZE	CALORIES	TOTAL FAT (G)	SAT FAT (G)	SODIUM (MG)	CARBS (G)	FIBER (G)	PROTEIN (G)
Blimpie Burger	1 burger	460	24	10	1280	42	1	21
Blimpie Dog	1 hot dog	510	29	12	1420	45	1	17
Grilled Chicken Caesar, on Ciabatta	1 sandwich	580	20	5	1480	62	3	34
Mediterranean, on Ciabatta	1 sandwich	450	8	2.5	1720	65	3	26
SALADS, W/O DRESSING								
Buffalo Chicken	1 salad	220	9	5	840	10	4	25
Tuna	1 salad	270	19	2.5	370	6	3	18
Ultimate Club	1 salad	270	14	7	1070	11	4	24
SANDWICHES, 12"								
Blimpie Best, Super Stacked	1 sandwich	1100	45	16	4180	104	6	71
BLT, Super Stacked	1 sandwich	1080	60	15	2840	86	5	44
Chicken Cheddar Bacon Ranch	1 sandwich	1200	59	19	3240	91	6	77
Club	1 sandwich	820	27	8	2110	97	6	47
Ham & Swiss	1 sandwich	820	28	10	2040	94	6	47
Hot Pastrami	1 sandwich	860	33	15	2790	81	3	61
Meatball	1 sandwich	1120	58	26	3640	94	7	57
Philly Steak & Onion	1 sandwich	1190	70	24	2860	89	3	53
Reuben	1 sandwich	1060	40	12	3480	105	6	67
Roast Beef & Provolone	1 sandwich	860	30	10	2030	88	6	60
Tuna	1 sandwich	920	42	6	1550	82	5	50
Turkey & Bacon Super Stacked	1 sandwich	1240	54	22	5420	99	6	84
Turkey & Cranberry	1 sandwich	700	7	1.5	2440	116	6	40
Veggie Supreme	1 sandwich	1090	56	28	3000	97	7	53

restaurants

	SERVING SIZE	CALORIES	TOTAL FAT (G)	SAT FAT (G)	SODIUM (MG)	CARBS (G)	FIBER (G)	PROTEIN (G)
Bojangles								
BISCUITS								
Bacon, Egg & Cheese	1 biscuit	550	37	21	1280	35	0	20
Country Ham & Egg	1 biscuit	480	29	14	1590	34	0	21
Egg & Cheese	1 biscuit	515	34	19	1100	35	0	17
Sausage	2 biscuits	840	54	24	1780	66	0	22
Sausage & Egg	1 biscuit	545	38	17	1040	34	0	17
Steak	1 biscuit	555	35	15	1270	44	0	16
CHICKEN								
Breast	1 breast	440	26	9	1230	12	0	40
Leg	1 leg	230	15	5	670	9	0	15
Roasted Chicken Bites	1 serving	280	11	3	1300	9	0	36
Supreme	1 piece	90	3	1	220	8	1	8
Thigh	1 thigh	370	26	9	1090	12	1	22
Wing	1 wing	200	13	4.5	580	10	0	10
FIXIN'S, INDIVIDUAL								
Bojangles' Dirty Rice	as served	165	6	1	551	24	0	4
Macaroni 'N Cheese	as served	240	7	3	660	33	1	11
Mashed Potatoes 'N Gravy	as served	150	6	1	614	21	0	3
Seasoned Fries	as served	215	14	3	741	20	2	2
SALADS								
Chicken Supremes	1 salad	460	18	8	850	33	4	42
Grilled Chicken	1 salad	305	11	6	4	11	3	40
SANDWICHES								
Cajun Filet	1 sandwich	495	27	5	680	43	3	20
Grilled Chicken	1 sandwich	375	15	2	910	33	3	27
Grilled Chicken Club	1 sandwich	520	27	10	1390	34	3	35
Boston Market								
GOURMET SIDES								
Cinnamon Apples	as served	210	3	0	15	47	3	0
Cornbread	as served	180	5	2	270	30	1	3
Creamed Spinach	as served	280	23	15	580	12	4	9
Loaded Mashed Potatoes	as served	300	15	8	800	30	3	9
Macaroni & Cheese	as served	300	11	7	1100	35	2	11
Sweet Potato Casserole	as served	460	16	4.5	270	77	3	4
INDIVIDUAL MEALS								
Beef Brisket, Regular	1 entrée	230	13	3.5	570	0	0	28

	SERVING SIZE	CALORIES	TOTAL FAT (G)	SAT FAT (G)	SODIUM (MG)	CARBS (G)	FIBER (G)	PROTEIN (G)
Meatloaf, Regular	1 entrée	480	30	13	1090	25	6	28
Pastry Top Chicken Pot Pie	1 entrée	800	48	24	1120	60	4	32
Pastry Top Turkey Pot Pie	1 entrée	790	46	23	1220	60	4	34
Turkey Breast, Regular	1 entrée	180	3	1	620	0	0	38
ROTISSERIE CHICKEN								
Half Chicken	as served	640	33	10	1380	2	0	84
Quarter White, w/Skin	as served	320	13	4	710	1	0	51
Three Piece Dark, w/Skin, 2 Thighs & 1 Drumstick	as served	540	36	11	1080	1	0	53
SALADS								
Caesar, w/Chicken	1 salad	660	43	11	1590	31	3	39
Caesar, w/o Chicken	1 salad	560	42	10	1340	31	3	16
Mediterranean	1 salad	640	44	10	1190	27	3	36
Southwest Santa Fe	1 salad	740	46	10	1250	50	5	36
SANDWICHES								
All White Rotisserie Chicken Salad	1 sandwich	1050	64	10	1700	87	11	39
Brisket Dip Carver	1 sandwich	840	45	12	1660	62	3	46
Homestyle Meatloaf Carver	1 sandwich	940	40	18	2430	96	10	46
Pulled BBQ Rotisserie Chicken	1 sandwich	690	17	6	1880	93	5	41
Rotisserie Chicken Carver	1 sandwich	770	36	9	1760	66	3	45

Bruegger's
BAGELS & BREADS

	SERVING SIZE	CALORIES	TOTAL FAT (G)	SAT FAT (G)	SODIUM (MG)	CARBS (G)	FIBER (G)	PROTEIN (G)
Bagel Bowl	1 item	720	9	3	152	136	8	30
Ciabatta	1 roll	250	0	0.0	560	54	2	8
Everything	1 bagel	310	3	0	710	62	4	12
Fortified Multi-Grain	1 bagel	340	3	0	500	66	6	12
Jalapeno Cheddar	1 bagel	450	9	3.5	650	75	10	20
Plain	1 bagel	300	2	0	530	60	4	12
Whole Wheat	1 bagel	310	4	0.0	560	61	7	13
BREAKFAST SANDWICHES								
Breakfast Bagel, Egg & Cheese	1 sandwich	430	18	6.0	970	63	4	22
Breakfast Bagel, Egg, Cheese & Sausage	1 sandwich	650	38	14.0	1280	64	4	30
Breakfast Bagel, Egg White on Sundried Tomato	1 sandwich	480	13	5.0	870	66	4	22
Classic Wrap, w/Bacon	1 wrap	770	50	18.0	1670	39	3	38
Classic Wrap, w/Sausage	1 wrap	730	47	18.0	1240	37	3	32
Smoked Salmon on Plain Bagel	1 sandwich	460	10	4.5	1520	66	4	26

restaurants

	SERVING SIZE	CALORIES	TOTAL FAT (G)	SAT FAT (G)	SODIUM (MG)	CARBS (G)	FIBER (G)	PROTEIN (G)
HOT PANINI								
Ham & Cheddar, on Honey Wheat	1 sandwich	600	17	8	1930	72	2	36
Primo Pesto Chicken, on Hearty White	1 sandwich	630	24	9	1860	57	0	49
Tuna & Cheddar Melt, on Honey Wheat	1 sandwich	800	44	11	1260	60	2	38
SANDWICHES								
Garden Veggie, on Wheat Bread	1 sandwich	360	3	0	540	67	4	13
Ham, on Honey Wheat	1 sandwich	540	16	6	2430	64	2	38
Leonardo da Veggie, on Plain Softwich	1 sandwich	560	15	8	1170	76	4	25
Roma Roast Beef, on Hearty White	1 sandwich	750	39	14	1820	63	0	51
Turkey, on Honey Wheat	1 sandwich	550	16	7	1990	60	2	39
SOFTWICHES								
Everything	1 item	350	2	0	740	64	4	12
Plain	1 item	330	3	0	640	67	4	12
Sesame	1 item	370	4	0	690	70	4	14
SOUPS & SALADS, W/O DRESSING								
Beef Chili	1 cup	190	8	3	880	18	6	10
Chicken Caesar	1 salad	260	11	4	840	12	2	26
Classic Cobb	1 salad	300	17	8	1210	7	2	25
Garden Salad, Café	1 salad	80	2	0	90	9	2	2
Mandarin Medley	1 salad	340	16	5	800	16	5	28

Buffalo Wild Wings

BURGERS, SERVED W/FRIES								
Big Jack Daddy	1 entrée	1680	98	38	3820	136	9	61
Black & Bleu	1 entrée	1340	88	31	2820	89	8	45
Cheeseburger, Cheddar Cheese	1 entrée	1330	82	33	3590	95	8	49
Honey BBQ Bacon	1 entrée	1430	86	34	3680	105	7	55
Screamin' Nacho	1 entrée	1390	93	33	2900	92	6	44
ENTRÉES								
Popcorn Shrimp, Tartar Sauce & Fries	1 entrée	970	60	19	2930	83	5	16
Ribs, 1/2 lb, Average of All Sauces	1 entrée	990	61	23	2470	50	0	54
Ribs & More Ribs, Average of All Sauces	1 entrée	2510	160	56	5400	143	6	112
Ribs & Traditional Wings, Average of All Sauces	1 entrée	2540	187	60	5620	111	6	87
Wings, Boneless & Traditional, Average of All Sauces	1 entrée	2150	164	50	5920	97	8	55
SANDWICHES & WRAPS								
Sandwich, Jerk Chicken & Fries	1 sandwich	1410	50	14	4250	105	9	41

	SERVING SIZE	CALORIES	TOTAL FAT (G)	SAT FAT (G)	SODIUM (MG)	CARBS (G)	FIBER (G)	PROTEIN (G)
Wrap, Buffalitos, Grilled Chicken, Average of All Sauces	1 wrap	980	41	19	4130	106	5	43
Wrap, Pepper Jack Steak	1 wrap	1360	77	24	4160	113	7	51
SIDES								
Buffalo Chips, w/Shredded Cheese	1 basket	1150	70	32	1280	98	10	31
French Fries	1 basket	840	50	18	1750	85	8	8
Onion Rings	1 basket	1820	130	33	3100	144	16	10
Potato Wedges, w/Shredded Cheese	1 basket	720	52	22	1670	50	6	18
STARTERS								
Jalapeno Pepper Bites	as served	680	45	12	2490	52	5	18
Naked Tenders (6), w/Fries, Average of All Sauces	as served	790	30	11	4610	61	4	60
Roasted Garlic Mushrooms	as served	640	48	11	1600	44	2	6
Slammers, Cheeseburger, w/Fries	as served	1580	97	40	2340	112	7	64
Slammers, Pulled Pork, w/Fries, Average of All Sauces	as served	1410	74	25	4240	135	8	43
The Sampler, Average of All Sauces	as served	2810	193	60	7180	194	14	62

Burger King
BK SALAD COLLECTION

	SERVING SIZE	CALORIES	TOTAL FAT (G)	SAT FAT (G)	SODIUM (MG)	CARBS (G)	FIBER (G)	PROTEIN (G)
Chicken Garden, Tendercrisp	1 salad	470	26	8	1170	26	2	31
Chicken Garden, Tendergrill	1 salad	290	12	6	1030	8	1	38
Garden, No Chicken	1 salad	130	8	5	200	6	1	8
BREAKFAST								
Biscuit, Bacon, Egg & Cheese	1 sandwich	470	28	17	1420	33	1	17
Biscuit, Sausage, Egg & Cheese	1 sandwich	570	37	19	1510	34	1	20
BK Wrapper, Cheesy Bacon	1 wrap	410	25	8	980	28	2	14
Breakfast Platter	1 platter	810	54	22	1790	57	4	25
Croissan'wich, Bacon, Egg & Cheese	1 sandwich	380	22	8	890	26	0	15
Croissan'wich, Sausage, Egg & Cheese	1 sandwich	490	31	11	990	27	0	18
Egg & Cheese Muffin	1 item	290	14	5	650	24	1	11
French Toast Sticks	3 pieces	230	11	2	260	29	1	3
Hash Browns, Medium	as served	500	33	7	810	48	7	4
Pancake Platter, w/Sausage, w/1 oz Breakfast Syrup	1 platter	670	34	9	1010	78	1	14
BURGERS & SANDWICHES								
Bacon Cheeseburger	1 burger	330	16	7	830	32	1	18
Big Fish Sandwich	1 sandwich	590	31	5	1480	57	3	21

restaurants

	SERVING SIZE	CALORIES	TOTAL FAT (G)	SAT FAT (G)	SODIUM (MG)	CARBS (G)	FIBER (G)	PROTEIN (G)
BK Double Stacker	1 burger	520	33	12	830	32	1	28
BK Single Stacker	1 burger	380	22	8	690	32	1	18
BK Triple Stacker	1 burger	670	44	18	1060	32	1	39
BK Veggie Burger, w/Cheese	1 burger	450	20	5	1250	44	7	24
Cheeseburger	1 burger	300	14	6	710	28	1	16
Double Bacon Cheeseburger	1 burger	520	31	14	1180	33	1	31
Double Cheeseburger	1 burger	450	26	12	960	29	1	26
Hamburger	1 burger	260	10	4	490	28	1	13
Original Chicken Sandwich	1 sandwich	630	39	7	1390	46	3	24
Tendercrisp Chicken Sandwich	1 sandwich	750	45	8	1560	58	3	30
Tendergrill Chicken Sandwich	1 sandwich	470	18	3.5	1330	39	2	37
Spicy Chick'n Crisp Sandwich	1 sandwich	460	30	5	810	34	2	13
Whopper	1 burger	670	40	11	980	51	3	29
Whopper, Junior, w/Cheese	1 burger	380	23	8	730	29	2	16
Whopper, Triple, w/Cheese	1 burger	1230	82	32	1550	53	3	71
Whopper, w/Cheese	1 burger	760	47	16	1410	53	3	33
SIDES								
Chicken Tenders	6 pieces	290	17	3	460	15	1	15
French Fries, Medium	as served	410	18	3	570	58	4	4
Onion Rings, Medium	as served	410	21	3.5	1080	53	4	4
Burgerville								
BEVERAGES, MEDIUM								
Chocolate Smoothie	16 fl oz	450	0	0	260	93	0	12
Northwest Cherry Chocolate Milkshake	16 fl oz	1030	47	29	360	138	3	18
Vanilla Milkshake	16 fl oz	810	33	21	290	117	0	13
BURGERS								
Double Beef, w/Cheese	1 burger	450	27	8	750	30	1	22
Half-Pound Colossal, w/Cheese	1 burger	750	45	15	1020	43	2	42
Original Cheeseburger	1 burger	380	20	3.5	750	30	1	18
Tillamook Cheeseburger	1 burger	640	39	14	900	42	2	30
SALADS & SANDWICHES								
Burgerville Spread, Cup	1 item	300	32	4	380	4	0	0
Halibut Fillet Sandwich	1 sandwich	490	27	2	750	43	2	17
Rogue River Smokey Blue Salad	1 salad	280	10	6	135	39	6	9
Rosemary Chicken Sandwich	1 sandwich	450	18	3.5	1010	44	1	28
Turkey Club	1 sandwich	590	38	11	940	33	2	31
Wild Smoked Salmon & Hazelnut Salad	1 salad	460	30	8	830	17	7	29

California Pizza Kitchen

APPETIZERS & SMALL CRAVINGS

	SERVING SIZE	CALORIES	TOTAL FAT (G)	SAT FAT (G)	SODIUM (MG)	CARBS (G)	FIBER (G)	PROTEIN (G)
Avocado Club Egg Rolls	as served	1224	n/a	22	2079	60	4	50
Crispy Mac 'N' Cheese	as served	401	n/a	12	659	27	1	16
Dynamite Shrimp	as served	547	n/a	5	661	40	2	30
Korean BBQ Steak Tacos	as served	440	n/a	3	369	53	9	20
Lettuce Wraps, w/Chicken	as served	543	n/a	2	1399	54	6	28
Mediterranean Focaccia	as served	656	n/a	6	1033	83	3	18
Mediterranean Plate	as served	368	n/a	4	690	36	3	8
Sesame Ginger Chicken Dumplings	as served	465	n/a	1	1801	63	0	25
Spinach Artichoke Dip	as served	850	n/a	20	1264	85	9	18
Tuscan Hummus	as served	862	n/a	4	1515	124	7	21

ENTRÉES

Chicken Milanese	1 entrée	1034	n/a	17	1341	29	3	58
Chicken Piccata	1 entrée	1247	n/a	24	1753	79	4	70
Norwegian Atlantic Salmon, w/Spaghettini	1 entrée	1261	n/a	26	1202	75	6	67

PASTA ENTRÉES

Asparagus & Spinach Spaghettini	1 entrée	1102	n/a	11	1203	118	9	38
Broccoli Sun-Dried Tomato Fusilli	1 entrée	1074	n/a	10	1147	121	9	37
Four Cheese Ravioli	1 entrée	1035	n/a	41	1475	64	4	33
Garlic Cream Fettuccine	1 entrée	1386	n/a	49	1121	111	5	32
Jambalaya	1 entrée	1235	n/a	16	2123	106	8	61
Pesto Cream Penne, w/Shrimp	1 entrée	1453	n/a	50	1169	92	5	52
Spaghetti Bolognese	1 entrée	929	n/a	8	999	117	5	33
Tomato Basil Spaghettini	1 entrée	1026	n/a	6	1427	123	9	21
Traditional Mac 'N' Cheese	1 entrée	1439	n/a	54	1674	105	4	39

PIZZA

BBQ Chicken, w/Applewood-Smoked Bacon	1 pizza	1162	n/a	19	2986	135	6	60
BLT	1 pizza	1191	n/a	19	2376	121	8	44
California Club	1 pizza	1401	n/a	21	2693	128	13	60
Hawaiian	1 pizza	1016	n/a	14	2558	131	7	44
Margherita, Thin Crust	1 pizza	1038	n/a	22	1952	98	5	47
Pepperoni	1 pizza	1109	n/a	19	2669	124	5	44
Thai Chicken	1 pizza	1223	n/a	14	3005	138	9	55

restaurants	SERVING SIZE	CALORIES	TOTAL FAT (G)	SAT FAT (G)	SODIUM (MG)	CARBS (G)	FIBER (G)	PROTEIN (G)
The Meat Cravers	1 pizza	1490	n/a	31	4163	124	6	70
The Original BBQ Chicken	1 pizza	1055	n/a	16	2561	135	6	53
The Works	1 pizza	1349	n/a	25	3341	130	7	55
Traditional Cheese	1 pizza	1004	n/a	16	2157	124	6	43
White	1 pizza	1080	n/a	20	2447	119	6	47
SALADS, FULL								
Classic Caesar	1 salad	505	n/a	15	687	20	8	15
CPK Cobb, w/Blue Cheese Dressing	1 salad	1007	n/a	21	1758	22	10	51
Field Greens	1 salad	805	n/a	9	593	56	12	10
Moroccan Chicken	1 salad	1370	n/a	12	1040	116	23	43
Original Chopped	1 salad	937	n/a	16	1865	18	6	42
Waldorf Chicken, w/Blue Cheese Dressing	1 salad	1347	n/a	28	1994	71	13	48
SANDWICHES ON HERB ONION FOCACCIA								
California Club, w/Chicken	1 sandwich	892	n/a	8	1645	91	7	35
Grilled Chicken Caesar	1 sandwich	963	n/a	9	1651	91	4	56
Grilled Vegetable	1 sandwich	788	n/a	8	1357	95	6	22

Captain D's
ENTRÉES

	SERVING SIZE	CALORIES	TOTAL FAT (G)	SAT FAT (G)	SODIUM (MG)	CARBS (G)	FIBER (G)	PROTEIN (G)
Batter Dipped Fish	1 piece	182	12	6	454	8	1	9
Bite Size Shrimp	1 entrée	460	21	9	840	51	2	16
Catfish	1 piece	105	6	2	233	6	0	7
Clam Platter, 1/2 pound	1 entrée	770	47	8	1450	64	6	22
Country Style Fish	1 piece	195	10	5	584	14	1	14
Crab Cake	1 piece	174	11	5	467	12	1	7
Oyster Dinner	1 entrée	320	18	8	710	31	1	10
Premium Shrimp	3 shrimp	154	6	3	323	0	0	8
Seasoned Tilapia	1 piece	130	3	2	520	1	0	24
SANDWICHES & SALADS								
Bite Size Shrimp Salad	1 salad	267	10	4	437	33	4	10
Great Little Fish Sandwich	1 sandwich	642	38	15	1456	56	2	17
The Captain	1 sandwich	1008	49	20	1565	28	2	19
Wild Alaskan Salmon Salad	1 salad	177	1	0	427	8	3	35
Wild Alaskan Salmon Sandwich	1 sandwich	520	18	2	980	48	2	42
SIDES & SAUCES								
Fried Okra	as served	230	14	6	410	23	2	3
Hush Puppies	as served	200	13	6	330	18	1	2
Macaroni & Cheese	as served	160	7	2	570	17	0	6

Caribou Coffee

BAKERY

	SERVING SIZE	CALORIES	TOTAL FAT (G)	SAT FAT (G)	SODIUM (MG)	CARBS (G)	FIBER (G)	PROTEIN (G)
Apple Fritter	1 fritter	500	16	7	660	86	11	9
Blueberry Muffin	1 muffin	410	18	3.5	370	55	1	7
Classic Milk Chocolate Chunk Cookie	1 cookie	340	16	8	160	41	1	4
Cinnamon Coffee Cake	1 cake	540	24	6	370	74	0	5
Lemon Poppyseed Bread	1 slice	470	26	5	450	56	1	6
Sandwich, Italian Chicken Melt	1 sandwich	470	21	11	990	41	7	35
Sandwich, Three Cheese Classic	1 sandwich	500	25	14	800	46	1	21
COOLERS, MEDIUM, W/O WHIPPED CREAM								
Caramel Cooler	16 fl oz	400	5	5	95	86	0	3
Coffee Cooler	16 fl oz	320	6	6	105	65	0	3
Espresso Cooler	16 fl oz	270	5	5	95	55	0	3
Mocha Cooler, Milk Chocolate	16 fl oz	550	13	8	180	98	0	10
Vanilla Cooler	16 fl oz	380	5	5	95	83	0	3
Hot Chocolate, Medium, 2% Milk, Milk Chocolate, w/o Whipped Cream	16 fl oz	440	22	14	170	49	1	15
LATTES, MEDIUM, 2% MILK, W/O WHIPPED CREAM								
Iced Latte	16 fl oz	90	4	2	85	8	0	7
Latte	16 fl oz	200	8	5	170	19	0	14
MOCHAS, MEDIUM, 2% MILK, MILK CHOCOLATE, W/O WHIPPED CREAM								
Campfire Mocha	16 fl oz	460	20	13	135	63	1	12
Iced Mocha	16 fl oz	350	11	5	160	51	0	12
Mocha	16 fl oz	390	20	13	135	43	1	12
Turtle Mocha	16 fl oz	480	20	13	135	67	1	12
OATMEAL								
Classic Oatmeal	1 bowl	260	3	0.5	170	47	7	15
Maple Brown Sugar Crunch Blend	1 bowl	320	4	1	200	57	7	15
Very Berry Blend	1 bowl	440	8	0.5	220	78	10	17
SMOOTHIES, MEDIUM, W/O WHIPPED CREAM								
Mango Orange Key Lime	16 fl oz	450	0	0	40	113	0	0
Strawberry Banana	16 fl oz	350	0	0	25	85	0	0
White Peach Berry	16 fl oz	300	0	0	50	75	0	0

restaurants

	SERVING SIZE	CALORIES	TOTAL FAT (G)	SAT FAT (G)	SODIUM (MG)	CARBS (G)	FIBER (G)	PROTEIN (G)
SNOWDRIFTS, MEDIUM, 2% MILK, MILK CHOCOLATE, W/O WHIPPED CREAM								
Cookies & Cream Snowdrift	16 fl oz	630	18	8	320	103	1	15
Mint Snowdrift	16 fl oz	510	13	6	180	84	0	14
SPECIALTY BEVERAGES, MEDIUM, W/O WHIPPED CREAM								
Cappuccino, 2% Milk	16 fl oz	70	3	2	70	6	0	6
Caramel High Rise, 2% Milk	16 fl oz	260	7	4.5	150	39	0	12
Hot Apple Blast	16 fl oz	300	0	0	45	74	0	0
Macchiato, 2% Milk	16 fl oz	20	1	0	30	1	0	3
Mint Condition, 2% Milk, Milk Chocolate	16 fl oz	480	20	13	135	66	1	12

Carinos
APPETIZERS

Baked Stuffed Mushrooms	as served	463	37	23	1095	20	2	13
Bruschetta	as served	1074	63	16	1665	104	7	25
Hand-Breaded Calamari	as served	1233	26	6	5264	176	7	68
Mozzarella w/Marinara	as served	922	53	24	2663	70	3	41
Sicilian Fire Sticks w/Ranch Dressing	as served	1564	94	32	4601	115	13	58
ENTRÉES, DINNER								
Angel Hair w/Artichokes & Chicken	1 entrée	754	15	1	1774	112	11	41
Chicken Penne Gorgonzola	1 entrée	1361	80	43	1812	106	6	52
Chicken Primavera	1 entrée	684	6	1	980	112	9	43
Florentine Pasta w/Chicken	1 entrée	1211	64	33	1660	106	6	48
Grilled Chicken Bowtie Festival	1 entrée	1185	63	31	1444	103	6	47
Lemon Pepper Mahi Mahi w/Angel Hair	1 entrée	859	53	21	1147	38	5	51
Lemon Pepper Salmon	1 entrée	937	70	25	1397	21	5	53
Lobster Ravioli	1 entrée	912	60	34	1905	64	5	26
Shredded Beef Pappardelle	1 entrée	1194	66	32	2938	94	8	46
Shrimp Scampi	1 entrée	1920	136	81	1115	114	7	46
Skilletini Combo	1 entrée	1280	78	16	2103	94	6	50
Spaghetti & Handmade Meatballs	1 entrée	1166	38	12	2609	138	12	56
Spicy Shrimp & Chicken	1 entrée	1259	66	34	1577	106	5	58
Stuffed Vegetable Rigatoni	1 entrée	886	40	19	2708	96	12	32
SALADS								
Chicken, Gorgonzola & Tomato	1 salad	627	36	9	1282	46	6	35
Classic Caesar, Shrimp & Artichokes	1 salad	515	33	8	1280	23	4	33
Pecan Crusted Chicken	1 salad	953	46	15	3216	86	6	44

	SERVING SIZE	CALORIES	TOTAL FAT (G)	SAT FAT (G)	SODIUM (MG)	CARBS (G)	FIBER (G)	PROTEIN (G)

Carl's Jr.

BREAKFAST

Bacon & Egg Burrito	1 burrito	560	32	12	1000	37	1	30
Bacon, Egg & Cheese Biscuit	1 biscuit	460	26	12	1130	37	2	17
French Toast Dips, w/o Syrup	5 pieces	460	21	4	570	60	3	9
Hash Brown Nuggets	as served	350	23	4	440	32	3	3
Loaded Breakfast Burrito	1 burrito	780	48	17	1460	51	3	35
Monster Biscuit	1 biscuit	740	50	21	1750	39	2	32
Sausage, Egg & Cheese Biscuit	1 biscuit	570	37	16	1350	38	2	20
Sourdough Breakfast Sandwich	1 sandwich	450	21	8	1470	38	1	29

BURGERS

Big Hamburger	1 burger	490	18	8	1000	59	3	25
Famous Star, w/Cheese	1 burger	680	39	14	1220	57	3	28
Guacamole Bacon Six Dollar Burger	1 burger	1060	72	24	2290	55	4	49
Low Carb Six Dollar Burger	1 burger	570	43	19	1390	9	1	38
Original Six Dollar Burger	1 burger	910	54	21	2030	63	3	45
Super Star, w/Cheese	1 burger	940	59	24	1560	59	3	48
Teriyaki Turkey Burger	1 burger	470	14	5	1120	55	3	32
Turkey Burger	1 burger	490	23	4.5	960	45	3	29
Western Bacon Cheeseburger	1 burger	740	34	14	1500	74	4	33
Western Bacon Six Dollar Burger	1 burger	1030	55	22	2440	81	4	53

CHICKEN & FISH

Carl's Catch Fish Sandwich	1 sandwich	700	37	6	1300	73	5	21
Charbroiled BBQ Chicken Sandwich	1 sandwich	390	7	1.5	990	50	3	30
Chicken Stars	6 pieces	260	16	3.5	540	18	2	12
Fish & Chips	1 entrée	710	38	6	1410	69	7	22
Honey Mustard HB Chicken Tender Wrapper	1 wrap	320	18	6	760	22	1	16
Spicy Chicken Sandwich	1 sandwich	460	26	5	1370	47	4	14

SALADS, W/O DRESSING

Cranberry Apple Walnut Grilled Chicken	1 salad	320	11	3.5	850	29	5	27
Original Grilled Chicken	1 salad	270	9	3	800	23	4	25

SIDES

CrissCut Fries	as served	450	29	5	900	42	4	5
Fried Zucchini	as served	330	18	3	610	36	2	6
Onion Rings	as served	530	28	4.5	590	61	3	8

restaurants

	SERVING SIZE	CALORIES	TOTAL FAT (G)	SAT FAT (G)	SODIUM (MG)	CARBS (G)	FIBER (G)	PROTEIN (G)
Carvel								
BLENDED DRINKS, SMALL								
Arctic Blender, Cookie Dough	16 fl oz	920	40	22	460	126	1	15
Arctic Blender, Fried Ice Cream	16 fl oz	670	31	18	330	85	2	13
Arctic Blender, Peanut Butter	16 fl oz	870	33	17	510	88	3	18
Carvelanche, Butterfinger	16 fl oz	850	45	28	400	104	1	11
Carvelanche, Cake Mix	16 fl oz	770	31	20	500	110	0	10
Carvelanche, Cookies & Cream	16 fl oz	860	45	26	550	103	2	11
Carvelanche, M&M'S	16 fl oz	890	49	32	280	100	0	11
Carvelanche, Reese's	16 fl oz	870	46	33	380	97	0	16
Carvelatte, Caramel Macchiato	16 fl oz	680	27	17	420	97	0	11
Carvelatte, Coffee	16 fl oz	670	32	20	340	84	0	14
Carvelatte, Mocha	16 fl oz	610	25	15	280	88	1	10
Float, Chocolate Ice Cream & Coke	16 fl oz	360	14	8	150	54	1	6
Float, Vanilla Ice Cream & Coke	16 fl oz	380	17	11	150	53	0	4
Iceberg, Barq's Root Beer	16 fl oz	550	27	18	290	67	0	10
Iceberg, Coke	16 fl oz	550	27	18	280	65	0	10
Iceberg, Fanta Orange	16 fl oz	550	27	18	280	65	0	10
Mint Chocolate Chip	16 fl oz	1230	64	36	480	157	8	14
Thick Chocolate Shake	16 fl oz	650	27	16	320	93	2	14
Thick Strawberry Shake	16 fl oz	600	31	20	280	70	1	11
Thick Vanilla Shake	16 fl oz	660	31	20	280	86	0	11
CLASSIC SUNDAES, SMALL								
Banana Barge	1 sundae	970	46	24	290	128	7	19
Caramel	1 sundae	700	36	25	370	84	0	8
Hot Fudge	1 sundae	540	30	22	220	60	2	7
DASHERS, SMALL								
Bananas Foster	12 fl oz	660	23	15	420	105	2	6
Fudge Brownie	12 fl oz	850	45	21	420	102	4	10
Peanut Butter Cup	12 fl oz	1060	60	20	670	95	7	22
The Cheesecake Factory								
APPETIZERS								
Ahi Carpaccio	as served	250	n/a	n/a	n/a	n/a	n/a	n/a
BLT Salad	as served	1400	n/a	n/a	n/a	n/a	n/a	n/a
Buffalo Wings	as served	1760	n/a	n/a	n/a	n/a	n/a	n/a
Chicken Pot Stickers	as served	460	n/a	n/a	n/a	n/a	n/a	n/a

	SERVING SIZE	CALORIES	TOTAL FAT (G)	SAT FAT (G)	SODIUM (MG)	CARBS (G)	FIBER (G)	PROTEIN (G)
Factory Nachos	as served	1530	n/a	n/a	n/a	n/a	n/a	n/a
French Country Salad	as served	510	n/a	n/a	n/a	n/a	n/a	n/a
Hot Spinach & Cheese Dip	as served	1270	n/a	n/a	n/a	n/a	n/a	n/a
Popcorn Shrimp	as served	630	n/a	n/a	n/a	n/a	n/a	n/a
Quesadilla w/Chicken	as served	1270	n/a	n/a	n/a	n/a	n/a	n/a
Southern Fried Chicken Sliders	as served	1420	n/a	n/a	n/a	n/a	n/a	n/a
BEVERAGES								
Chocolate, Vanilla, or Strawberry Milkshake	as served	1200	n/a	n/a	n/a	n/a	n/a	n/a
Frozen Iced Berry	as served	240	n/a	n/a	n/a	n/a	n/a	n/a
Oreo Milkshake	as served	1390	n/a	n/a	n/a	n/a	n/a	n/a
Strawberry Cheesecake Milkshake	as served	1360	n/a	n/a	n/a	n/a	n/a	n/a
Strawberry Fruit Smoothie	as served	340	n/a	n/a	n/a	n/a	n/a	n/a
Tropical Smoothie	as served	340	n/a	n/a	n/a	n/a	n/a	n/a
CHEESECAKES								
Brownie Sundae	1 slice	1480	n/a	n/a	n/a	n/a	n/a	n/a
Chocolate Chip Cookie Dough	1 slice	1210	n/a	n/a	n/a	n/a	n/a	n/a
Chocolate Mousse	1 slice	960	n/a	n/a	n/a	n/a	n/a	n/a
Chocolate Raspberry Truffle	1 slice	1070	n/a	n/a	n/a	n/a	n/a	n/a
Dulce de Leche Caramel	1 slice	1120	n/a	n/a	n/a	n/a	n/a	n/a
Fresh Strawberry	1 slice	750	n/a	n/a	n/a	n/a	n/a	n/a
Godiva Chocolate	1 slice	1040	n/a	n/a	n/a	n/a	n/a	n/a
Hershey's Chocolate Bar	1 slice	1310	n/a	n/a	n/a	n/a	n/a	n/a
Key Lime	1 slice	880	n/a	n/a	n/a	n/a	n/a	n/a
Lemon Raspberry	1 slice	840	n/a	n/a	n/a	n/a	n/a	n/a
Low Carb	1 slice	540	n/a	n/a	n/a	n/a	n/a	n/a
Original	1 slice	710	n/a	n/a	n/a	n/a	n/a	n/a
Reese's Peanut Butter Chocolate Cake	1 slice	1560	n/a	n/a	n/a	n/a	n/a	n/a
Tiramisu	1 slice	800	n/a	n/a	n/a	n/a	n/a	n/a
Ultimate Red Velvet Cake	1 slice	1570	n/a	n/a	n/a	n/a	n/a	n/a
EGGS & OMELETTES								
Brioche Breakfast Sandwich	1 entrée	1790	n/a	n/a	n/a	n/a	n/a	n/a
California Omelette	1 omelette	2080	n/a	n/a	n/a	n/a	n/a	n/a
Energy Breakfast	1 entrée	720	n/a	n/a	n/a	n/a	n/a	n/a
Mini Egg Breakfast	1 entrée	1140	n/a	n/a	n/a	n/a	n/a	n/a
Morning Quesadilla	1 entrée	2120	n/a	n/a	n/a	n/a	n/a	n/a

	SERVING SIZE	CALORIES	TOTAL FAT (G)	SAT FAT (G)	SODIUM (MG)	CARBS (G)	FIBER (G)	PROTEIN (G)
FACTORY COMBINATIONS, W/MASHED POTATOES								
Chicken Madeira & Steak Diane	1 entrée	2170	n/a	n/a	n/a	n/a	n/a	n/a
Herb-Crusted Salmon & Shrimp Scampi	1 entrée	2020	n/a	n/a	n/a	n/a	n/a	n/a
Shrimp Scampi & Steak Diane	1 entrée	2230	n/a	n/a	n/a	n/a	n/a	n/a
FISH & SEAFOOD, W/SIDES								
Bar-B-Que Salmon	1 entrée	1220	n/a	n/a	n/a	n/a	n/a	n/a
Fried Shrimp Platter	1 entrée	1410	n/a	n/a	n/a	n/a	n/a	n/a
Miso Salmon	1 entrée	1770	n/a	n/a	n/a	n/a	n/a	n/a
New Orleans Shrimp	1 entrée	1030	n/a	n/a	n/a	n/a	n/a	n/a
GLAMBURGERS & SANDWICHES, W/FRENCH FRIES								
BBQ Pulled Pork	1 entrée	1770	n/a	n/a	n/a	n/a	n/a	n/a
Chicken Parmesan Sandwich	1 entrée	2150	n/a	n/a	n/a	n/a	n/a	n/a
Farmhouse Cheeseburger	1 entrée	1860	n/a	n/a	n/a	n/a	n/a	n/a
Grilled Cheese Sandwich	1 entrée	1640	n/a	n/a	n/a	n/a	n/a	n/a
Grilled Chicken & Bacon Club Sandwich	1 entrée	2220	n/a	n/a	n/a	n/a	n/a	n/a
Kobe Burger	1 entrée	1540	n/a	n/a	n/a	n/a	n/a	n/a
Old Fashioned Burger	1 entrée	1350	n/a	n/a	n/a	n/a	n/a	n/a
Smokehouse BBQ Burger	1 entrée	1760	n/a	n/a	n/a	n/a	n/a	n/a
Spicy Crispy Chicken Sandwich	1 entrée	1670	n/a	n/a	n/a	n/a	n/a	n/a
The Club Sandwich	1 entrée	1690	n/a	n/a	n/a	n/a	n/a	n/a
The Incredible Eggplant Sandwich	1 entrée	1790	n/a	n/a	n/a	n/a	n/a	n/a
Veggie Burger	1 entrée	1630	n/a	n/a	n/a	n/a	n/a	n/a
Wild Mushroom Burger	1 entrée	1850	n/a	n/a	n/a	n/a	n/a	n/a
PASTAS								
Bistro Shrimp	1 entrée	3020	n/a	n/a	n/a	n/a	n/a	n/a
Cajun Jambalaya	1 entrée	1210	n/a	n/a	n/a	n/a	n/a	n/a
Fettuccini Alfredo	1 entrée	2300	n/a	n/a	n/a	n/a	n/a	n/a
Louisiana Chicken	1 entrée	2430	n/a	n/a	n/a	n/a	n/a	n/a
Pasta Carbonara, w/Chicken	1 entrée	2630	n/a	n/a	n/a	n/a	n/a	n/a
Pasta, w/Meat Sauce	1 entrée	1210	n/a	n/a	n/a	n/a	n/a	n/a
Shrimp, w/Angel Hair	1 entrée	1140	n/a	n/a	n/a	n/a	n/a	n/a
Tomato Basil	1 entrée	1700	n/a	n/a	n/a	n/a	n/a	n/a
PIZZA								
Cheese	1 pizza	1260	n/a	n/a	n/a	n/a	n/a	n/a
Pepperoni	1 pizza	1500	n/a	n/a	n/a	n/a	n/a	n/a

	SERVING SIZE	CALORIES	TOTAL FAT (G)	SAT FAT (G)	SODIUM (MG)	CARBS (G)	FIBER (G)	PROTEIN (G)
Roasted Vegetable & Goat Cheese	1 pizza	1390	n/a	n/a	n/a	n/a	n/a	n/a
Spicy Meat	1 pizza	1680	n/a	n/a	n/a	n/a	n/a	n/a
SALADS								
Barbeque Ranch Chicken	1 salad	1810	n/a	n/a	n/a	n/a	n/a	n/a
Carlton	1 salad	1000	n/a	n/a	n/a	n/a	n/a	n/a
Chicken Caesar	1 salad	1440	n/a	n/a	n/a	n/a	n/a	n/a
Chinese Chicken	1 salad	1660	n/a	n/a	n/a	n/a	n/a	n/a
Herb-Crusted Salmon	1 salad	800	n/a	n/a	n/a	n/a	n/a	n/a
Santa Fe	1 salad	1900	n/a	n/a	n/a	n/a	n/a	n/a
Seared Tuna Tataki	1 salad	580	n/a	n/a	n/a	n/a	n/a	n/a
SIDE DISHES								
Corn Succotash	as served	300	n/a	n/a	n/a	n/a	n/a	n/a
French Fries	as served	560	n/a	n/a	n/a	n/a	n/a	n/a
Macaroni & Cheese	as served	1600	n/a	n/a	n/a	n/a	n/a	n/a
Mashed Potatoes	as served	570	n/a	n/a	n/a	n/a	n/a	n/a
Sweet Potato Fries	as served	950	n/a	n/a	n/a	n/a	n/a	n/a
SMALL PLATES & SNACKS								
Ahi Tartare	as served	250	n/a	n/a	n/a	n/a	n/a	n/a
Crispy Artichoke Hearts	as served	650	n/a	n/a	n/a	n/a	n/a	n/a
Greek Salad	as served	450	n/a	n/a	n/a	n/a	n/a	n/a
Hand-Battered Onion Rings	as served	520	n/a	n/a	n/a	n/a	n/a	n/a
Sausage & Ricotta Flatbread	as served	460	n/a	n/a	n/a	n/a	n/a	n/a
White Bean Hummus, w/Flatbread	as served	960	n/a	n/a	n/a	n/a	n/a	n/a
SPECIALTIES, W/SIDES								
Chicken Bellagio	1 entrée	2000	n/a	n/a	n/a	n/a	n/a	n/a
Chicken Madeira	1 entrée	1660	n/a	n/a	n/a	n/a	n/a	n/a
Crispy Chicken Costoletta	1 entrée	2560	n/a	n/a	n/a	n/a	n/a	n/a
Factory Burrito Grande	1 entrée	1700	n/a	n/a	n/a	n/a	n/a	n/a
Famous Factory Meatloaf	1 entrée	1810	n/a	n/a	n/a	n/a	n/a	n/a
Fish & Chips	1 entrée	1500	n/a	n/a	n/a	n/a	n/a	n/a
Salisbury Chopped Steak	1 entrée	1410	n/a	n/a	n/a	n/a	n/a	n/a
Shepherd's Pie	1 entrée	1780	n/a	n/a	n/a	n/a	n/a	n/a
Stuffed Chicken Tortillas	1 entrée	1910	n/a	n/a	n/a	n/a	n/a	n/a
White Chicken Chili	1 entrée	585	n/a	n/a	n/a	n/a	n/a	n/a
SPECIALTY DESSERTS								
Black-Out Cake	1 slice	1560	n/a	n/a	n/a	n/a	n/a	n/a
Chocolate Tower Truffle Cake	1 slice	1700	n/a	n/a	n/a	n/a	n/a	n/a

	SERVING SIZE	CALORIES	TOTAL FAT (G)	SAT FAT (G)	SODIUM (MG)	CARBS (G)	FIBER (G)	PROTEIN (G)
Chris's Outrageous Chocolate Cake	1 slice	1550	n/a	n/a	n/a	n/a	n/a	n/a
Tiramisu	1 slice	1000	n/a	n/a	n/a	n/a	n/a	n/a
Warm Apple Crisp	1 slice	1430	n/a	n/a	n/a	n/a	n/a	n/a
STEAKS & CHOPS, W/SIDES								
Chargrilled Coulotte Steak	1 entrée	1400	n/a	n/a	n/a	n/a	n/a	n/a
Filet Mignon	1 entrée	1200	n/a	n/a	n/a	n/a	n/a	n/a
Grilled Pork Chop	1 entrée	1500	n/a	n/a	n/a	n/a	n/a	n/a
Hibachi Steak	1 entrée	1770	n/a	n/a	n/a	n/a	n/a	n/a
Steak Diane	1 entrée	1660	n/a	n/a	n/a	n/a	n/a	n/a
SUNDAY BRUNCH								
Brunch Combo	1 entrée	1330	n/a	n/a	n/a	n/a	n/a	n/a
Buttermilk Pancakes, w/Blueberries	1 entrée	1250	n/a	n/a	n/a	n/a	n/a	n/a
Eggs Benedict, w/Ham & Hollandaise	1 entrée	1950	n/a	n/a	n/a	n/a	n/a	n/a
French Toast Napoleon	1 entrée	2530	n/a	n/a	n/a	n/a	n/a	n/a
Giant Belgian Waffle, w/Strawberries, Pecans & Chantilly Cream	1 entrée	1020	n/a	n/a	n/a	n/a	n/a	n/a
Monte Crisco Sandwich	1 sandwich	2830	n/a	n/a	n/a	n/a	n/a	n/a
Smoked Salmon Platter	as served	730	n/a	n/a	n/a	n/a	n/a	n/a

Chick-Fil-A
BREAKFAST

	SERVING SIZE	CALORIES	TOTAL FAT (G)	SAT FAT (G)	SODIUM (MG)	CARBS (G)	FIBER (G)	PROTEIN (G)
Chicken Biscuit	1 sandwich	440	20	8	1230	47	3	17
Chicken Burrito	1 burrito	450	20	8	990	43	2	24
Chicken, Egg & Cheese Bagel	1 sandwich	490	20	6	1230	49	3	29
Chick-N-Minis	4 pieces	370	14	3.5	870	41	2	21
Multigrain Oatmeal, w/Toppings	1 oatmeal	280	11	0.5	45	44	5	6
Sausage, Egg & Cheese Biscuit	1 sandwich	680	47	19	1470	43	2	24
Yogurt Parfait, w/Strawberries & Granola	1 parfait	290	6	2	85	53	1	7

CHICKEN

	SERVING SIZE	CALORIES	TOTAL FAT (G)	SAT FAT (G)	SODIUM (MG)	CARBS (G)	FIBER (G)	PROTEIN (G)
Chargrilled Chicken Cool Wrap	1 wrap	410	12	4	1290	50	9	33
Chargrilled Chicken Sandwich	1 sandwich	290	4	1	1030	36	3	29
Chicken Deluxe Sandwich	1 sandwich	490	22	6	1660	41	3	33
Chicken Nuggets	8 pieces	260	12	2.5	990	11	1	28
Chicken Salad Sandwich	1 sandwich	490	19	3	1130	55	5	28
Chicken Sandwich	1 sandwich	430	17	3.5	1410	38	3	30
Chick-N-Strips	3 pieces	360	17	3.5	1230	17	1	34
Spicy Chicken Sandwich	1 sandwich	480	20	4.5	1660	44	3	31

	SERVING SIZE	CALORIES	TOTAL FAT (G)	SAT FAT (G)	SODIUM (MG)	CARBS (G)	FIBER (G)	PROTEIN (G)
SALADS & SIDES								
Chargrilled & Fruit Salad	1 entrée	220	6	3.5	640	22	4	22
Chick-N-Strips Salad	1 entrée	460	22	6	1350	26	5	40
Hearty Breast of Chicken Soup, Medium	1 serving	140	4	1	1110	19	2	7
Southwest Chargrilled Salad	1 entrée	240	9	4	820	18	5	26
Waffle Potato Fries, Medium	as served	390	21	3	180	47	5	5

Chili's
APPETIZERS

	SERVING SIZE	CALORIES	TOTAL FAT (G)	SAT FAT (G)	SODIUM (MG)	CARBS (G)	FIBER (G)	PROTEIN (G)
Boneless Buffalo Wings, w/Bleu Cheese	as served	1490	88	16	4590	94	2	76
Bottomless Tostada Chips, w/Salsa	as served	1020	51	10	1210	125	11	12
Classic Nachos, Large	as served	1410	96	50	2580	77	11	61
Classic Nachos, w/Chicken, Large	as served	1640	101	51	2830	80	12	105
Fire-Grilled Corn Guacamole, w/Chips	as served	1400	84	15	2250	151	25	17
Hot Spinach & Artichoke Dip, w/Chips	as served	1610	103	42	1610	139	14	33
Loaded Potato Skins	as served	1050	84	38	1540	36	3	44
Skillet Queso, w/Chips	as served	1710	101	37	3490	147	13	45
Southwestern Eggrolls, w/Avocado Ranch	as served	780	41	10	1830	81	7	24
Wings Over Buffalo Honey-Roasted, w/Bleu Cheese	as served	690	53	11	2100	7	1	46
BURGERS ON A WHITE BUN W/FRIES, UNLESS STATED								
Avocado Burger, Wheat Bun	1 entrée	1570	90	29	3170	138	15	54
Big Mouth Bites, w/Ranch	1 entrée	2120	133	38	4810	163	7	66
Classic Bacon Burger	1 entrée	1570	91	28	3690	125	9	61
Oldtimer Burger	1 entrée	1310	65	20	3230	128	10	51
Shiner Bock BBQ Burger	1 entrée	1680	87	27	4050	166	10	58
Southern Smokehouse Burger, w/Ancho Chile BBQ	1 entrée	2290	139	46	6500	163	11	93
CHICKEN & SEAFOOD								
Cajun Pasta, w/Grilled Chicken	1 entrée	1500	76	36	4130	124	6	79
Chicken Crispers, w/Honey Mustard	1 entrée	1350	68	13	3910	129	11	61
Crispy Honey-Chipotle Chicken Crispers, w/Ranch	1 entrée	1660	76	13	4110	196	13	54
Grilled Salmon, w/Garlic & Herbs	1 entrée	560	25	7	1640	37	5	49
Margarita Grilled Chicken	1 entrée	550	14	3.5	1870	62	8	46

restaurants

	SERVING SIZE	CALORIES	TOTAL FAT (G)	SAT FAT (G)	SODIUM (MG)	CARBS (G)	FIBER (G)	PROTEIN (G)
Monterey Chicken	1 entrée	890	48	20	2920	51	8	66
LIGHTER CHOICES								
Classic Sirloin	1 entrée	260	7	2.5	1630	14	4	40
Grilled Chicken Salad	1 salad	420	22	6	660	21	5	38
Grilled Chicken Sandwich, w/Steamed Broccoli	1 entrée	610	13	5	1320	78	8	43
Grilled Salmon, w/Garlic & Herbs	1 entrée	480	17	4.5	1590	37	5	49
Margarita Grilled Chicken	1 entrée	550	14	3.5	1870	62	8	46
Santa Fe Chicken Wrap, w/Steamed Broccoli	1 entrée	680	25	8	2120	80	8	37
Sweet & Spicy Chicken	1 entrée	670	18	6	2740	95	6	37
RIBS, SLOW-SMOKED IN-HOUSE								
Memphis Dry-Rub Ribs	1 entrée	1990	111	37	6180	137	17	119
Original Ribs	1 entrée	2170	123	44	6510	137	20	133
Shiner Bock BBQ Ribs	1 entrée	2310	123	44	6340	168	20	134
SALADS, W/DRESSING								
Boneless Buffalo Chicken	1 salad	990	68	14	4330	48	8	47
Caribbean, w/Grilled Chicken	1 salad	610	25	4	820	65	6	34
Quesadilla Explosion	1 salad	1300	86	28	2070	75	9	62
SANDWICHES, W/FRIES								
Buffalo Chicken Ranch Sandwich, White Bun	1 sandwich	1410	68	12	3940	143	12	52
California Club Sandwich	1 sandwich	1490	76	20	3950	147	15	46
Classic Turkey Sandwich	1 sandwich	1340	64	17	3140	138	11	41
Grilled Chicken Sandwich, White Bun	1 sandwich	1280	63	15	2580	121	9	57
Santa Fe Chicken Wrap, w/Ancho-Chile Ranch	1 wrap	1320	73	20	3200	126	11	46
SOUPS & CHILI, W/O CRACKERS								
Chicken Enchilada	1 cup	190	12	5	770	11	1	10
Chili's Terlingua Chili, w/Toppings	1 cup	180	10	5	580	9	3	14
Southwest Chicken & Sausage	1 cup	160	10	4	850	13	2	7
SOUTHWEST GRILL								
Bacon Ranch Quesadilla, Average of Chicken & Steak	as served	1475	103	39	3030	71	4	70
Beef Fajitas, w/Tortillas & Condiments	as served	880	40	18	3060	77	12	54
Chicken Club Quesadilla	as served	1240	88	35	2560	62	9	59

	SERVING SIZE	CALORIES	TOTAL FAT (G)	SAT FAT (G)	SODIUM (MG)	CARBS (G)	FIBER (G)	PROTEIN (G)
Chicken Fajitas, w/Tortillas & Condiments	as served	850	36	16	2440	74	12	61
Crispy Chicken Tacos	as served	1500	74	22	3910	151	12	59
Crispy Shrimp Tacos	as served	1370	65	20	4340	154	10	47
Fajita Trio, w/Tortillas & Condiments	as served	990	43	18	3430	80	13	73
STEAKS								
Classic Ribeye, 12 oz	1 entrée	1520	110	46	3510	56	7	78
Classic Sirloin, 10 oz	1 entrée	1060	57	20	3530	60	7	79
STUPENDOUSLY SWEET ENDINGS								
Brownie Sundae	as served	1290	61	30	930	195	8	14
Chocolate Chip Paradise Pie	as served	1250	64	33	660	163	4	15
Frosty Chocolate Shake	as served	690	33	21	210	92	0	8
Molten Chocolate Cake	as served	1020	46	27	710	144	5	11

Chipotle Mexican Grill
INGREDIENTS

	SERVING SIZE	CALORIES	TOTAL FAT (G)	SAT FAT (G)	SODIUM (MG)	CARBS (G)	FIBER (G)	PROTEIN (G)
Barbacoa	4 oz	170	7	2.5	510	2	0	24
Black Beans	4 oz	120	1	0	250	23	11	7
Carnitas	4 oz	190	8	2.5	540	1	0	27
Chicken	4 oz	190	6.5	2	370	1	0	32
Cilantro Lime Rice, White	4 oz	170	4	1	200	31	0	2.5
Fajita Vegetables	2-1/2 oz	20	0.5	0	170	4	1	1
Flour Tortilla (Burrito)	1 tortilla	290	9	3	670	44	2	7
Flour Tortilla (Taco)	1 tortilla	270	7.5	3	600	39	3	6
Fresh Tomato Salsa	3-1/2 oz	20	0	0	470	4	<1	1
Guacamole	3-1/2 oz	150	13	2	190	8	6	2
Sour Cream	2 oz	120	10	7	30	2	0	2
Steak	4 oz	190	6.5	2	320	2	0	30

Chuck E. Cheese
COMPLEMENTS

	SERVING SIZE	CALORIES	TOTAL FAT (G)	SAT FAT (G)	SODIUM (MG)	CARBS (G)	FIBER (G)	PROTEIN (G)
Breadsticks	1 stick	175	9	2	412	18	1	6
Buffalo Wings	1 wing	75	5	1	327	4	1	4
French Fries, w/Ketchup & Light Ranch	as served	420	20	2	929	55	6	6
Hot Dog, w/Relish & Mustard	1 hot dog	310	19	7	1084	35	2	11
Mozzarella Sticks	1 stick	93	6	2	211	6	0	4
DESSERTS								
Apple Dessert Pizza	1 slice	192	5	2	164	33	1	2
Cake, Chocolate, 1/4 Sheet	1 slice	310	14	5	200	41	2	3

	SERVING SIZE	CALORIES	TOTAL FAT (G)	SAT FAT (G)	SODIUM (MG)	CARBS (G)	FIBER (G)	PROTEIN (G)
Cinnamon Sticks	1 stick	70	2	1	87	11	0	1
PIZZA, MEDIUM								
All Meat Combo	1 slice	215	11	4	608	21	1	9
BBQ Chicken	1 slice	185	6	2	460	24	1	8
Cheese	1 slice	155	5	2	360	21	1	6
Super Combo	1 slice	185	8	3	453	22	1	7
PIZZA, SMALL								
Cheese, Individual	1 pizza	540	19	8	1255	69	3	21

Church's Chicken
MAIN COURSES

	SERVING SIZE	CALORIES	TOTAL FAT (G)	SAT FAT (G)	SODIUM (MG)	CARBS (G)	FIBER (G)	PROTEIN (G)
Boneless Wing, w/Sauce, Average of All Flavors	1 piece	95	5	1	340	18	1	6
Chicken Fried Steak	1 entrée	470	28	7	1620	36	1	21
Double Chicken N Cheese	1 sandwich	740	38	12	2570	63	4	32
Original Breast	1 entrée	200	11	3	440	3	1	22
Original Chicken Sandwich	1 sandwich	360	18	4	660	35	3	14
Original Leg	1 entrée	110	6	1.5	280	3	0	10
Original Thigh	1 entrée	330	23	6	680	8	1	21
Original Wing	1 entrée	300	18	5	540	7	3	27
Spicy Breast	1 entrée	320	20	5	760	12	2	21
Spicy Leg	1 entrée	180	11	3	470	8	1	12
Spicy Thigh	1 entrée	480	35	9	1040	20	2	22
Spicy Wing	1 entrée	430	27	7	1020	17	2	29
SMALL SIDES								
Honey-Butter Biscuit	1 piece	240	12	3	540	28	1	3
Jalapeño Cheese Bombers	4 pieces	160	8	1	680	20	0	8

Cici's
ADDITIONAL ITEMS

	SERVING SIZE	CALORIES	TOTAL FAT (G)	SAT FAT (G)	SODIUM (MG)	CARBS (G)	FIBER (G)	PROTEIN (G)
Chicken Noodle Soup	1/2 cup	60	2	0	520	8	0	3
Garlic Bread Sticks	1 piece	100	5	1.5	120	10	0	4
Mild Wings	4 pieces	320	26	6	980	1	0	22
DESSERT								
Apple Dessert	1 slice	240	6	1	290	43	< 1	5
Cinnamon Rolls	1 roll	140	5	1	100	20	0	2
Fudge Brownies	1 slice	140	6	1	125	23	< 1	1
PIZZA, 12″ (BUFFET)								
Alfredo	1 slice	120	4	1.5	270	19	< 1	4

	SERVING SIZE	CALORIES	TOTAL FAT (G)	SAT FAT (G)	SODIUM (MG)	CARBS (G)	FIBER (G)	PROTEIN (G)
Buffalo Chicken	1 slice	140	5	1.5	460	19	< 1	6
Cheese	1 slice	150	4	2	330	20	< 1	6
Deep Dish Pepperoni	1 slice	180	6	3	340	19	< 1	7
Pepperoni	1 slice	160	5	2	370	20	< 1	6
Philly Cheesesteak	1 slice	120	4	1	280	19	< 1	4
Sausage	1 slice	170	6	2.5	350	19	1	6
Zesty Veggie	1 slice	120	3	2	320	20	< 1	4

Claim Jumper
APPETIZERS

Artichoke Spinach Dip	as served	677	n/a	22	1249	57	9	18
Hand-Battered Onion Rings	as served	992	n/a	10	2782	127	8	22
Range Rattlers (6)	as served	1407	n/a	39	5361	62	3	73
Southwest Eggrolls	as served	1192	n/a	9	2284	114	9	64

FAVORITES

Chicken Pot Pie	1 entrée	2078	n/a	26	3210	170	10	57
Chicken Tenderloin Dinner	1 entrée	1166	n/a	12	3078	94	3	88
Country Fried Steak	1 entrée	2032	n/a	49	5399	189	8	79
Giant Stuffed Chicken Baker	1 entrée	990	n/a	18	951	118	11	53
Meatloaf & Mashed Potatoes	1 entrée	1301	n/a	34	3038	117	11	40
Sourdough Steak Chili	1 entrée	1233	n/a	19	2828	154	11	54

PASTA

Black Tie Chicken	1 entrée	1533	n/a	41	2572	126	5	72
Parmesan Crusted Chicken	1 entrée	977	n/a	20	1925	83	4	55
Shrimp Fresca	1 entrée	1998	n/a	74	2809	121	6	71

SALADS

California Citrus Chicken	1 entrée	865	n/a	14	966	58	13	39
Chopped Cobb	1 entrée	678	n/a	20	1662	13	7	53
Seared Ahi Spinach	1 entrée	571	n/a	8	1241	28	4	47

SANDWICHES & BURGERS

BBQ Chicken	1 sandwich	1151	n/a	15	2691	134	7	71
Classic Cheeseburger	1 burger	900	n/a	19	1964	51	3	57
Clubhouse	1 sandwich	1200	n/a	16	3351	107	4	61
Original Tri Tip Dip	1 sandwich	1067	n/a	19	1797	68	2	78
Widow Maker	1 burger	1149	n/a	21	2571	79	8	63

SEAFOOD

Fried Shrimp	1 entrée	1048	n/a	14	3382	71	4	44
Lobster Tail Dinner	1 entrée	595	n/a	26	1111	16	4	30

	SERVING SIZE	CALORIES	TOTAL FAT (G)	SAT FAT (G)	SODIUM (MG)	CARBS (G)	FIBER (G)	PROTEIN (G)
Norwegian Salmon BBQ	1 entrée	663	n/a	10	2021	46	4	42
Shrimp Fresca Pasta	1 entrée	1998	n/a	74	2809	121	6	71
Tilapia Bianca	1 entrée	1046	n/a	28	1518	30	5	48
SOUPS								
French Onion	1 bowl	390	n/a	13	1807	22	2	19
Sourdough New England Clam Chowder	1 bowl	1219	n/a	41	2326	116	5	26
Sourdough Steak Chili	1 bowl	1233	n/a	19	2828	154	11	54
SPECIALTIES & COMBOS								
BBQ Baby Back Ribs, Full Rack	1 entrée	1743	n/a	39	3665	111	4	75
Pork & Beef Ribs Combo	1 entrée	2004	n/a	58	3571	109	4	70
Rib & Chicken Combo	1 entrée	1092	n/a	23	1958	63	4	53
Tri Tip & Shrimp Combo	1 entrée	763	n/a	16	1369	16	4	66
Whiskey-Apple Glazed Chicken	1 entrée	1216	n/a	26	591	66	7	67
SWEETS								
Chocolate Motherload Cake	1 slice	2768	n/a	54	1466	340	11	27
Italian Lemon Cake	1 slice	1238	n/a	41	569	158	1	13
Red Velvet Motherload Cake	1 slice	2988	n/a	67	2381	333	4	29

Cold Stone Creamery
ICE CREAM

Cake Batter	love it	550	30	19	280	66	0	8
Cheesecake	love it	510	30	20	140	57	0	6
Chocolate	love it	520	32	20	160	53	2	9
Coffee	love it	530	31	20	125	54	0	8
Cookie Batter	love it	580	33	19	430	68	1	7
Mint	love it	227	30	19	120	57	0	8
Strawberry	love it	510	30	19	120	55	0	8
Strawberry Cheesecake	love it	520	33	18	85	63	0	8
Vanilla Bean	love it	530	31	19	120	52	0	8
MIX-INS, CANDY								
Butterfinger Candy	1/2 bar	140	6	3	65	22	<1	2
Chocolate Chips	1 oz	130	7	4.5	0	16	1	1
Heath Toffee Bar	1 bar	110	7	3.5	75	12	0	<1
Kit Kat Wafer Bar	1/2 bar	110	5	3.5	15	13	0	1
M&M'S	1 oz	170	7	4.5	20	25	<1	2
Nestlé Crunch Bar	1/2 bar	130	7	4	35	16	<1	2
Peanut M&M'S	1 oz	150	8	3.5	30	18	<1	3

	SERVING SIZE	CALORIES	TOTAL FAT (G)	SAT FAT (G)	SODIUM (MG)	CARBS (G)	FIBER (G)	PROTEIN (G)
Reese's Peanut Butter Cups	1 piece	190	11	4	110	19	1	4
Reese's Pieces Candy	1 oz	180	9	6	70	21	1	4
Snickers Candy Bar	1/2 bar	170	9	3	95	21	<1	3
Whoppers Candy	1 oz	120	4	3.5	85	19	0	1
SHAKES								
Cake 'n Shake	love it	1320	69	43	910	164	2	19
Cherry Cheeseshake	love it	1190	64	43	330	146	1	16
Cream de Menthe	love it	1250	77	50	320	131	4	16
Lotta Caramel Latte	love it	1310	71	47	450	160	1	18
Milk & Cookies	love it	1300	78	48	570	144	2	19
Oh Fudge!	love it	1360	78	52	540	161	5	24
PB&C	love it	1510	103	54	630	131	8	36
Savory Strawberry	love it	1130	66	43	320	128	3	17
Very Vanilla	love it	1210	66	44	380	145	1	16
SORBET								
Lemon	love it	250	0	0	25	64	0	0
Raspberry	love it	260	0	0	30	67	0	0
YOGURT								
Cake Batter	love it	330	1	0	380	74	0	7
Cheesecake	love it	290	0	0	230	67	0	7
Chocolate	love it	280	1	0	240	64	2	8
Coffee	love it	280	0	0	240	63	0	7
Strawberry, Sweet & Tart	love it	300	0	0	230	69	1	7
Vanilla	love it	280	0	0	240	63	0	7

Cousins Subs
DESSERTS

	SERVING SIZE	CALORIES	TOTAL FAT (G)	SAT FAT (G)	SODIUM (MG)	CARBS (G)	FIBER (G)	PROTEIN (G)
Chocolate Chip Cookie	1 cookie	210	11	4	120	26	0	2
Peanut Butter Crispy Bar	1 cookie	290	13	5	260	38	2	6
Snickerdoodle Cookie	1 cookie	190	9	5	60	25	0	2
SOUPS & SALADS								
Almond Berry Chicken Salad	1 salad	440	20	6	560	37	8	34
Cheddar Cheese Soup, Large	1 bowl	316	18	10	1705	29	1	11
Chicken w/Wild Rice Soup, Large	1 bowl	344	14	3	1416	21	6	19
Chili, Large	1 bowl	344	12	7	1691	41	25	25
Gourmet Garden Salad, w/Chicken Breast	1 salad	340	15	8	610	21	5	37
Turkey Bacon Delight	1 salad	370	21	10	1330	23	5	23

restaurants	SERVING SIZE	CALORIES	TOTAL FAT (G)	SAT FAT (G)	SODIUM (MG)	CARBS (G)	FIBER (G)	PROTEIN (G)
Vegetable Beef, Large	1 bowl	110	3	0	1389	18	3	6
SUBS, 7-1/2" ON ITALIAN BREAD								
BLT	1 sub	591	38	9	1116	47	1	19
Cheese Steak	1 sub	680	32	15	1580	50	1	46
Chicken Cheddar Deluxe	1 sub	669	39	10	1693	51	1	34
Club	1 sub	646	35	8	1925	51	1	36
Double Cheese Steak	1 sub	1090	63	31	2460	50	1	80
Garden Provolone	1 sub	880	54	21	1620	65	3	39
Ham & Provolone	1 sub	630	35	9	1690	50	3	32
Italian Special	1 sub	817	51	16	2115	50	1	36
Meatball & Provolone	1 sub	723	38	18	1706	54	2	40
Pepperoni Melt	1 sub	722	45	13	1936	50	1	31
Roast Beef & Cheddar	1 sub	710	35	9	1100	52	1	41
Tuna	1 sub	670	40	6	1110	49	3	33
Turkey Breast	1 sub	531	28	4	1544	50	1	25
Culvers								
BUTTERBURGERS, SANDWICHES & FAVORITES								
Beef Pot Roast Sandwich	1 sandwich	363	16	8	948	33	1	24
ButterBurger Cheese, Single	1 burger	423	21	9	990	38	1	22
ButterBurger "The Original," Double	1 burger	484	23	8	700	37	1	33
ButterBurger "The Original," Single	1 burger	346	15	6	670	36	1	19
Cheddar ButterBurger, w/Bacon, Single	1 burger	541	32	14	1015	31	1	30
Crispy Chicken Filet Sandwich	1 sandwich	578	34	12	1056	50	2	21
Grilled Reuben Melt	1 sandwich	588	30	13	2010	42	2	39
Mushroom & Swiss Burger, Double	1 burger	661	39	16	752	35	1	45
The Culver's Bacon Deluxe, Double	1 burger	791	53	24	1481	35	1	44
Wisconsin Swiss Melt, Double	1 burger	616	34	16	720	35	2	46
DINNERS								
Beef Pot Roast Dinner	1 entrée	745	36	25	1710	73	8	34
Butterfly Jumbo Shrimp, 10 Pieces	1 entrée	1560	79	14	2606	172	10	42
Chicken Basket, 2 pieces, w/Fries	1 basket	1265	67	16	2336	84	4	82
Fresh Fried Chicken, 4 Pieces	1 entrée	2220	121	29	3616	159	6	124
North Atlantic Cod Filet, 3 Pieces	1 entrée	2156	139	21	2378	148	8	76
SALADS, W/O DRESSING								
Chicken Cashew, w/Flame-Roasted Chicken	1 salad	443	24	7	925	19	6	38

	SERVING SIZE	CALORIES	TOTAL FAT (G)	SAT FAT (G)	SODIUM (MG)	CARBS (G)	FIBER (G)	PROTEIN (G)
Classic Caesar, w/Flame-Roasted Chicken	1 salad	340	16	6	1445	14	3	34
Garden Fresco	1 salad	229	10	4	375	19	4	16
SIDES & SOUPS								
Chili Cheddar Fries	1 side	607	29	8	482	72	5	15
George's Chili Supreme	1 bowl	458	29	14	822	26	5	24
Onion Rings, Breaded	1 side	630	36	4	1070	70	3	7
Wisconsin Cheese Curds	1 side	670	38	15	1740	54	3	28

Currito
BURRITOS, MEATLESS, REGULAR SIZE

	SERVING SIZE	CALORIES	TOTAL FAT (G)	SAT FAT (G)	SODIUM (MG)	CARBS (G)	FIBER (G)	PROTEIN (G)
Bangkok	1 burrito	655	20	4.1	2013	106	5	16
Buffalo	1 burrito	811	44	15.5	2025	92	3	14
Cajun	1 burrito	805	25	10.8	5425	126	11	23
Classic Burrito	1 burrito	784	28	11.9	2879	105	7	26
Mediterranean	1 burrito	828	34	10.6	3027	107	9	23
Summer	1 burrito	837	28	11.8	2596	115	10	28
Teriyaki	1 burrito	650	16	3	2206	111	8	15
SMOOTHIES, LARGE								
Berry Blitz	20 fl oz	349	1	0.2	34	87	7	1
Cape Codder	20 fl oz	426	1	0.1	62	103	5	4
Jimmy Carter	20 fl oz	765	21	4.5	466	120	4	29
Mango Passion	20 fl oz	401	1	0.1	74	95	3	5
Milkshake	20 fl oz	595	1	0.3	364	122	0	23
Soy Smoothie	20 fl oz	326	7	0.9	46	62	10	11
Strawbana	20 fl oz	369	2	1	72	89	5	2
Triathlete	20 fl oz	282	1	0.2	39	70	5	2

Daily Grill
APPETIZERS

	SERVING SIZE	CALORIES	TOTAL FAT (G)	SAT FAT (G)	SODIUM (MG)	CARBS (G)	FIBER (G)	PROTEIN (G)
Fried Calamari	as served	665	46	8	1052	32	2	30
Grilled Artichoke	as served	639	56	8	871	24	10	7
Jumbo Lump Crab Cake	as served	281	20	10	497	6	0	16
Seared Ahi Tuna Sashimi	as served	477	14	1	1578	15	4	69
Spinach Artichoke Dip	as served	553	27	19	1017	43	3	28
BREAKFAST								
Belgian Waffle	1 entrée	517	15	5	1515	83	0	7
Buttermilk Pancakes	1 entrée	451	8	1	1296	76	0	12
Corned Beef Hash	1 entrée	655	29	10	2507	51	6	41
Denver Omelette	1 entrée	643	35	15	1760	29	4	47

restaurants

	SERVING SIZE	CALORIES	TOTAL FAT (G)	SAT FAT (G)	SODIUM (MG)	CARBS (G)	FIBER (G)	PROTEIN (G)
Egg White Omelette	1 entrée	421	29	10	638	12	6	24
Eggs Benedict	1 entrée	735	46	24	1070	47	3	31
French Toast	1 entrée	659	17	4	932	96	4	28
Good Start Breakfast	1 entrée	562	8	3	253	116	10	10
Three Eggs w/Bacon	1 entrée	420	24	8	939	22	2	26
Three Eggs w/Country Sausage	1 entrée	915	75	26	1554	22	2	32
ENTRÉE SALADS, W/DRESSING								
Blackened Ahi Tuna	1 salad	1026	71	8	1495	46	15	53
Daily Grill Cobb, Dinner	1 salad	1504	116	31	2654	25	11	84
Grilled Lime Chicken, Dinner	1 salad	1072	95	14	576	43	16	10
Grilled Skirt Steak	1 salad	1134	88	26	2350	29	7	46
Parmesan Crusted Chicken Caesar	1 salad	1123	81	19	1221	36	5	60
ENTRÉES								
Angel Hair Pasta Pomodoro	1 entrée	837	37	3	1807	108	9	21
Blackened Mahi Mahi	1 entrée	331	7	1	951	22	4	45
Blackened Steak Quesadilla	1 entrée	1951	117	53	3697	146	19	79
Cedar Plank Salmon	1 entrée	675	16	2	1051	73	12	60
Charbroiled Filet Mignon	1 entrée	1052	69	32	1036	39	5	63
Charbroiled Rib Eye, 16 oz	1 entrée	1634	95	33	1379	53	11	134
Chicken Piccata	1 entrée	1223	75	47	1324	72	12	58
Double-Cut Pork Chop	1 entrée	1187	72	35	4432	63	7	58
Fish & Chips	1 entrée	1375	82	15	1444	106	9	54
Loaded Mac & Cheese	1 entrée	1206	65	33	2581	89	4	64
Meatloaf	1 entrée	1438	90	43	3279	106	9	39
New York Pepper Steak	1 entrée	1357	81	28	1605	64	14	90
Pan-Seared Salmon	1 entrée	1009	87	35	818	9	1	47
SIDES								
Garlic Mashed Potatoes	as served	507	28	18	801	54	6	8
Macaroni & Cheese	as served	839	32	20	892	97	5	37
Shoestring Fries	as served	303	18	4	767	33	3	3
Sweet Potato Fries	as served	286	13	1	333	40	5	2
SPECIALTY SANDWICHES								
Ahi Tuna Wrap	1 wrap	748	34	7	1542	66	11	46
Charbroiled Chicken Breast Sandwich	1 sandwich	888	40	11	1325	81	4	44
Classic Cheeseburger w/Cheddar Cheese	1 burger	1528	92	30	2450	104	8	66
Classic Chicken Burger	1 burger	1413	83	25	3162	110	12	55

	SERVING SIZE	CALORIES	TOTAL FAT (G)	SAT FAT (G)	SODIUM (MG)	CARBS (G)	FIBER (G)	PROTEIN (G)
Classic Hamburger	1 burger	1420	83	25	2268	104	8	59
Crab Cake Sandwich	1 sandwich	960	52	13	1635	83	4	34
Original Beef Dip Sandwich	1 sandwich	623	4	1	1667	88	2	52
Santa Fe Chicken Wrap	1 wrap	941	36	10	1630	102	14	51

Dairy Queen
BASKETS

Chicken Quesadilla	1 basket	1160	60	25	2930	110	6	44
Chicken Strips (6), w/Country Gravy	1 basket	1260	66	11	3500	121	12	49
Popcorn Shrimp	1 basket	1000	49	22	3650	116	8	19
Veggie Quesadilla	1 basket	1100	59	25	2500	110	6	31

BLIZZARD TREATS

Banana Split	1 medium	770	28	17	520	117	1	14
Butterfinger	1 medium	740	26	16	350	114	0	16
Chocolate Xtreme	1 medium	960	45	26	610	130	4	17
Cookie Dough	1 medium	1020	40	24	580	148	2	17
French Silk Pie	1 medium	900	42	26	440	120	2	15
Heath	1 medium	920	41	26	490	126	1	16
M&M's Chocolate Candy	1 medium	840	30	19	270	127	2	16
Oreo Cookies	1 medium	680	25	12	530	100	1	14
Reese's Peanut Butter Cups	1 medium	740	31	16	400	101	2	18
Snickers	1 medium	850	33	17	400	123	2	18
Strawberry CheeseQuake	1 medium	690	28	18	380	92	0	15
Turtle Pecan Cluster	1 medium	1070	56	29	450	129	4	17

BURGERS

1/2 lb. FlameThrower GrillBurger	1 burger	1000	74	26	1610	40	2	46
1/2 lb. GrillBurger, w/Cheese	1 burger	800	51	20	1280	44	3	40
1/4 lb. Bacon Cheese GrillBurger	1 burger	630	37	13	1250	44	2	30
1/4 lb. Mushroom Swiss GrillBurger	1 burger	570	35	11	820	39	2	24
Original Cheeseburger	1 burger	400	18	9	930	34	1	19
Original Double Cheeseburger	1 burger	630	34	18	1230	34	1	34

HOT DOGS

All-Beef Chili Cheese Dog	1 hot dog	380	24	11	900	23	1	16
All-Beef Foot-Long Chili Cheese Dog	1 hot dog	670	43	19	1720	40	2	28
All-Beef Hot Dog	1 hot dog	290	17	7	900	22	1	11

MOOLATTE FROZEN BLENDED

Cappuccino	1 medium	570	19	15	200	84	0	10
Caramel	1 medium	650	20	15	250	103	0	10

restaurants

	SERVING SIZE	CALORIES	TOTAL FAT (G)	SAT FAT (G)	SODIUM (MG)	CARBS (G)	FIBER (G)	PROTEIN (G)
French Vanilla	1 medium	630	19	14	190	101	0	10
Mocha	1 medium	660	25	16	250	96	0	11
OTHER FROZEN TREATS								
Arctic Rush, All Flavors	1 medium	260	0	0	70	70	0	0
Arctic Rush Float, All Flavors	1 medium	420	7	4.5	115	82	0	6
Arctic Rush Freeze, All Flavors	1 medium	470	12	8	170	80	0	10
Chocolate Cone	1 medium	340	10	7	160	54	0	9
Dipped Cone, Chocolate	1 medium	470	22	18	150	61	1	9
Lemonade Chiller, Classic	1 medium	380	0	0	0	87	0	0
Lemonade Chiller, Strawberry	1 medium	420	0	0	10	96	0	0
Sundae, Banana	1 medium	330	10	6	130	53	1	8
Sundae, Caramel	1 medium	430	11	7	210	74	0	9
Sundae, Chocolate	1 medium	400	12	7	170	70	1	8
Sundae, Hot Fudge	1 medium	440	15	11	200	67	1	9
Sundae, Pineapple	1 medium	340	10	6	140	54	0	8
Sundae, Strawberry	1 medium	350	10	6	140	56	0	8
Vanilla Cone	1 medium	330	10	6	140	53	0	9
Waffle Bowl Sundae, Chocolate Coated	1 sundae	540	21	13	190	77	1	10
Waffle Bowl Sundae, Chocolate Covered Strawberry	1 sundae	760	38	30	170	96	2	10
Waffle Bowl Sundae, Fudge Brownie Temptation	1 sundae	940	48	22	440	121	2	13
Waffle Bowl Sundae, Plain Waffle Cone w/Soft Serve	1 sundae	420	13	7	135	67	0	10
Waffle Bowl Sundae, Turtle	1 sundae	810	35	18	300	115	2	11
SANDWICHES, SALADS & WRAPS								
Salad, Crispy Chicken	1 salad	470	26	9	1240	29	7	30
Salad, Grilled Chicken	1 salad	330	15	8	1200	13	4	36
Sandwich, Classic Club, Iron Grilled	1 sandwich	600	24	8	1950	55	3	33
Sandwich, Crispy Chicken	1 sandwich	600	30	4.5	1250	59	7	24
Sandwich, Crispy FlameThrower Chicken	1 sandwich	830	51	11	2160	63	8	34
Sandwich, Supreme BLT Iron Grilled	1 sandwich	600	34	9	1380	40	2	28
Wrap, Crispy FlameThrower Chicken	1 wrap	360	22	5	870	30	2	12
SIDE ITEMS								
Chili Cheese Fries	as served	1020	51	15	2360	117	9	25

	SERVING SIZE	CALORIES	TOTAL FAT (G)	SAT FAT (G)	SODIUM (MG)	CARBS (G)	FIBER (G)	PROTEIN (G)
French Fries, Regular	as served	310	13	2	640	43	3	4
Onion Rings	as served	360	16	2	840	47	2	6

Daphne's California Greek

3-COURSE DINNER

Falafel & Spanakopita	1 entrée	410	26	6	640	32	7	12
Fresh-Carved Gyros Street Pita & Grilled Chicken Kabob	1 entrée	530	30	9	1200	30	2	36
Grilled Chicken Kabob & Crispy Shrimp	1 entrée	270	11	2	970	11	1	33
Grilled Chicken Kabob & Lemon Chicken Soup	1 entrée	290	14	4	1580	15	1	28
Two Fresh-Carved Gyros Street Pitas	1 entrée	760	52	17	1280	52	3	23

FLATBREAD PIZZAS

Margherita	1 pizza	500	32	10	970	41	3	18
Rustic Greek	1 pizza	460	25	12	1280	45	3	19

SALADS, W/O DRESSING

California Greek	1 salad	500	30	8	990	29	12	34
Classic Greek, Crispy Shrimp	1 salad	350	19	6	1130	28	5	19
Classic Greek, Fresh-Carved Gyros	1 salad	620	47	20	1270	28	5	24
Classic Greek, Grilled Chicken	1 salad	330	15	6	1130	21	5	32
Tabouli	1 salad	80	1	0	230	17	1	3

SANDWICHES, CLASSIC PITA

Crispy Shrimp	1 sandwich	390	19	3	880	40	2	15
Falafel	1 sandwich	510	28	4	860	54	8	12
Fire-Roasted Vegetables	1 sandwich	350	18	5	890	39	4	10
Fresh-Carved Gyros	1 sandwich	660	47	16	1025	40	2	21
Grilled Chicken	1 sandwich	370	15	2	880	33	2	28
Original Pita, w/Tzatziki Sauce	1 serving	230	9	3	400	30	1	5

STARTERS

Fire Feta & Multigrain Pita Chips	1 serving	290	15	5	630	30	5	10
Original Hummus, w/Pita	1 serving	300	15	2	520	37	3	6
Pesto Hummus, w/Pita	1 serving	360	22	3	580	38	3	7
Starter Sampler	1 serving	510	29	6	1120	52	11	15

Davanni's

CALZONES

Chicken & Tomato	1 calzone	847	44	n/a	1278	80	5	36

restaurants

	SERVING SIZE	CALORIES	TOTAL FAT (G)	SAT FAT (G)	SODIUM (MG)	CARBS (G)	FIBER (G)	PROTEIN (G)
Pepperoni & Sausage	1 calzone	959	56	n/a	1676	80	5	35
Three Cheese	1 calzone	926	53	n/a	1336	79	5	35
HOT HOAGIES								
BLT	1/2 sandwich	644	44	n/a	1342	40	1	25
Chicken Parmigiana	1/2 sandwich	447	16	n/a	938	40	1	38
Italian Sausage	1/2 sandwich	621	38	n/a	1355	46	3	24
Meatball	1/2 sandwich	564	33	n/a	1298	49	2	25
Roast Beef	1/2 sandwich	468	25	n/a	882	39	1	25
Salami	1/2 sandwich	621	43	n/a	1402	39	1	23
Turkey	1/2 sandwich	455	24	n/a	1022	39	1	25
Veggie	1/2 sandwich	445	24	n/a	669	43	2	14
PIZZA								
Cheese, Thin Crust	1 slice	178	7	4	365	18	1	9
Cheese, Traditional Crust	1 slice	224	8	4	450	28	1	11
Chicken & Roma Tomato, Light Cheese on Traditional Crust	1 slice	202	5	2	433	29	1	12
Five Meat, Traditional Crust	1 slice	567	33	n/a	1952	30	1	34
The Works, Deep Dish	1 slice	324	16	8	711	28	1	15
Veggie, Traditional Crust	1 slice	266	10	n/a	599	29	1	13

Del Taco
BURRITO

	SERVING SIZE	CALORIES	TOTAL FAT (G)	SAT FAT (G)	SODIUM (MG)	CARBS (G)	FIBER (G)	PROTEIN (G)
1 lb Macho Burrito, Beef	1 burrito	1010	44	19	2140	82	6	61
1 lb Macho Burrito, Combo	1 burrito	990	36	19	3460	110	15	50
1/2 lb Bean & Cheese Burrito, Red or Green	1 burrito	440	9	4	2080	54	12	18
Del Beef Burrito	1 burrito	470	19	8	1060	24	2	29
Del Combo Burrito	1 burrito	475	14	6	1980	47	10	26
Spicy Chicken Burrito	1 burrito	610	13	4	2450	82	7	27
Veggie Works Burrito	1 burrito	620	14	6	2200	83	9	18
CHEESEBURGERS								
Bacon Double Del Cheeseburger	1 burger	770	52	20	1440	40	1	34
Double Del Cheeseburger	1 burger	720	48	18	1270	40	1	31
Triple Del Cheeseburger	1 burger	950	66	27	1660	40	1	44
DESSERTS								
Caramel Cheesecake Bites	4 bites	940	59	21	600	84	0	12
Churro, w/Cinnamon & Sugar	as served	180	9	2	0	21	0	2
FRIES								
Chili Cheddar Fries	as served	550	32	10	930	42	5	16

	SERVING SIZE	CALORIES	TOTAL FAT (G)	SAT FAT (G)	SODIUM (MG)	CARBS (G)	FIBER (G)	PROTEIN (G)
Deluxe Chili Cheddar Fries	as served	590	35	12	940	44	5	17
Fries, Macho	as served	515	30	4	630	56	6	6
NACHOS & SALADS								
Deluxe Taco Salad	1 salad	845	47	17	2470	69	14	34
Macho Nachos	as served	1000	56	15	3050	94	14	33
Nachos	as served	370	22	4	530	28	1	5
QUESADILLA								
Cheddar Quesadilla	1 quesadilla	480	25	16	840	36	2	23
Chicken Cheddar Quesadilla	1 quesadilla	570	29	16	1180	38	2	34
Spicy Jack Quesadilla	1 quesadilla	480	25	13	820	38	2	23
TACOS								
Big Fat Taco, Chicken	1 taco	330	14	3	690	34	1	16
Big Fat Taco, Steak	1 taco	390	18	6	790	33	1	15
Chicken Soft Taco	1 taco	220	12	3	490	16	2	12
Classic Soft Taco	1 taco	220	11	5	470	16	2	14
Classic Taco	1 taco	200	12	5	320	10	1	13
Crispy Fish Taco	1 taco	300	17	2	320	29	3	8
Deluxe Taco	1 taco	170	10	4	260	11	1	8
Taco al Carbon, Chicken	1 taco	150	4	0	300	19	2	10
Taco al Carbon, Steak	1 taco	210	8	2	400	18	2	9
Denny's **AMERICAN DINNER CLASSICS, W/O SIDES UNLESS INDICATED**								
Chicken Strips, w/Bread	1 entrée	760	29	6	1830	84	3	44
Country-Fried Steak, w/Gravy	1 entrée	1170	74	25	2920	74	7	55
Fit Fare Sweet & Tangy BBQ Chicken, w/Broccoli & Corn	1 entrée	630	13	4	1230	56	6	78
Fit Fare Tilapia Ranchero	1 entrée	450	19	6	930	40	3	53
Lemon Pepper Grilled Tilapia, w/Bread	1 entrée	800	35	15	1740	59	3	58
Prime Rib & Chicken Sizzlin' Skillet	1 entrée	940	43	16	2400	67	8	69
Slow-Cooked Pot Roast	1 entrée	670	33	9	2070	80	3	50
Sweet & Tangy BBQ Chicken, w/Bread & Veggies	1 entrée	900	33	9	1790	99	4	80
T-Bone Steak & Breaded Shrimp, w/Bread	1 entrée	1000	59	17	3210	47	3	72
Tilapia Ranchero, w/Bread	1 entrée	630	27	7	1280	60	4	57
APPETIZERS								
Basket of Puppies, w/o Syrup	10 pieces	510	11	2	1640	100	4	11

restaurants

	SERVING SIZE	CALORIES	TOTAL FAT (G)	SAT FAT (G)	SODIUM (MG)	CARBS (G)	FIBER (G)	PROTEIN (G)
Cheese Burger Flatbread	as served	890	54	22	1620	53	6	38
Chicken Strips, w/Sweet & Tangy BBQ Sauce, w/o Dipping Sauce	as served	820	30	0	2160	83	2	58
Chicken Wings, w/Sweet & Tangy BBQ Sauce, w/o Dipping Sauce	as served	450	18	5	1400	40	1	35
Grilled Shrimp Skewer	1 skewer	90	4	1	160	1	0	14
Sampler, w/o Sauce	as served	1380	71	6	3710	139	6	53
Smothered Cheese Fries	as served	860	53	17	990	75	7	21
BREAKFAST, W/O SIDES UNLESS INDICATED								
All-American Slam	as served	800	68	25	1410	5	1	40
Bacon Avocado Burrito, w/Hash Browns	as served	1010	59	15	2210	91	8	29
Bacon Lover's BLT	1 sandwich	810	47	12	1690	66	3	29
Bacon Slamburger	1 burger	1010	58	24	1730	56	3	56
Banana Pecan Pancake Breakfast	as served	780	15	4	1610	130	10	33
Belgian Waffle Slam	as served	820	64	27	1270	32	2	30
Country-Fried Steak & Eggs	as served	660	43	15	1620	29	3	39
Fit Fare Omelette	as served	390	18	8	870	25	4	34
Fit Fare Veggie Skillet	as served	330	9	1.5	1450	44	9	20
Fit Slam	as served	390	12	4	850	46	5	27
Harvest Oatmeal Breakfast	as served	530	11	5	600	93	9	19
Meat Lover's Omelette, w/Hash Browns	as served	1060	75	24	2710	39	4	56
Moons Over My Hammy	as served	760	41	15	2320	51	2	44
Prime Rib Skillet	as served	585	38	12.5	1460	15	3	33
Sausage Slam	as served	1260	63	25	2840	139	6	34
Southwestern Steak Burrito, w/Hash Browns	as served	1120	63	16	2565	101	7	36
The Grand Slamwich, w/Hash Browns	as served	1520	101	44	3550	97	5	53
Ultimate Skillet	as served	740	56	17	1470	34	6	27
Veggie-Cheese Omelette	as served	460	33	12	680	9	2	28
Western Omelette, w/Hash Browns	as served	700	46	13	2180	32	2	38
BURGERS & SANDWICHES, W/O SIDES UNLESS INDICATED								
Chicken Avocado Sandwich, w/Fit Fare Fresh Veggies	1 entrée	520	16	5	2040	48	6	46

	SERVING SIZE	CALORIES	TOTAL FAT (G)	SAT FAT (G)	SODIUM (MG)	CARBS (G)	FIBER (G)	PROTEIN (G)
Classic Cheeseburger	1 burger	820	44	21	1450	47	4	47
Double Cheeseburger	1 burger	1400	87	41	2680	49	4	87
Hickory Grilled Chicken Sandwich	1 sandwich	900	47	12	1370	67	5	50
Patty Melt	1 burger	1040	73	29	2180	41	4	50
Prime Rib Philly Melt	1 sandwich	670	36	11	1770	52	3	35
Spicy Buffalo Chicken Melt	1 sandwich	860	48	12	3760	76	3	32
The Super Bird	1 sandwich	610	29	9	2320	54	2	34
Veggie Burger, w/Balsamic Vinaigrette & Veggies	1 entrée	540	13	5	1340	76	11	31
Western Burger	1 burger	1010	55	22	1450	69	6	50
SOUPS, SALADS & SIDES								
Chicken Deluxe Salad, w/Grilled Chicken	1 salad	340	13	6	530	13	4	44
Clam Chowder	12 fl oz	270	17	12	1840	24	1	5
Cranberry Apple Chicken Salad, w/Balsamic Vinaigrette, w/o Bread	1 salad	370	12	3	610	32	3	36
French Fries, Salted	as served	430	23	5	95	50	5	5
French Fries, Seasoned	as served	630	47	9	1010	48	5	6
Loaded Baked Potato Soup	13 fl oz	420	32	16	1710	23	2	9
Onion Rings	as served	520	36	2	980	48	3	6
Vegetable Beef Soup	12 fl oz	140	5	0	1290	17	3	7
Dippin' Dots								
Candy Bar Crunch w/Snickers	1/2 cup	200	11	7	60	23	0	4
Caramel Brownie Sundae	1/2 cup	190	10	6	90	22	0	3
Chocolate Chip Cookie Dough	1/2 cup	210	11	6	80	25	0	3
Cookies 'n Cream w/Oreo	1/2 cup	200	10	6	105	24	2	3
Moose Tracks	1/2 cup	210	12	8	55	23	0	3
Average of All Other Flavors	1/2 cup	180	10	6	100	22	0	3
NO SUGAR ADDED ICE CREAM								
Low-Fat Fudge	1/2 cup	90	2	1	85	27	0	4
Reduced-Fat Vanilla	1/2 cup	120	5	3	80	28	0	4
SHERBET								
Average of All Flavors	1/2 cup	110	1	0.5	20	31	0	1
Domino's **CHEESE PIZZA, LARGE 14"**								
Brooklyn	1 slice	270	12	6	650	28	1	13
Deep Dish	1 slice	350	16	7	860	39	4	14

restaurants	SERVING SIZE	CALORIES	TOTAL FAT (G)	SAT FAT (G)	SODIUM (MG)	CARBS (G)	FIBER (G)	PROTEIN (G)
Hand Tossed	1 slice	290	11	5.5	640	35	2	12
Thin Crust	1 slice	230	12	5	460	20	1	9
PASTA & SALADS								
Pasta in a Breadbowl, Chicken Alfredo	1/2 bowl	700	26	11	1040	93	3	25
Pasta in a Breadbowl, Italian Sausage Marinara	1/2 bowl	730	27	10	1380	97	4	26
Pasta in a Breadbowl, Mac-N-Cheese	1/2 bowl	730	28	14	1390	95	3	27
Pasta in a Breadbowl, Pasta Primavera	1/2 bowl	670	24	11	880	94	4	20
Pasta in a Dish, Chicken Alfredo	1 bowl	600	29	16	1080	58	2	27
Pasta in a Dish, Italian Sausage Marinara	1 bowl	670	32	15	1760	66	5	28
Pasta in a Dish, Pasta Primavera	1 bowl	540	27	16	770	59	3	16
Salad, Garden Fresh	1/2 salad	70	4	2.5	80	5	2	4
Salad, Grilled Chicken Caesar	1/2 salad	90	4	1.5	290	5	2	9
PEPPERONI PIZZA, LARGE 14"								
Brooklyn	1 slice	300	16	6.5	810	27	1	14
Deep Dish	1 slice	350	17	6.5	890	38	4	13
Hand Tossed	1 slice	300	13	5.5	700	34	2	12
Thin Crust	1 slice	240	13	5	520	19	1	9
SANDWICHES								
Buffalo Chicken w/Blue Cheese	1 sandwich	830	41	16	2690	74	3	42
Chicken Bacon Ranch	1 sandwich	870	45	16	2380	72	2	45
Chicken Parm	1 sandwich	750	30	16	2200	73	3	47
Italian	1 sandwich	820	41	20	2700	70	3	41
Italian Sausage	1 sandwich	730	27	10	35	1380	97	4
Mediterranean Veggie	1 sandwich	680	29	1	2050	72	4	32
Philly Cheese Steak	1 sandwich	690	28	15	2120	70	3	39
Sweet & Spicy Chicken Habanero	1 sandwich	800	32	17	2170	83	3	46
SAUSAGE & PEPPERONI PIZZA, LARGE 14"								
Brooklyn	1 slice	350	20	8.5	930	28	1	16
Deep Dish	1 slice	375	20	7.5	985	39	4	14
Hand Tossed	1 slice	335	16	6.5	795	35	2	13
Thin Crust	1 slice	275	16	6	615	20	1	10
SIDES								
Barbeque Buffalo Wings	2 pieces	230	14	3.5	410	6	0	17
Breadsticks	1 piece	110	6	1.5	100	11	0	6

	SERVING SIZE	CALORIES	TOTAL FAT (G)	SAT FAT (G)	SODIUM (MG)	CARBS (G)	FIBER (G)	PROTEIN (G)
Buffalo Chicken Kickers	2 pieces	100	5	1	280	7	1	9
Cheesy Bread	1 piece	120	6	2	140	11	0	4
Cinna Stix	1 piece	120	6	1	85	14	1	2
Hot Buffalo Wings	2 pieces	200	14	3.5	690	2	0	16
SPECIALTY PIZZA, LARGE 14", ON HAND-TOSSED CRUST								
Bacon Cheeseburger Feast	1 slice	380	19	9	830	36	2	17
Buffalo Chicken	1 slice	350	17	8.5	880	32	1	17
Cali Chicken Bacon Ranch	1 slice	430	25	9	900	33	1	19
Deluxe Feast	1 slice	320	14	6	730	36	2	13
ExtravaganZZa Feast	1 slice	390	19	8	1020	37	2	17
Fiery Hawaiian (Hot Sauce)	1 slice	350	16	6.5	1030	36	2	15
MeatZZa Feast	1 slice	380	19	8	1030	36	2	18
Memphis BBQ Chicken	1 slice	360	15	7.5	680	37	1	16
Pacific Veggie	1 slice	320	14	6.5	640	34	2	13
Philly Cheese Steak	1 slice	330	16	8	690	32	1	15
Ultimate Pepperoni Feast	1 slice	360	18	8	880	34	2	15
Wisconsin 6 Cheese	1 slice	340	16	7.5	690	34	2	15
VEGETABLE PIZZA (ONIONS, MUSHROOMS, GREEN PEPPERS, BLACK OLIVES), LARGE 14"								
Brooklyn	1 slice	260	12	5	630	27	1	12
Deep Dish	1 slice	310	14	5	760	38	4	11
Hand Tossed	1 slice	270	10	4	570	34	2	10
Thin Crust	1 slice	210	11	3.5	390	19	1	7

Don Pablo's
APPETIZERS, W/O SIDES

	SERVING SIZE	CALORIES	TOTAL FAT (G)	SAT FAT (G)	SODIUM (MG)	CARBS (G)	FIBER (G)	PROTEIN (G)
Cantina Nachos	as served	901	39	19	2202	104	12	35
Fajita Nachos, Mesquite-Grilled Chicken	as served	1321	76	41	2398	89	110	72
Fajita Nachos, Mesquite-Grilled Steak	as served	1394	81	46	2372	74	10	92
Flautas	as served	507	29	14	1274	40	7	27
Quesadillas, Mesquite-Grilled Chicken, Large	as served	1557	93	42	2798	119	5	61
Quesadillas, Mesquite-Grilled Steak, Large	as served	1630	99	47	2772	104	5	82
BURRITOS, CARNITAS & CHIMICHANGAS, W/O SIDES								
Bean Burrito	1 entrée	1188	56	28	2783	127	13	43

restaurants

	SERVING SIZE	CALORIES	TOTAL FAT (G)	SAT FAT (G)	SODIUM (MG)	CARBS (G)	FIBER (G)	PROTEIN (G)
Carnita, Pork	1 entrée	789	31	11	2330	82	11	49
Chimichanga, Chicken	1 entrée	991	59	20	2907	69	7	47
Chimichanga, Spicy Beef De Oro	1 entrée	1358	79	28	2509	89	15	72
COMBOS, W/O SIDES								
Cinco Combo	1 entrée	1222	69	33	3300	71	8	80
Conquistador	1 entrée	1572	86	31	3861	117	12	84
El Matador	1 entrée	1059	62	30	2904	65	9	62
Mexicano	1 entrée	736	45	20	1728	59	6	53
Numero Uno Favorito	1 entrée	979	54	23	2660	77	7	49
Presidente	1 entrée	1068	60	29	3297	72	6	61
San Angelo	1 entrée	1100	57	27	3333	90	7	58
Tejas	1 entrée	707	43	21	1797	39	5	42
ENCHILADAS, W/O SIDES								
Four Amigos	1 entrée	1028	65	32	3004	57	6	55
Mama's Skinny	1 entrée	465	22	9	1710	30	3	36
Three Amigos	1 entrée	671	42	21	2090	27	3	45
MESQUITE-GRILLED FAVORITES, W/O SAUCES OR SIDES								
Grilled Chicken & Shrimp	1 entrée	470	26	4	2362	39	2	23
Steak & Enchiladas	1 entrée	1331	101	47	3144	20	2	80
PRIMO TACOS, W/O SIDES								
Chipotle Pork Taco Trio	1 entrée	808	39	18	1962	69	5	46
Crispy Chicken Taco Trio	1 entrée	1005	54	190	2200	93	6	40
Fried Fish Tacos	1 entrée	1018	56	16	2326	77	4	53
SALADS, W/O DRESSING								
Original Caesar Salad, w/Chicken	1 salad	874	32	6	1285	114	11	34
Red River Salad	1 salad	479	21	3	1842	51	8	25
Sizzling Fajita Salad, Chicken, w/o Salsa	1 salad	841	45	15	1268	81	14	36
Sizzling Fajita Salad, Steak, w/o Salsa	1 salad	895	49	19	1248	69	14	52
Southwest Salad, w/Buffalo Sauce	1 salad	950	57	15	4877	73	11	45
Southwest Salad, w/Chipotle-Honey BBQ Sauce	1 salad	1214	67	17	3219	118	12	46
Taco Salad, Beef, w/Fried Tortilla Shell, w/o Salsa	1 salad	1380	73	32	2593	102	18	79
SIZZLIN' FAJITAS, W/SIDES								
Mesquite-Grilled Chicken	1 entrée	572	27	4	1283	58	3	29
Mesquite-Grilled Steak	1 entrée	681	36	11	1244	36	3	59

	SERVING SIZE	CALORIES	TOTAL FAT (G)	SAT FAT (G)	SODIUM (MG)	CARBS (G)	FIBER (G)	PROTEIN (G)
Pecos Valley Veggie	1 entrée	334	20	3	315	39	8	7
TASTES OF TEXAS, W/O SIDES								
Rio Grande Ribs, Full Rack, w/BBQ Sauce	1 entrée	1001	85	25	3878	32	1	58
Texas Two Step	1/2 entrée	842	53	14	3551	57	2	51
The Ultimate Tex-Mex Combo, Steak, w/Peppers & Onions	1 entrée	947	68	19	2570	44	4	60

Donatos
PIZZA, BAKERY

	SERVING SIZE	CALORIES	TOTAL FAT (G)	SAT FAT (G)	SODIUM (MG)	CARBS (G)	FIBER (G)	PROTEIN (G)
Pepperoni	2 slices	690	28	12	1580	75	5	35
The Works	2 slices	750	31	13	1770	79	6	38
Vegy	2 slices	640	22	10	1770	80	6	31
PIZZA, HAND TOSSED								
Pepperoni	2 slices	499	27	12	1439	65	5	23
The Works	2 slices	669	31	14	1622	68	6	28
Vegy	2 slices	550	19	10	1489	70	6	22
PIZZA, THICKER CRUST, LARGE								
Pepperoni	1/4 pizza	710	32	14	1710	69	5	36
Serious Cheese	1/4 pizza	700	30	15	1750	69	5	38
The Works	1/4 pizza	760	35	15	1910	74	6	39
Vegy	1/4 pizza	620	22	10	1910	75	7	30
PIZZA, THIN CRUST, LARGE								
Pepperoni	1/4 pizza	627	34	15	1471	50	2	32
Serious Cheese	1/4 pizza	710	31	15	1800	69	5	38
The Works	1/4 pizza	689	37	15	1716	56	4	35
Vegy	1/4 pizza	544	24	11	1675	57	4	26
STARTERS								
Buffalo Wings, Hot	5 wings	597	48	11	2236	11	0	34
Buffalo Wings, Mild	5 wings	618	48	10	2355	13	0	34
Buffalo Wings, Plain	5 wings	552	43	10	1297	10	0	34
STROMBOLI								
Cheese	1 stromboli	693	31	15	1773	66	5	35
Deluxe	1 stromboli	613	25	10	1588	68	5	28
Pepperoni	1 stromboli	716	34	14	1775	67	5	34
Vegy	1 stromboli	606	24	10	1877	69	5	27

Dunkin' Donuts
BAGELS

	SERVING SIZE	CALORIES	TOTAL FAT (G)	SAT FAT (G)	SODIUM (MG)	CARBS (G)	FIBER (G)	PROTEIN (G)
Blueberry	1 bagel	320	1	0	570	68	4	11

restaurants

	SERVING SIZE	CALORIES	TOTAL FAT (G)	SAT FAT (G)	SODIUM (MG)	CARBS (G)	FIBER (G)	PROTEIN (G)
Cinnamon Raisin	1 bagel	320	1	0	500	66	4	12
Everything	1 bagel	340	3	0	630	67	5	12
Multigrain	1 bagel	330	6	0.5	500	58	7	13
Plain	1 bagel	310	1	0	620	64	4	11
Poppy Seed	1 bagel	350	4	0.5	630	66	5	12
Wheat	1 bagel	280	1	0	500	56	4	13
BEVERAGES, MEDIUM								
Coffee Coolatta, w/Milk	24 fl oz	360	6	3.5	130	75	0	6
Hot Chocolate	16 fl oz	320	11	10	400	58	2	3
Iced Coffee, w/Skim Milk & Splenda	24 fl oz	40	0	0	35	8	0	3
Latte Lite	16 fl oz	120	0	0	170	19	0	10
Mocha Coffee, w/Cream	14 fl oz	260	9	6	45	41	2	3
Peach-Flavored Sweetened Iced Tea	16 fl oz	90	0	0	0	21	0	0
Strawberry Fruit Coolatta	24 fl oz	350	0	0	55	86	0	0
Tropicana Orange Coolatta	24 fl oz	310	0	0	20	81	0	2
Vanilla Bean Coolatta	24 fl oz	630	9	5	220	138	0	4
Vanilla Chai	14 fl oz	330	8	8	180	53	1	11
BREAKFAST SANDWICHES								
Bacon, Egg & Cheese on Bagel	1 sandwich	520	17	6	1310	67	4	24
Bacon, Egg & Cheese on Croissant	1 sandwich	550	34	14	1050	41	2	20
Bacon, Egg & Cheese on English Muffin	1 sandwich	370	6	0	1030	34	1	18
Big N' Toasted	1 sandwich	530	28	10	1360	43	1	26
Egg & Cheese on Bagel	1 sandwich	470	14	5	1090	67	4	20
Egg & Cheese on Croissant	1 sandwich	500	30	12	840	40	2	16
Egg & Cheese on English Muffin	1 sandwich	320	15	5	820	34	1	14
Ham, Egg & Cheese on English Muffin	1 sandwich	350	16	6	1110	34	1	19
Sausage, Egg & Cheese on English Muffin	1 sandwich	530	34	13	1340	34	1	23
DONUTS								
Bavarian Kreme	1 doughnut	270	15	7	350	31	1	4
Boston Kreme	1 doughnut	310	16	7	370	39	1	3
Chocolate Frosted	1 doughnut	270	15	7	340	31	1	3
Chocolate Glazed Cake	1 doughnut	370	24	11	390	35	1	3
Éclair	1 pastry	390	19	8	360	52	2	5
Glazed Cake	1 doughnut	360	22	10	300	44	1	3
Glazed Cake Stick	1 stick	370	18	8	420	48	1	4

	SERVING SIZE	CALORIES	TOTAL FAT (G)	SAT FAT (G)	SODIUM (MG)	CARBS (G)	FIBER (G)	PROTEIN (G)
Jelly Filled	1 doughnut	290	14	7	340	36	1	3
Old-Fashioned Cake	1 doughnut	320	22	10	300	33	1	3
Powdered Cake	1 doughnut	340	22	10	300	38	1	4
Vanilla Kreme	1 doughnut	380	23	10	370	42	1	4
MUFFINS								
Blueberry	1 muffin	460	15	3	450	76	2	6
Blueberry, Reduced-Fat	1 muffin	410	10	2	620	75	2	7
Corn	1 muffin	460	16	3	470	72	1	6
MUNCHKINS								
Glazed	1 piece	70	4	1.5	65	8	0	1
Glazed Chocolate Cake	1 piece	70	4	1.5	85	8	0	1
Jelly Filled	1 piece	80	4	2	85	9	0	1
Plain Cake	1 piece	60	4	1.5	65	6	0	1
Powdered Cake	1 piece	60	4	1.5	65	7	0	1
WAKE-UP WRAP								
Egg & Cheese	1 wrap	180	11	4	470	14	1	8
Egg White & Turkey Sausage	1 wrap	150	5	2.5	400	14	1	11
Egg White & Veggie	1 wrap	150	6	3	340	14	1	10
Sausage, Egg & Cheese	1 wrap	290	20	8	730	14	1	12

Eat 'N Park
APPETIZERS

	SERVING SIZE	CALORIES	TOTAL FAT (G)	SAT FAT (G)	SODIUM (MG)	CARBS (G)	FIBER (G)	PROTEIN (G)
Appetizer Platter	as served	1338	88	n/a	2236	76	5	61
Grilled Chicken Quesadilla	as served	907	55	n/a	1131	51	6	53
Hand-Breaded Zucchini	as served	478	26	n/a	630	50	4	14
Onion Rings Basket	as served	366	24	n/a	338	34	1	8
Spinach Artichoke Dip	as served	637	42	n/a	1171	42	5	25
BREAKFAST								
All-American Scrambler, w/Bacon	as served	619	29	n/a	1650	55	2	34
Buttermilk Pancakes	3 pancakes	223	3	n/a	703	43	2	6
Grilled Stickies & Eggs	as served	790	47	n/a	1334	65	2	19
Ground Sirloin & Eggs Smile	as served	807	60	n/a	602	22	1	55
Home Fries	as served	208	12	n/a	177	24	3	2
Meat Lover's Omelette	as served	726	55	n/a	2070	3	0	51
Oatmeal, w/Milk	as served	202	4	n/a	56	33	4	10
Skinny Scrambler	as served	354	13	n/a	1147	33	4	27
Veggie Omelette	as served	415	30	n/a	752	8	2	28

restaurants

	SERVING SIZE	CALORIES	TOTAL FAT (G)	SAT FAT (G)	SODIUM (MG)	CARBS (G)	FIBER (G)	PROTEIN (G)
BURGERS & SANDWICHES								
Black Angus American Grill Burger	1 burger	612	37	n/a	711	31	2	38
Black Angus BBQ Bacon & Cheddar Burger	1 burger	865	53	n/a	1908	53	2	44
Black Angus Mushroom & Onion Burger	1 burger	712	41	n/a	1486	45	2	40
Black Angus Superburger	1 burger	1086	73	n/a	1477	28	2	75
Chargrilled Chicken Sandwich	1 sandwich	318	6	n/a	394	32	1	31
Chicken BLT	1 sandwich	542	28	n/a	984	26	4	46
Classic Gardenburger	1 burger	292	5	n/a	940	44	5	19
Original Superburger	1 burger	563	38	n/a	1039	27	2	26
Philly Steak & Cheese	1 sandwich	839	48	n/a	1331	50	3	51
Santa Fe Turkey & Bacon Sandwich	1 sandwich	878	60	n/a	3476	45	2	40
Whale of a Cod Fish Sandwich	1 sandwich	882	41	n/a	1192	76	3	49
Whitefish Sandwich	1 sandwich	446	14	n/a	523	53	3	25
DESSERT								
Grilled Stickies à la Mode	as served	727	39	n/a	1267	81	2	9
DINNERS								
Beef Liver & Onions	1 entrée	299	11	n/a	94	13	1	35
Chargrilled Sockeye Salmon	1 entrée	287	15	n/a	88	0	0	36
Chicken & Broccoli Alfredo	1 entrée	630	19	n/a	702	66	5	46
Chicken Parmigiana, w/Marinara Sauce	1 entrée	959	37	n/a	1581	100	7	56
Chicken Stir-Fry	1 entrée	392	8	n/a	124	47	6	34
Mile-High Meatloaf	1 entrée	897	56	n/a	1717	58	3	41
Seafood Pasta Bake	1 entrée	855	53	n/a	1342	38	2	34
Sesame Pork Chops, 2 chops	1 entrée	400	23	n/a	1290	3	0	43
Smothered Ground Sirloin Steak	1 entrée	447	27	n/a	371	8	1	41
T-Bone Steak	1 entrée	576	39	n/a	104	1	1	51
SALADS, W/O DRESSING								
Buffalo Chicken	1 salad	609	35	n/a	2387	42	7	34
Grilled Chicken	1 salad	444	19	n/a	217	30	5	37
Grilled Chicken Portobella	1 salad	320	11	n/a	499	23	5	33
Steak	1 salad	740	46	n/a	290	33	8	49
Strawberry Chicken	1 salad	215	6	n/a	134	13	8	29
Einstein Bros. Bagels								
BAGEL THIN SINGLES								
Everything	1 bagel	160	2	0	400	29	1	6

	SERVING SIZE	CALORIES	TOTAL FAT (G)	SAT FAT (G)	SODIUM (MG)	CARBS (G)	FIBER (G)	PROTEIN (G)
Honey Whole Wheat	1 bagel	140	2	0	120	28	4	6
Oatmeal	1 bagel	150	1	0	0	32	2	4
Plain	1 bagel	140	1	0	240	29	1	5
CLASSIC BAGELS								
Everything	1 bagel	270	2	0	620	56	2	9
Honey Whole Wheat	1 bagel	250	1	0	440	56	3	9
Plain	1 bagel	260	1	0	460	56	2	9
GOURMET BAGELS								
Power Bagel	1 bagel	310	5	0.5	280	61	4	11
Spinach Florentine	1 bagel	320	6	3.5	570	56	2	13
SIGNATURE BAGELS								
Asiago Cheese	1 bagel	310	5	3	630	56	2	14
Cinnamon Raisin	1 bagel	290	1	0	450	63	3	10
Garlic	1 bagel	270	3	0	460	56	2	9
Good Grains	1 bagel	270	3	0	440	57	3	10
Onion	1 bagel	270	1	0	460	59	2	9
Poppy	1 bagel	280	3	0	460	56	2	9
Sesame	1 bagel	280	3	0	460	56	2	10
EGG SANDWICHES								
Bacon & Cheddar	1 sandwich	510	19	8	840	58	2	28
Ham & Swiss	1 sandwich	490	16	6	1180	59	2	32
Nova Lox & Bagel	1 sandwich	480	18	9	930	62	3	23
Turkey Sausage & Cheddar	1 sandwich	540	20	8	890	59	2	33
SIGNATURE SANDWICHES								
Club Mex, on Challah	1 sandwich	540	23	6	1760	53	2	34
Tasty Turkey, on Asiago Bagel	1 sandwich	540	18	10	1440	65	3	36
Veg Out, on Sesame Seed Bagel	1 sandwich	400	11	5	610	66	5	14

El Pollo Loco
BOWLS, SALADS & SOUPS

	SERVING SIZE	CALORIES	TOTAL FAT (G)	SAT FAT (G)	SODIUM (MG)	CARBS (G)	FIBER (G)	PROTEIN (G)
Chicken Tostada Salad, w/o Dressing	1 salad	900	43	12	1490	86	7	41
Grilled Chicken Salad, w/o Dressing	1 salad	230	7	2	520	18	3	26
Original Pollo Bowl	1 bowl	680	11	2	1870	106	12	40
Ultimate Pollo Bowl	1 bowl	1040	34	14	2500	110	14	70
BURRITOS								
Califresco	1 burrito	853	35	12	2494	87	7	47
El Tradicional	1 burrito	785	31	11	1860	86	7	40
Poblano	1 burrito	910	39	12	2340	93	9	49

restaurants

	SERVING SIZE	CALORIES	TOTAL FAT (G)	SAT FAT (G)	SODIUM (MG)	CARBS (G)	FIBER (G)	PROTEIN (G)
Spicy Chipotle	1 burrito	845	35	14	2136	83	6	48
FLAME-GRILLED CHICKEN								
Chicken Breast	1 breast	220	9	2.5	620	0	0	36
Chicken Breast, Skinless	1 breast	180	4	1	560	0	0	35
Leg	1 leg	90	1	0	170	0	0	12
Thigh	1 thigh	220	15	4.5	320	0	0	21
Wing	1 wing	90	5	1.5	290	0	0	11
LOCO VALUE MENU								
Chicken Taquito, w/Avocado Salsa	1 serving	230	12	2.5	590	20	2	10
Crunchy Chicken Taco	1 taco	190	8	2.5	480	16	2	12
Taco al Carbón	1 taco	160	6	1.4	290	17	1	10
SIDES								
BBQ Black Beans	as served	200	3	0.4	520	36	4	7
French Fries (Small)	as served	330	17	3	680	42	4	4
Macaroni & Cheese	as served	280	17	11	770	28	0	11

Famous Dave's
BARBECUE CLASSICS, W/CORNBREAD MUFFIN & CORN ON THE COB

	SERVING SIZE	CALORIES	TOTAL FAT (G)	SAT FAT (G)	SODIUM (MG)	CARBS (G)	FIBER (G)	PROTEIN (G)
Barbeque Chicken	as served	880	54	16	4470	26	0	73
BBQ Chicken Wings Platter, w/Blue Cheese Dipping Sauce	as served	940	61	14	3160	31	3	68
Georgia Chopped Pork	as served	530	21	7	2860	38	1	47
St. Louis Style, Baby Back Ribs, Big Baby	as served	1150	67	24	2380	35	2	103
St. Louis Style, Memphis, Baby Back Ribs, Big Baby	as served	1010	60	21	2750	12	2	107
St. Louis Style, XXL Ribs, "The Big Slab"	as served	1810	117	45	2800	54	3	139
Texas Beef Brisket	as served	840	50	20	3100	30	< 1	66
RIB-N-RIB COMBO, W/CORNBREAD MUFFIN & CORN ON THE COB								
Baby Back Ribs	1/2 slab	570	34	12	1190	17	< 1	52
Memphis Baby Ribs	1/2 slab	500	30	10	1370	6	1	53
St. Louis Ribs	1/2 slab	900	58	22	1400	27	< 1	69
SIDE DISHES								
Dave's Cheesy Mac & Cheese	as served	240	14	5	630	23	2	9
Famous Fries	as served	540	21	4.5	810	89	9	9
Garlic Red-Skin Mashed Potatoes	as served	100	4	1.5	290	14	1	2
Wilbur Beans	as served	150	4	1	450	26	4	8

	SERVING SIZE	CALORIES	TOTAL FAT (G)	SAT FAT (G)	SODIUM (MG)	CARBS (G)	FIBER (G)	PROTEIN (G)
Fatburger								
BURGERS & SANDWICHES								
Bacon & Egg Sandwich	1 sandwich	350	16	5	970	37	1	18
Crispy Chicken Sandwich	1 sandwich	560	27	5	1540	53	2	26
Fatburger, Large	1 burger	850	41	13	1490	69	4	50
Fish Sandwich	1 sandwich	560	31	5	850	55	2	20
Sausage & Egg Sandwich	1 sandwich	780	53	21	1810	47	1	27
Spicy Chicken Sandwich	1 sandwich	520	21	6	2160	58	2	26
Turkeyburger	1 burger	480	21	4.5	1270	50	3	26
Veggieburger	1 burger	510	20	4.5	1560	60	11	33
HOT DOGS								
Chili Cheese	1 hot dog	480	27	11	1150	35	2	24
Regular	1 hot dog	320	15	6	780	32	1	13
SHAKES & FLOATS								
Big Fat Float	16 fl oz	390	12	8	140	73	0	3
Shakes, Average of Chocolate, Vanilla, & Strawberry	16 fl oz	893	44	30	370	113	1	14
SIDES								
Chili Cheese Fat Fries	as served	590	33	11	590	53	6	21
Chili Fat Fries	as served	480	24	6	410	52	6	14
Fat Fries	as served	380	18	4	40	47	5	6
Onion Rings	as served	540	29	6	490	64	4	7
Skinny Fries	as served	390	15	3.5	730	58	4	4
Fazoli's								
FRESH CHOPPED SALADS, W/DRESSING								
Cherry Almond Chicken	1 salad	480	25	6	1190	38	5	26
Citrus Apple & Roasted Chicken	1 salad	510	30	9	1700	30	6	31
Pasta Ranch Italia	1 salad	770	50	14	2290	44	4	38
OVEN-BAKED PASTA & SPECIALTY PASTA								
Baked Spaghetti, w/Meatballs	1 entrée	890	39	20	2040	86	7	41
Cheesy Baked Ziti	1 entrée	670	27	15	1630	71	7	34
Chicken Carbonara	1 entrée	800	27	13	1790	88	4	42
Chicken Parmigano	1 entrée	1000	39	15	2550	108	8	51
Four Cheese Lasagna	1 entrée	1000	49	27	2560	79	5	59
Penne Romano	1 entrée	880	44	20	2460	76	7	44
Penne w/Creamy Basil Chicken	1 entrée	980	51	25	2400	72	4	51

restaurants

	SERVING SIZE	CALORIES	TOTAL FAT (G)	SAT FAT (G)	SODIUM (MG)	CARBS (G)	FIBER (G)	PROTEIN (G)
PICK YOUR PASTA								
Fettuccine, w/Alfredo	1 entrée	800	26	15	1480	108	5	26
Ravioli, w/Meat Sauce	1 entrée	570	24	12	2190	58	7	32
PIZZA								
Pepperoni Classico	1 slice	300	13	6	810	32	2	14
Triple Cheese	1 slice	290	12	6	730	32	2	14
SAMPLERS								
Classic	1 entrée	890	25	11	2270	122	9	39
Italian	1 entrée	980	29	12	2100	122	9	51
Ultimate	1 entrée	1130	34	16	2740	153	12	49

Finagle a Bagel
BAGELS

	SERVING SIZE	CALORIES	TOTAL FAT (G)	SAT FAT (G)	SODIUM (MG)	CARBS (G)	FIBER (G)	PROTEIN (G)
100% Whole Wheat	1 bagel	320	4	1	444	62	6	14
Blueberry	1 bagel	299	2	0	391	66	4	9
Chocolate Chip	1 bagel	329	4	3	391	66	4	10
Cinnamon Raisin	1 bagel	300	1	0	350	67	5	8
Egg	1 bagel	293	2	0.5	480	61	5	12
Jalapeño	1 bagel	267	1	0	418	61	4	10
Onion	1 bagel	300	1	0	380	65	4	9
Plain	1 bagel	290	1	0	410	63	4	8
Sesame	1 bagel	310	5	1.5	380	60	5	10
CREAM CHEESE								
Garden Scallion, Light	2 tbsp	60	6	3	120	1	0	2
Nova Scotia Salmon	2 tbsp	90	9	6	160	2	0	3

Firehouse Subs
SUBS, MEDIUM, ON WHITE

	SERVING SIZE	CALORIES	TOTAL FAT (G)	SAT FAT (G)	SODIUM (MG)	CARBS (G)	FIBER (G)	PROTEIN (G)
Beef Brisket	1 sub	890	59	19	1690	64	2	30
Beef Brisket, Double Meat	1 sub	1170	84	29	2400	64	2	46
Chicken	1 sub	690	38	9	1750	55	3	37
Club, Double Meat	1 sub	990	51	14	2940	74	3	66
Engine Company	1 sub	700	36	9	1750	57	4	36
Engineer	1 sub	690	35	8	1910	61	3	39
Hero	1 sub	770	37	9	2170	64	3	48
Hook & Ladder	1 sub	700	36	9	1660	64	3	35
Italian	1 sub	910	57	16	2430	64	3	38
Roast Beef	1 sub	710	36	9	1820	54	3	39
Steak	1 sub	770	46	12	1720	56	3	38

	SERVING SIZE	CALORIES	TOTAL FAT (G)	SAT FAT (G)	SODIUM (MG)	CARBS (G)	FIBER (G)	PROTEIN (G)
Steamer	1 sub	720	43	10	2360	51	2	33
Tuna	1 sub	1000	68	12	1610	67	4	36
Turkey	1 sub	670	34	8	1850	58	3	37
Veggie	1 sub	720	45	13	1520	60	4	25

Five Guys Burgers and Fries
BURGERS

	SERVING SIZE	CALORIES	TOTAL FAT (G)	SAT FAT (G)	SODIUM (MG)	CARBS (G)	FIBER (G)	PROTEIN (G)
Bacon Burger	1 burger	780	50	22.5	690	39	2	43
Bacon Cheeseburger	1 burger	920	62	29.5	1310	40	2	51
Cheeseburger	1 burger	840	55	26.5	1050	40	2	47
Hamburger	1 burger	700	43	19.5	430	39	2	39
DOGS								
Bacon Cheese Dog	1 hot dog	695	48	22	1700	40	2	26
Bacon Dog	1 hot dog	625	42	18.5	1390	40	2	22
Cheese Dog	1 hot dog	615	41	19	1440	40	2	22
Hot Dog	1 hot dog	545	35	15.5	1130	40	2	18
Fries, Regular	1/2 order	310	15	3	45	39	3	5
LITTLE BURGERS								
Little Bacon Burger	1 burger	560	33	14.5	640	39	2	27
Little Bacon Cheeseburger	1 burger	630	39	18	950	40	2	31
Little Cheeseburger	1 burger	550	32	15	690	40	2	27
Little Hamburger	1 burger	480	26	11.5	380	39	2	23
OTHER SANDWICHES								
Grilled Cheese	1 sandwich	470	26	9	715	41	2	11
Veggie Sandwich	1 sandwich	440	15	6	1040	60	2	16

Freshens
BLENDED FRUIT CLASSIC SMOOTHIES

	SERVING SIZE	CALORIES	TOTAL FAT (G)	SAT FAT (G)	SODIUM (MG)	CARBS (G)	FIBER (G)	PROTEIN (G)
Citrus Mango	1 smoothie	490	7	4.5	60	108	1	2
Orange Sunrise	1 smoothie	360	3	1.5	45	82	2	3
Peach Sunset	1 smoothie	270	0	0	20	67	1	1
Strawberry Kiwi	1 smoothie	320	0	0	15	81	1	0
Tropical Pineapple	1 smoothie	310	4	3	20	97	1	0
BREAKFAST CREPES								
Egg White Florentine	1 crepe	270	8	4.5	710	24	2	22
Wake Up	1 crepe	420	22	11	660	23	1	28
DESSERT CREPES								
Nutella Supreme	1 crepe	600	22	8	160	88	5	14

restaurants	SERVING SIZE	CALORIES	TOTAL FAT (G)	SAT FAT (G)	SODIUM (MG)	CARBS (G)	FIBER (G)	PROTEIN (G)
The Guilty Pleasure	1 crepe	540	13	3	200	91	5	16
FRO-YO BLAST								
Oreo Overload	1 blast	430	4	1	370	83	1	12
Reese's Pieces & Peanut Butter	1 blast	680	19	7	390	105	3	20
INDULGENT SHAKES								
Oreo Cream	1 shake	610	7	3	460	115	1	16
Vanilla	1 shake	510	4	2.5	280	99	0	15
SAVORY CREPES								
Fajita Chicken	1 crepe	500	13	7	1310	58	6	32
Greek Salad	1 crepe	370	9	3.5	660	52	5	15
Harvest Salad	1 crepe	520	12	4	1060	73	6	30
Honey Mustard Chicken	1 crepe	470	14	6	1160	52	3	31
Philly Cheese Steak	1 crepe	650	30	12	1470	55	6	36
Southwest Chicken	1 crepe	610	27	8	1290	57	5	32
Tomato, Cheese & Basil	1 crepe	460	18	11	710	49	5	24
SMOOTHIES								
High Protein, Peanut Butter	1 smoothie	540	12	2.5	350	84	2	26
Low Calorie, Strawberry Oasis, No Sugar Added	1 smoothie	70	0	0	10	50	1	0
Friendly's **BIG BEEF BURGERS**								
All American Burger	1 entrée	1060	60	18	1110	92	7	39
BBQ Fronion Burger	1 entrée	1520	90	30	1690	129	8	51
Grilled Cheese Burger	1 entrée	1540	92	35	2490	124	9	55
Patty Melt	1 entrée	1290	71	26	1120	111	8	52
Swiss 'N' Mushroom Bacon Burger	1 entrée	1450	94	32	1840	97	6	56
CREATE YOUR OWN, TOPPINGS								
Caramel Topping	as served	130	2	1	130	28	0	0
Hot Fudge Topping	as served	110	4	4	46	18	1	2
Marshmallow Topping	as served	70	0	0	7	18	0	0
No-Sugar-Added Fudge Topping	as served	90	0	0	0	25	2	1
Peanut Butter Topping	as served	210	17	3	130	7	3	7
Whipped Topping	as served	80	6	4	21	6	0	1
ENTRÉES								
Bourbon BBQ Chicken	1 entrée	1480	73	27	3230	121	9	87
Chicken Strips Basket, 6 Pieces, w/Honey Mustard	1 entrée	1330	80	12	1720	112	8	43

	SERVING SIZE	CALORIES	TOTAL FAT (G)	SAT FAT (G)	SODIUM (MG)	CARBS (G)	FIBER (G)	PROTEIN (G)
Honey BBQ Chicken Strips, 6 Strips	1 entrée	1680	81	13	2430	196	8	45
Kickin' Buffalo Chicken Strips, 6 Strips	1 entrée	1650	116	16	3040	105	8	46
FOUNTAIN BEVERAGES								
Barq's Float	as served	590	21	14	150	98	0	6
Original Fribble, Chocolate	as served	720	20	13	390	119	1	17
Original Fribble, Coffee	as served	640	20	12	360	102	0	16
Original Fribble, Strawberry	as served	650	20	12	460	103	0	16
Original Fribble, Vanilla	as served	640	20	12	360	100	0	16
FRIEND-Z								
Birthday Cake	as served	690	29	13	270	100	0	9
Butterfinger	as served	820	32	19	430	122	3	11
Chips Ahoy!	as served	580	25	12	350	80	1	10
Heath	as served	680	34	19	410	88	0	9
Kit Kat	as served	790	31	20	280	115	2	12
M&M's	as served	670	24	14	260	103	2	10
Oreo	as served	580	23	12	470	84	2	9
Reese's Peanut Butter Cup	as served	860	45	19	500	95	5	19
Strawberry Banana	as served	430	14	9	220	69	1	8
Strawberry Shortcake	as served	470	17	9	260	72	1	8
ICE CREAM, SINGLE SCOOP								
Black Raspberry	1 scoop	120	5	4	35	15	0	2
Butter Pecan	1 scoop	130	8	4	37	13	0	2
Chocolate	1 scoop	110	6	4	41	10	0	2
Chocolate Chip Cookie Dough	1 scoop	140	7	4	42	17	0	2
Coffee	1 scoop	110	6	4	35	13	0	2
Cookies 'N Cream	1 scoop	130	6	4	55	16	0	2
Peanut Butter Cup	1 scoop	160	9	4	70	16	1	3
Soft Serve, Average of All Flavors	8 oz	107	5	3	35	14	1	3
Strawberry	1 scoop	110	5	3	35	14	0	2
Vanilla	1 scoop	120	6	4	35	14	0	2
MUNCHIES & STARTERS								
Chicken Quesadilla	as served	570	35	15	1330	29	3	35
Kickin' Buffalo Chicken Strips	as served	1090	88	21	2740	39	4	35
Loaded Waffle Fries	as served	1670	114	28	4780	123	9	31
Mini Mozzarella Cheese Sticks	as served	680	40	14	1850	56	3	25
SALADS, W/O DRESSING								
Apple Harvest Chicken	1 salad	570	33	9	2370	31	5	38

restaurants

	SERVING SIZE	CALORIES	TOTAL FAT (G)	SAT FAT (G)	SODIUM (MG)	CARBS (G)	FIBER (G)	PROTEIN (G)
Bleu Moon Sirloin	1 salad	750	37	11	2800	62	8	44
Kickin' Buffalo Chicken	1 salad	1180	95	19	2090	45	7	35
SANDWICHES								
Buffalo Chicken Wrap	1 entrée	1520	94	21	2650	124	9	42
Crispy Chicken Wrap	1 entrée	1140	55	10	1620	133	9	31
Fishamajig	1 entrée	990	51	15	1580	104	6	30
Friendly Frank	1 entrée	750	44	14	1070	74	5	15
Grilled Cheese	1 entrée	800	37	14	1280	96	6	20
SUNDAE CREATIONS, LAVA CAKES & MORE								
Butterfinger Sundae	1 sundae	830	36	23	370	117	2	9
Caramel Cone Crunch Sundae	1 sundae	700	33	20	280	91	3	11
Caramel Fudge Oreo Brownie Sundae	1 sundae	1410	66	40	620	186	2	19
Forbidden Chocolate Lava Cake Sundae	1 sundae	1280	51	30	660	186	6	19
Forbidden Fudge Oreo Brownie Sundae	1 sundae	940	41	51	320	129	6	13
Giant Crowd Pleaser	1 sundae	2470	118	65	920	317	5	41
Happy Ending Hot Fudge Sundae	1 sundae	330	17	11	110	40	1	5
Reese's Peanut Butter Cup (5 Scoops)	1 sundae	1190	70	62	460	123	7	21
Reese's Pieces Sundae (5 Scoops)	1 sundae	1330	71	38	460	152	4	23
Royal Banana Split	1 sundae	870	35	19	200	127	3	10
Strawberry Shortcake Sundae	1 sundae	580	27	16	190	79	2	8
Ultimate Cookies 'N' Cream	1 sundae	680	33	20	320	85	2	11
SUPERMELT SANDWICHES								
Reuben	1 entrée	1140	56	19	2900	106	6	53
Tuna	1 entrée	1110	63	13	1390	99	7	36
Turkey Club	1 entrée	1010	48	15	2280	103	6	43

Godfather's Pizza
GLUTEN-FREE, SMALL

	SERVING SIZE	CALORIES	TOTAL FAT (G)	SAT FAT (G)	SODIUM (MG)	CARBS (G)	FIBER (G)	PROTEIN (G)
Cheese	1 slice	140	5	2	380	18	1	5
Meat Combo	1 slice	190	8	3.5	570	18	1	9
GOLDEN CRUST, LARGE								
All Meat Combo	1 slice	340	16	6	760	29	2	17
Cheese	1 slice	250	9	3.5	440	28	1	11
Pepperoni	1 slice	290	12	4.5	560	28	1	12
Veggie	1 slice	260	10	3.5	500	30	2	11
MOZZARELLA LOADED CRUST, LARGE								
All Meat Combo	1 slice	390	21	8	890	30	2	20

	SERVING SIZE	CALORIES	TOTAL FAT (G)	SAT FAT (G)	SODIUM (MG)	CARBS (G)	FIBER (G)	PROTEIN (G)
Cheese	1 slice	300	14	6	560	29	1	13
Pepperoni	1 slice	340	17	7	690	29	1	14
Veggie	1 slice	310	14	6	630	30	2	13
ORIGINAL CRUST, LARGE								
All Meat Combo	1 slice	410	17	7	920	37	2	22
Cheese	1 slice	290	9	4	530	36	2	14
Pepperoni	1 slice	330	12	5	650	36	2	15
Veggie	1 slice	300	9	4	610	38	2	14
THIN CRUST, LARGE								
All Meat Combo	1 slice	300	17	6	610	19	1	16
Cheese	1 slice	210	10	3.5	270	17	1	9
Pepperoni	1 slice	240	13	5	400	18	1	10
Veggie	1 slice	220	10	3.5	340	19	1	9

Gold Star Chili
BURRITOS & BURRITO BOWLS

	SERVING SIZE	CALORIES	TOTAL FAT (G)	SAT FAT (G)	SODIUM (MG)	CARBS (G)	FIBER (G)	PROTEIN (G)
Chili Beef Burrito	1 entrée	968	33	n/a	1434	126	9	41
Gold Star Chili Burrito Bowl	1 entrée	898	33	n/a	1244	112	10	36
Veggie Chili Burrito	1 entrée	948	33	n/a	1381	126	7	7
Veggie Chili Burrito Bowl	1 entrée	878	33	n/a	1191	112	8	34
CHILI CLASSICS								
2-Way, Regular	1 entrée	394	10	n/a	1120	54	5	22
2-Way, Veggie, Regular	1 entrée	364	10	n/a	1040	54	7	14
3-Way, Regular	1 entrée	679	34	n/a	1560	55	5	39
3-Way, Veggie, Regular	1 entrée	650	34	n/a	1480	55	7	32
4-Way, Bean, Regular	1 entrée	827	34	n/a	1830	81	14	49
4-Way, Onion, Regular	1 entrée	697	34	n/a	1561	59	6	40
5-Way, Regular	1 entrée	795	34	n/a	1948	77	13	46
CONEYS								
Cheese Coney	1 entrée	310	19	n/a	765	21	1	14
Coney	1 entrée	225	12	n/a	633	21	1	9
DOUBLE DECKERS								
Beef & Bacon	1 entrée	627	31	n/a	1768	49	6	38
Ham & Bacon	1 entrée	513	29	n/a	943	40	6	22
Turkey & Bacon	1 entrée	591	30	n/a	1513	44	7	35
FRIES								
Chili Cheese Fries	as served	679	36	n/a	1364	63	9	27
Original	as served	401	16	n/a	467	58	7	7

restaurants

Good Times Burgers

	SERVING SIZE	CALORIES	TOTAL FAT (G)	SAT FAT (G)	SODIUM (MG)	CARBS (G)	FIBER (G)	PROTEIN (G)
BURGERS								
BBQ Bacon Double Craver	1 burger	600	27	10	1470	45	2	38
Bacon Cheeseburger	1 burger	830	38	11	2110	69	2	51
Big Daddy Bacon Cheeseburger	1 burger	1490	76	24	4060	100	3	98
Cheesy Double Craver	1 burger	460	23	10	740	30	1	29
Double Good Time Cheeseburger	1 burger	890	52	19	1530	46	2	60
Good Time Deluxe Cheeseburger	1 burger	590	30	10	1220	46	2	34
Mushroom Swiss Burger	1 burger	520	24	9	980	40	2	34
CHICKEN SANDWICHES								
BBQ Bacon Crispy Chicken	1 sandwich	850	31	6	2770	98	3	47
Buffalo Crispy Chicken	1 sandwich	510	19	2	1520	59	2	26
Crispy Chicken	1 sandwich	440	13	1	1050	57	2	26
Guacamole Bacon Chicken	1 sandwich	700	20	2	2460	77	7	54
Kickin' Chicken Craver	1 sandwich	230	6	1	380	33	1	11
FROZEN CUSTARD HANDSPUN CUPS								
Butter Pecan	as served	540	32	10	320	55	2	8
Chocolate	as served	360	14	9	210	52	0	6
Chocolate Chocolate Chip	as served	540	26	19	230	71	1	8
Cotton Candy	as served	380	15	9	150	56	0	6
Mint Chocolate Chip	as served	530	26	19	170	69	1	7
New York Cheesecake	as served	420	19	11	420	53	0	7
Peanut Butter	as served	450	28	11	250	41	1	12
Vanilla	as served	380	18	11	200	48	0	7
Verry Cherry	as served	410	14	9	160	64	0	6
SIDES								
Thick Cut, Beer-Battered Onion Rings	as served	530	29	7	850	62	5	5
Wild Fries, Regular	as served	260	13	4	560	32	3	3
SPOONBENDERS								
Caramel Toffee Crunch	16 oz	1270	63	35	740	167	0	14
Chocolate Cookie Dough	16 oz	970	43	23	500	132	0	15
Cookies & Cream	16 oz	1010	44	24	630	137	0	16
Peanut Butter Chocolate Crunch	16 oz	970	43	23	500	132	0	15
Strawberry Cheesecake Addiction	16 oz	1070	44	26	740	148	5	17
Turtle	16 oz	1310	75	28	490	140	3	19
SUNDAES & HANDSPUN SHAKES & MALTS								
Banana Malt	24 oz	1420	55	32	820	200	2	30

	SERVING SIZE	CALORIES	TOTAL FAT (G)	SAT FAT (G)	SODIUM (MG)	CARBS (G)	FIBER (G)	PROTEIN (G)
Banana Shake	24 oz	1130	48	29	540	152	0	20
Chocolate Malt	24 oz	1350	52	30	650	197	3	25
Chocolate Shake	24 oz	1290	50	29	600	190	3	23
Hot Fudge Peak Sundae	1 sundae	720	37	21	250	84	2	12
Root Beer Float	24 oz	710	28	17	340	107	0	11
Strawberry Shortcake Sundae	1 sundae	340	11	8	125	56	5	1
Turtle Sundae	1 sundae	950	46	21	410	120	1	13
Vanilla Shake	24 oz	1030	51	30	550	121	0	23

Great Steak and Potato Company

BAKED POTATOES

	SERVING SIZE	CALORIES	TOTAL FAT (G)	SAT FAT (G)	SODIUM (MG)	CARBS (G)	FIBER (G)	PROTEIN (G)
Broccoli & Cheese	1 potato	300	12	8	950	35	4	13
Cheese & Bacon	1 potato	430	23	12	730	29	3	25
Great Potato, Chicken	1 potato	500	22	11	1310	37	4	32
Great Potato, Steak	1 potato	520	26	11	1250	37	4	35
King	1 potato	490	29	16	740	31	3	26

BREAKFAST SANDWICHES

Bacon, Egg & Cheese	1 sandwich	600	36	11	1300	39	2	29
Egg & Cheese	1 sandwich	500	29	9	890	39	2	23
Ham, Egg & Cheese	1 sandwich	570	32	10	1540	42	2	31
Sausage, Egg & Cheese	1 sandwich	700	47	15	1300	39	2	30

BURGERS

Cheese	1 burger	600	39	11	730	33	2	29
Cheese, w/Bacon	1 burger	680	45	13	1050	33	2	34
Chili	1 burger	550	27	9	800	47	9	33
Hamburger	1 burger	550	34	8	470	32	2	26
Philly	1 burger	530	28	9	500	39	3	31

FRIES & SIDES

Cheese Fries, Large	as served	620	35	11	2060	63	7	15
Chili	as served	440	24	14	1480	34	19	27
Coney Island Fry, Large	as served	740	39	14	2630	77	15	24
Great Fry, Large	as served	540	25	4	1360	72	8	8
King Fry, Large	as served	880	55	21	2790	66	7	31
Nacho Fry, Large	as served	650	35	11	3520	67	7	15
Potato Skins	as served	390	26	12	1070	24	2	17

SALADS, NO DRESSING

Chef	1 salad	260	11	6	1320	15	4	28

restaurants

	SERVING SIZE	CALORIES	TOTAL FAT (G)	SAT FAT (G)	SODIUM (MG)	CARBS (G)	FIBER (G)	PROTEIN (G)
Great, w/Grilled Chicken	1 salad	380	18	8	460	18	5	31
Great, w/Grilled Steak	1 salad	400	23	7	590	18	5	33
SANDWICHES (7") & WRAPS								
Bacon Cheddar Cheesesteak	1 sandwich	720	32	12	1930	62	5	45
Buffalo Chicken Philly	1 sandwich	660	24	10	2420	65	5	37
Chicagoland Cheesesteak	1 sandwich	680	29	11	2480	63	5	43
Chicken Bacon Ranch	1 sandwich	990	56	18	1160	66	6	55
Great Steak Cheesesteak	1 sandwich	740	37	9	1270	62	5	41
Great Steak Cheesesteak Wrap	1 wrap	820	43	11	1400	67	5	40
Kansas City, BBQ Cheesesteak	1 sandwich	680	26	10	1740	71	5	40
Original Chicken Philly Wrap	1 wrap	700	28	11	1800	67	4	36
Original Philly Cheesesteak	1 sandwich	650	26	10	2570	62	5	40
Pepper Steak	1 sandwich	880	50	11	1370	67	6	42
Super Steak Cheesesteak Wrap	1 wrap	930	54	13	1500	69	5	41
Teriyaki Chicken Philly	1 sandwich	740	32	9	2280	65	5	40
Ultimate Chicken Philly Wrap	1 wrap	810	39	13	1720	69	5	36
Veggie Delight	1 sandwich	510	19	6	950	64	5	18
Green Burrito								
BURRITOS								
Bean & Cheese	1 burrito	470	19	8	1150	54	5	18
Bean & Cheese, Average of Chicken, Ground Beef & Steak	1 burrito	470	20	9	1290	49	4	24
Grilled Chicken	1 burrito	860	44	13	2070	77	3	35
The Green, Chicken	1 burrito	820	28	10	2690	100	9	42
The Green, Steak	1 burrito	850	31	12	2910	102	8	42
NACHOS, SUPER								
Chicken	as served	920	47	10	1670	90	10	34
Ground Beef	as served	1000	56	14	1720	93	13	30
Steak	as served	950	50	12	1890	92	10	34
QUESADILLAS								
Cheese	1 quesadilla	380	18	10	810	36	1	16
Chicken	1 quesadilla	470	20	10	1270	38	1	34
Steak	1 quesadilla	500	22	12	1500	41	1	33
TACO SALAD								
Chicken	1 salad	810	44	12	1730	64	9	40
Ground Beef	1 salad	880	53	16	1780	67	12	36
Steak	1 salad	840	47	14	1950	67	9	39

	SERVING SIZE	CALORIES	TOTAL FAT (G)	SAT FAT (G)	SODIUM (MG)	CARBS (G)	FIBER (G)	PROTEIN (G)
TACOS								
Fish	1 taco	320	15	2.5	500	36	4	9
Hard, Chicken	1 taco	190	8	3	350	14	2	14
Hard, Ground Beef	1 taco	210	12	5	340	15	3	11
Nacho	1 taco	180	9	3	380	16	3	8
Soft, Ground Beef	1 taco	220	11	5	570	19	2	12
Soft, Southwest Chicken	1 taco	300	19	6	680	17	1	15

Hardee's
BREAKFAST

	SERVING SIZE	CALORIES	TOTAL FAT (G)	SAT FAT (G)	SODIUM (MG)	CARBS (G)	FIBER (G)	PROTEIN (G)
Bacon, Egg & Cheese Biscuit	1 sandwich	400	25	8	1190	38	1	15
Big Country Breakfast Platter, w/Bacon	1 platter	810	40	10	1620	74	5	26
Biscuit 'N' Gravy	as served	410	23	6	1370	50	2	9
Chicken Fillet Biscuit	1 sandwich	500	26	5	1420	50	2	24
Country Fried Steak Biscuit	1 sandwich	470	29	8	1150	46	2	13
Country Ham Biscuit	1 sandwich	300	18	5	1590	38	1	15
Frisco Breakfast Sandwich	1 sandwich	430	19	7	1510	41	2	23
Ham, Egg & Cheese Biscuit	1 sandwich	400	22	7	1400	38	1	19
Hash Rounds, Medium	as served	390	26	4.5	490	36	4	3
Loaded Breakfast Burrito	1 burrito	770	49	21	1790	39	2	39
Loaded Omelet Biscuit	1 sandwich	490	31	11	1410	38	1	20
Low-Carb Breakfast Bowl	as served	650	54	20	1620	2		39
Monster Biscuit	1 sandwich	640	44	16	2130	40	1	30
Sausage & Egg Biscuit	1 sandwich	470	32	9	1160	38	1	16
Sunrise Croissant, w/Ham	1 sandwich	430	27	11	1090	27	1	21
FRIED CHICKEN								
Breast	1 breast	370	15	4	1190	29	0	29
Hand-Breaded Chicken Tenders	5 pieces	440	21	4.5	1290	21	3	41
Leg	1 leg	170	7	2	570	15	0	13
Thigh	1 thigh	330	15	4	1000	30	0	19
Wing	1 wing	200	8	2	740	23	0	10
SIDES								
Beer-Battered Onion Rings	as served	410	24	4.5	470	45	3	3
Crispy Curls, Medium	as served	410	20	5	1020	52	4	5
Natural-Cut French Fries, Medium	as served	430	19	4	960	60	4	5
THICKBURGERS & SANDWICHES								
1/3 lb Bacon Cheese Thickburger	1 burger	840	56	18	1560	49	3	38
1/3 lb Cheeseburger Thickburger	1 burger	620	33	13	1590	51	3	35

restaurants

	SERVING SIZE	CALORIES	TOTAL FAT (G)	SAT FAT (G)	SODIUM (MG)	CARBS (G)	FIBER (G)	PROTEIN (G)
1/3 lb Low Carb Thickburger	1 burger	470	36	13	1050	9	1	28
1/3 lb Original Thickburger	1 burger	860	58	17	1630	52	4	35
2/3 lb Monster Thickburger	1 burger	1290	92	35	2840	47	3	70
Charbroiled BBQ Chicken Sandwich	1 sandwich	380	6	1	1220	58	4	26
Charbroiled Chicken Club Sandwich	1 sandwich	610	30	8	1640	55	4	33
Jumbo Chili Dog	1 item	380	25	8	1130	24	1	15
Little Thick Cheeseburger	1 burger	430	23	9	1090	34	3	24
Low Carb It Charbroiled Chicken Club Sandwich	1 sandwich	340	21	6	1200	14	1	25
Original Turkey Burger	1 burger	460	17	4	930	47	4	31
Spicy Chicken Sandwich	1 sandwich	440	21	5	1140	41	3	11
Six Dollar Thickburger	1 burger	930	63	23	1810	59	4	34

Harvey's
BURGERS & CHICKEN

Chicken Strips	3 strips	320	15	1.5	780	27	2	20
Great Canadian, w/Cheese	1 burger	650	31	15	1270	54	3	38
Great Canadian, w/Cheese & Bacon	1 burger	690	35	16	1430	54	3	40
Original Bacon Cheeseburger	1 burger	500	26	12	1290	39	2	28
Original Cheeseburger	1 burger	460	23	11	1130	39	2	25
Original Hamburger	1 burger	380	16	7	980	37	2	20

DESSERTS

Apple Pie	1 item	220	8	4	310	34	1	2
Milkshake, Chocolate	14 fl oz	730	33	21	520	91	5	17

HOT DOGS

Hot Dog, w/Bacon & Cheese	1 hot dog	410	21	10	1040	33	3	22
Hot Dog, w/Bun	1 hot dog	290	12	4.5	730	31	2	14

SALADS

Warm Grilled Chicken	1 salad	170	3	1	550	9	4	30
Warm Grilled Chicken BLT	1 salad	230	7	2.5	760	9	4	33

SANDWICHES

Crispy Chicken	1 sandwich	470	16	2	1320	51	1	29
Grilled Chicken, on a Whole Wheat Bun	1 sandwich	290	5	1.5	810	28	4	34

SIDES

Fries, Large	as served	410	16	1	1190	61	5	4
Frings	as served	520	24	2	1510	69	5	6

	SERVING SIZE	CALORIES	TOTAL FAT (G)	SAT FAT (G)	SODIUM (MG)	CARBS (G)	FIBER (G)	PROTEIN (G)
Homefries	as served	300	19	2.5	530	29	3	3
Onion Rings, Large	as served	550	29	2.5	1580	65	4	6
Poutine	as served	840	43	15	2210	87	8	25

Hot Dog on a Stick
BEVERAGES, REGULAR

Original Frozen Lemonade	16 fl oz	210	n/a	n/a	15	53	n/a	n/a
Original Lemonade	16 fl oz	150	n/a	n/a	15	38	n/a	n/a
Sugar-Free Lemonade	16 fl oz	13	n/a	n/a	18	3	n/a	n/a

HOT DOGS

American Cheese on a Stick	1 hot dog	260	16	7	640	21	1	9
Beef Hot Dog on a Bun	1 hot dog	470	29	12	1220	36	2	15
Turkey Dog on a Stick	1 hot dog	250	14	3	700	22	1	9
Veggie Dog on a Stick	1 hot dog	220	8	1.5	570	24	2	12

PLATTERS

Fish	1 platter	320	21	3.5	410	24	1	11
Fish & Zucchini	1 platter	560	37	6	718	42	1	20
Zucchini	1 platter	780	68	11	700	35	5	6

SIDES

French Fries	as served	400	21	3.5	75	49	5	4
Funnel Cake Sticks	as served	210	8	1.5	200	31	<1	2

Houlihan's
APPETIZERS & SMALL PLATES

Calamari, w/o Sauce	as served	381	12	3	1010	35	2	33
Cheese Burger Slider, Single	as served	390	24	9	469	20	1	23
Chicken Wings—Buffalo Style, w/o Sauce	as served	782	62	11	2180	14	0	43
Chipotle Chicken Nachos	as served	1939	126	61	3031	98	14	88
Disco Fries	as served	1253	79	43	2584	65	7	52
Goat Cheese & Artichoke Bites	as served	779	49	17	1858	59	4	27
Lettuce Wraps	as served	627	18	4	2069	92	4	25
Spinach Dip Mini, w/ Tortilla Chips	as served	683	35	16	857	72	7	17

BURGERS & SANDWICHES

Brentwood Chicken Sandwich	1 sandwich	883	49	17	2561	51	2	58
Build Your Own Burger, w/o Toppings	1 burger	754	39	14	1535	50	3	48
French Dip	1 sandwich	897	30	12	2829	68	2	90
Southwest Grilled Chicken Wrap	1 wrap	806	56	14	1612	45	4	31
Veggie Burger	1 burger	840	42	18	2206	81	9	29

restaurants

	SERVING SIZE	CALORIES	TOTAL FAT (G)	SAT FAT (G)	SODIUM (MG)	CARBS (G)	FIBER (G)	PROTEIN (G)
ENTRÉE SALADS								
Buffalo Bleu, w/ Creamy Garlic Ranch Dressing	1 salad	1452	100	26	3038	66	8	69
Chicken Asian Chop Chop, w/ Napa Dressing	1 salad	1164	57	9	2792	129	10	35
Chicken Caesar, w/ Caesar Dressing	1 salad	1246	100	22	2547	34	6	47
Heartland Chicken—Fried, w/ Creamy Garlic Ranch Dressing	1 salad	1241	79	19	2055	53	8	75
Heartland Chicken—Grilled, w/ Creamy Garlic Ranch Dressing	1 salad	1064	80	20	2110	28	6	57
Mango Grilled Shrimp, w/ Caesar Dressing	1 salad	719	31	5	976	72	12	37
Prime Steak & Wedge, w/ Bleu Cheese Dressing	1 salad	1258	96	35	2123	28	6	51
ENTREES								
Atlantic Salmon, 5 oz	1 entrée	728	50	22	1065	33	7	34
Chicken Fettucini Alfredo	1 entrée	1474	77	40	2635	114	5	71
Chicken Parmesan	1 entrée	1475	60	21	3058	161	11	69
BBQ Baby Back Ribs – Full Slab, w/o Sides	1 entrée	1120	55	20	3665	86	5	68
Huge Panko Breaded Shrimp	1 entrée	946	31	8	2395	114	10	51
Creekstone Farms Meatloaf	1 entrée	1095	67	34	2449	76	10	38
Stuffed Chicken Breast	1 entrée	1409	88	44	3209	96	14	52
Tuscany Lemon Chicken Pasta	1 entrée	1608	83	40	1834	112	6	77

Hungry Howie's
HOWIE BREADS

	SERVING SIZE	CALORIES	TOTAL FAT (G)	SAT FAT (G)	SODIUM (MG)	CARBS (G)	FIBER (G)	PROTEIN (G)
Cajun	1/4 bread	300	9	1.9	239	46	1	9
Cinnamon	1/4 bread	313	9	1.9	239	59	1	9
Howie	1/4 bread	300	9	1.9	239	46	1	9
Three Cheeser	1/4 bread	370	14	4.9	384	47	1	15
OVEN-BAKED SUBS								
Deluxe Italian	1/2 sub	506	18	8.4	1005	61	2	24
Pizza	1/2 sub	689	34	14.3	1722	67	3	30
Pizza Special	1/2 sub	606	24	10.6	1584	68	3	29
Steak & Cheese	1/2 sub	491	15	6.7	914	64	2	27
Vegetarian	1/2 sub	530	21	10.7	895	64	3	22
PIZZA, LARGE								
Cheese	1 slice	200	5	2.7	314	25	1	12
Meat Eaters	1 slice	284	11	4.7	676	26	1	17

	SERVING SIZE	CALORIES	TOTAL FAT (G)	SAT FAT (G)	SODIUM (MG)	CARBS (G)	FIBER (G)	PROTEIN (G)
Pepperoni	1 slice	222	7	3.5	390	25	1	13
Veggie	1 slice	217	6	2.8	374	27	2	13
SALADS, SMALL								
Antipasto	1/2 salad	115	7	3.9	554	3	2	9
Chef	1/2 salad	114	7	3.5	396	4	2	9
Greek	1/2 salad	126	7	5	581	8	2	7
THIN CRUST PIZZA, LARGE								
Cheese Only	1 slice	124	5	2.7	314	11	< 1	12
Meat Eaters	1 slice	208	11	4.7	676	11	< 1	17
Pepperoni	1 slice	146	7	3.5	390	11	< 1	13
Veggie	1 slice	141	6	3.6	374	13	1	13

Husman's
CHIPS

	SERVING SIZE	CALORIES	TOTAL FAT (G)	SAT FAT (G)	SODIUM (MG)	CARBS (G)	FIBER (G)	PROTEIN (G)
Bar-B-Q	13 chips	150	10	2	280	14	1	2
Honey Bar-B-Q	17 chips	150	9	1.5	230	16	< 1	1
Kettle Cooked, Average of All Flavors	13 chips	148	9	2	278	15	1	2
Original	18 chips	150	10	2	125	14	1	2
Vlasic Dill Pickle	17 chips	150	10	1.5	280	14	1	1
Wavy Cheddar & Sour Cream	16 chips	150	10	2	260	14	1	2
OTHER SNACKS								
Baked Cheese Curls	1-1/3 cups	170	13	2	230	12	0	2
Bar-B-Q Pork Skins	1/2 oz	80	5	1.5	210	0	0	8

IHOP
BREAKFAST COMBOS

	SERVING SIZE	CALORIES	TOTAL FAT (G)	SAT FAT (G)	SODIUM (MG)	CARBS (G)	FIBER (G)	PROTEIN (G)
Belgian Waffle Combo	1 entrée	660	40	17	890	49	2	26
Big Two-Egg Breakfast	1 entrée	900	52	14	1990	79	6	30
Biscuits & Gravy Combo w/ Country Gravy	1 entrée	1440	92	30	3240	112	6	44
Breakfast Sampler	1 entrée	1220	76	23	3380	82	6	52
Chicken-Fried Chicken & Eggs w/ Country Gravy	1 entrée	1270	71	18	3080	104	9	54
Classic Skillets	1 entrée	1570	101	34	2710	115	9	52
Corned Beef Hash & Eggs	1 entrée	1160	64	22	3100	92	6	54
Country Chicken-Fried Steak & Eggs w/ Country Gravy	1 entrée	1750	107	30	4210	138	8	59
Eggs Benedict	1 entrée	1020	58	22	3340	78	5	43
Huevos Rancheros	1 entrée	1160	70	24	2080	80	11	53
Sirloin Tips & Eggs	1 entrée	1360	78	20	3300	100	8	66

restaurants

	SERVING SIZE	CALORIES	TOTAL FAT (G)	SAT FAT (G)	SODIUM (MG)	CARBS (G)	FIBER (G)	PROTEIN (G)
South-of-the-Border Burrito	1 entrée	1390	75	27	3530	127	10	52
Split Decision Breakfast	1 entrée	1100	69	24	2430	76	4	45
T-Bone Steak (10 oz.) & Eggs	1 entrée	1270	70	24	2660	76	4	83
FRENCH TOAST								
Cinn-A-Stack French Toast	1 entrée	940	38	13	1050	129	9	22
Create Your Own Vive La French Toast Combo, Original	1 entrée	1070	62	17	1560	94	8	35
Our Original French Toast	1 entrée	720	30	11	930	92	7	21
Stuffed French Toast Combo	1 entrée	990	56	16	1290	91	5	29
HEARTY OMELETTES								
Bacon Temptation	1 omelette	1100	87	32	2450	15	2	62
Corned Beef Hash & Cheese	1 omelette	1060	81	31	1960	29	3	55
Country	1 omelette	1220	90	31	2200	45	5	55
Create Your Own, Plain	1 omelette	530	43	11	590	7	1	27
Create Your Own, Plain w/ Egg Substitute	1 omelette	140	4	0.5	320	2	0	23
Garden	1 omelette	920	77	25	950	14	3	44
Spinach & Mushroom	1 omelette	1000	82	27	1630	22	4	46
OUR WORLD FAMOUS PANCAKES								
Cinn-A-Stacks	4 pancakes	890	29	10	2260	138	8	19
Double Blueberry	4 pancakes	690	17	5	2110	118	8	18
Original Buttermilk	3 pancakes	470	15	5	1590	69	4	13
Pick-A-Pancake Combo, Original Buttermilk	1 entrée	900	52	14	1990	79	6	30
Three Eggs & Pancakes w/ Hash Browns	1 entrée	1170	65	17	2670	103	8	44
Two x Two x Two	1 entrée	580	32	10	1400	48	3	27
Whole Wheat Pancakes with Blueberries	4 pancakes	600	14	3	1600	103	10	16
SIMPLE & FIT BREAKFASTS								
Blueberry Harvest Grain 'N Nut Combo	1 entrée	440	18	2.5	890	48	5	22
Seasonal Mixed Fruit Crepes	1 entrée	570	24	4.5	440	80	6	12
Two-Egg Breakfast	1 entrée	340	8	1.5	710	44	6	25

In-N-Out Burger
BURGERS

	SERVING SIZE	CALORIES	TOTAL FAT (G)	SAT FAT (G)	SODIUM (MG)	CARBS (G)	FIBER (G)	PROTEIN (G)
Cheeseburger, w/Onion	1 burger	480	27	10	1000	39	3	22
Double-Double, w/Onion	1 burger	670	41	18	1440	39	3	37
Hamburger, w/Onion	1 burger	390	19	5	650	39	3	16
SHAKES								
Average of All Flavors	15 fl oz	587	29	19	340	73	0	9

	SERVING SIZE	CALORIES	TOTAL FAT (G)	SAT FAT (G)	SODIUM (MG)	CARBS (G)	FIBER (G)	PROTEIN (G)
SIDES								
French Fries	as served	395	18	5	245	54	2	7

Jack in The Box
BURGERS & MORE

	SERVING SIZE	CALORIES	TOTAL FAT (G)	SAT FAT (G)	SODIUM (MG)	CARBS (G)	FIBER (G)	PROTEIN (G)
Bacon Ultimate Cheeseburger	1 burger	920	63	27	1840	45	2	44
Big Cheeseburger	1 burger	570	34	14	1050	43	2	23
Hamburger Deluxe	1 burger	340	16	5	540	33	2	15
Jumbo Jack, w/Cheese	1 burger	580	34	15	1190	45	2	23
Sirloin Cheeseburger	1 burger	900	60	19	1870	52	3	40
Sirloin Cheeseburger, w/Bacon	1 burger	990	66	21	2280	52	3	47
Sourdough Jack	1 burger	660	44	16	1210	40	3	28
Sourdough Ultimate Cheeseburger	1 burger	870	63	26	1370	38	3	37
Ultimate Cheeseburger	1 burger	830	57	25	1430	44	2	36
CHICKEN & MORE								
Chicken Fajita Pita, Whole Grain, w/Salsa	1 pita	330	11	5	990	35	4	24
Chicken Sandwich, w/Bacon	1 sandwich	470	25	5	1160	42	2	21
Chicken Strips, Crispy	4 pieces	560	24	3	1580	53	3	33
Chicken Strips, Grilled	4 pieces	250	7	1.5	1070	5	0	43
Homestyle Ranch Chicken Club	1 sandwich	730	35	8	2010	65	3	39
Jack's Spicy Chicken, w/Cheese	1 sandwich	610	26	7	1200	61	3	32
Sourdough Grilled Chicken Club	1 sandwich	540	26	7	1490	38	3	39
SALADS, W/O DRESSING								
Club Salad, w/Crispy Chicken Strips	1 salad	520	28	9	1230	37	5	32
Club Salad, w/Grilled Chicken Strips	1 salad	370	20	8	970	13	4	38
Southwest Salad, w/Crispy Chicken Strips	1 salad	500	23	7	1260	53	8	29
Southwest Salad, w/Grilled Chicken Strips	1 salad	350	15	6	1010	29	7	34
SHAKES & DESSERT								
Cake, Chocolate Overload	1 slice	300	7	1.5	350	57	2	4
Cake, New York-Style Cheesecake	1 slice	310	17	9	260	32	1	7
Mini Churros	10 pieces	690	37	7	550	84	4	7
Shake, Average of All Other Flavors	24 fl oz	1090	54	36	393	131	1	18
Shake, Oreo Cookie, w/Whipped Topping	24 fl oz	1170	61	38	560	134	2	19
SNACKS & SIDES								
Bacon Cheddar Potato Wedges	as served	680	42	10	1270	58	5	18
Beef Taco	1 taco	190	11	3	320	17	2	6

	SERVING SIZE	CALORIES	TOTAL FAT (G)	SAT FAT (G)	SODIUM (MG)	CARBS (G)	FIBER (G)	PROTEIN (G)
Chiquita Apple Bites, w/Caramel	as served	70	0	0	55	17	2	0
Egg Roll	3 pieces	440	22	5	950	46	7	16
French Fries, Medium	as served	450	21	2	820	61	4	5
Mozzarella Cheese Sticks	6 sticks	560	33	11	1190	43	3	24
Onion Rings	as served	450	28	2	620	45	3	6
Seasoned Curly Fries, Medium	as served	430	25	2	940	46	4	5
Stuffed Jalapeños	7 pieces	510	29	10	1690	49	3	14

Jack's
BREAKFAST

Bacon, Egg & Cheese Biscuit	1 sandwich	420	26	8	1150	31	1	17
Bacon, Egg & Cheese Wrap	1 wrap	320	18	6	870	24	1	17
Deluxe Breakfast, w/Bacon	1 entrée	1040	63	17	2390	91	3	25
Deluxe Breakfast, w/Sausage	1 entrée	1270	85	22	2480	93	3	33
Egg & Cheese Biscuit	1 sandwich	360	21	6	880	31	1	12
Gravy Biscuit, Single	as served	420	24	6	1140	40	1	9
Grits, w/Butter	as served	230	12	2	1150	27	5	3
Hash Browns, Large	as served	650	40	11	770	66	0	6
Pancakes	1 entrée	330	8	1.5	450	57	0	8
Sausage, Egg & Cheese Biscuit	1 sandwich	520	35	10	1120	32	1	20
Sausage, Egg & Cheese Wrap	1 wrap	310	17	6	630	24	1	14

BURGERS & SANDWICHES

Big Bacon	1 burger	610	41	13	940	31	2	29
Big Jack	1 burger	530	33	9	830	35	2	23
Big Jack, Double Cheese	1 burger	850	59	21	1310	35	2	44
Cheese	1 burger	380	21	7	680	31	1	16
Cheese, Double	1 burger	540	33	13	920	31	1	27
Chicken Fillet	1 sandwich	490	24	4.5	1160	40	3	27
Grilled Chicken	1 sandwich	380	16	3	750	32	2	27
Hamburger	1 burger	340	18	5	510	31	1	14

CHICKEN

3 Piece Combo, w/Fries	1 entrée	610	27	4	1490	56	2	36
4 Piece Combo, w/Fries	1 entrée	720	32	4.5	1870	60	2	47
Breast, Fried	1 breast	480	29	8	660	20	0	35
Fingers	3 fingers	300	14	0.5	1170	14	2	32
Leg, Fried	1 leg	150	10	3	200	7	0	10
Thigh, Fried	1 thigh	390	30	7	430	13	0	18
Wing, Fried	1 wing	200	13	3.5	240	9	0	11

	SERVING SIZE	CALORIES	TOTAL FAT (G)	SAT FAT (G)	SODIUM (MG)	CARBS (G)	FIBER (G)	PROTEIN (G)
Fries, Large	as served	440	19	5	460	61	0	7
MILKSHAKES, SMALL								
Chocolate Peanut Butter	16 fl oz	450	25	15	180	44	0	13
Cookies 'n Cream	16 fl oz	510	26	15	280	55	0	13
Homemade Vanilla	16 fl oz	450	23	13	200	47	0	13
Strawberry	16 fl oz	440	21	12	170	52	0	11
SALADS								
Crispy Chicken	1 salad	380	18	6	990	25	6	30
Grilled Chicken	1 salad	270	10	5	580	16	5	30
Spring	1 salad	160	7	4.5	190	15	5	9
Jamba Juice								
ALL FRUIT SMOOTHIES, ORIGINAL								
Five Fruit Frenzy	22 fl oz	340	1	0	30	82	6	2
Peach Perfection	22 fl oz	300	1	0	30	75	5	2
Pomegranate Paradise	22 fl oz	340	1	0	35	85	5	2
Strawberry Whirl	22 fl oz	300	1	0	25	75	6	2
BEVERAGES								
Blueberry Pomegranate Peaks	12 fl oz	140	0	0	80	33	4	4
Carrot Juice	12 fl oz	100	1	0	170	22	0	3
Orange Juice	12 fl oz	170	1	0	0	39	1	3
The Chillbuster	12 fl oz	180	0	0	20	45	1	0
CLASSIC SMOOTHIES, ORIGINAL								
Aloha Pineapple	22 fl oz	410	2	0.5	55	97	4	6
Banana Berry	22 fl oz	400	2	0.5	90	94	4	4
Caribbean Passion	22 fl oz	360	2	0.5	50	82	3	3
Mango-a-Go-Go	22 fl oz	400	2	0.5	45	94	3	3
Orange-A-Peel	22 fl oz	370	0	0	125	85	3	7
Peach Pleasure	22 fl oz	370	2	1	50	88	4	3
Pomegranate Pick-Me-Up	22 fl oz	370	2	0.5	50	88	4	3
Razzmatazz	22 fl oz	390	2	1	55	91	4	3
Strawberries Wild	22 fl oz	370	0	0	140	87	3	5
Strawberry Surf Rider	22 fl oz	430	2	0.5	10	103	4	3
CREAMY TREATS, ORIGINAL								
Apple Cinnamon Cheer	22 fl oz	420	1	0	120	97	4	6
Chocolate Moo'd	22 fl oz	570	5	2.5	380	116	3	15
Matcha Green Tea Blast	22 fl oz	420	0	0	210	91	2	10
Orange Dream Machine	22 fl oz	470	2	1	200	103	1	10

	SERVING SIZE	CALORIES	TOTAL FAT (G)	SAT FAT (G)	SODIUM (MG)	CARBS (G)	FIBER (G)	PROTEIN (G)
Peanut Butter Moo'd	22 fl oz	770	20	4.5	490	126	5	20
Pumpkin Smash	22 fl oz	550	1	0	460	118	2	14
JAMBA LIGHT SMOOTHIES, ORIGINAL								
Berry Fulfilling	22 fl oz	230	1	0	190	49	5	7
Mango Mantra	22 fl oz	250	1	0	170	56	4	8
Strawberry Nirvana	22 fl oz	230	1	0	180	51	4	7
PRE-BOOSTED SMOOTHIES, ORIGINAL								
Acai Super-Antioxidant	22 fl oz	380	6	2	55	98	5	5
Protein Berry Workout	22 fl oz	380	1	0	200	74	5	20
The Coldbuster	22 fl oz	350	2	1	25	82	3	5
SMOOTHIES, ORIGINAL								
Orange Carrot Karma	22 fl oz	270	1	0	120	66	4	4
Peach Mango	22 fl oz	400	5	1	90	79	7	13
Strawberries Alive Smoothie	22 fl oz	330	0	0	190	67	3	13
Strawberry Raspberry Banana	22 fl oz	390	5	1	85	75	9	13
Vibrant Blueberry Smoothie	22 fl oz	310	1	0	190	62	4	13

Jersey Mike's Subs
COLD SUBS, WHEAT, REGULAR

	SERVING SIZE	CALORIES	TOTAL FAT (G)	SAT FAT (G)	SODIUM (MG)	CARBS (G)	FIBER (G)	PROTEIN (G)
Club Sub, w/Mayonnaise	1 sub	890	52	15	2260	66	5	43
Club Supreme, w/Mayonnaise	1 sub	940	52	14	1560	66	5	56
Original Italian	1 sub	680	27	11	2250	68	5	45
Turkey Breast & Provolone	1 sub	540	16	6	1590	64	5	41
Veggie	1 sub	720	33	18	900	65	6	45
COLD WRAPS, FLOUR TORTILLA								
American Classic	1 wrap	580	22	10	1980	63	7	35
BLT	1 wrap	590	29	12	1460	60	7	23
Super Sub	1 wrap	600	22	10	1820	65	7	38
HOT SUBS, WHEAT, REGULAR								
Big Kahuna	1 sub	670	28	14	2070	65	5	43
Chicken Parmesan	1 sub	650	22	7	1590	77	5	37
Chipotle Steak	1 sub	900	55	16	2180	66	4	42
Grilled Chicken	1 sub	670	33	5	1290	60	4	34
Meatball & Cheese	1 sub	890	52	21	1950	72	6	39
Reuben	1 sub	700	27	9	2680	72	5	41
Steak Philly	1 sub	620	24	11	1700	64	4	41
SOUPS & SALADS								
Cape Cod Clam Chowder	1 cup	140	6	21	1110	17	0	4

	SERVING SIZE	CALORIES	TOTAL FAT (G)	SAT FAT (G)	SODIUM (MG)	CARBS (G)	FIBER (G)	PROTEIN (G)
Grilled Chicken Caesar Salad	1 salad	510	35	9	1480	11	2	34
Italian Wedding Soup	1 cup	120	5	2.5	1000	13	1	5
Tuna Salad	1 salad	690	60	9	740	15	5	24

Jimmy John's
GIANT CLUB

	SERVING SIZE	CALORIES	TOTAL FAT (G)	SAT FAT (G)	SODIUM (MG)	CARBS (G)	FIBER (G)	PROTEIN (G)
Beach	1 sandwich	729	31	8	1519	71	2	36
Billy	1 sandwich	800	34	9	1958	68	1	47
Bootlegger	1 sandwich	684	25	4	1660	67	1	42
Country	1 sandwich	768	31	8	1908	69	1	44
Gourmet Smoked Ham	1 sandwich	775	32	9	1877	69	1	41
Gourmet Veggie	1 sandwich	773	38	12	1235	71	2	30
Hunter's	1 sandwich	807	35	10	1781	67	1	52
Italian Night	1 sandwich	948	51	12	2166	70	1	44
Lulu	1 sandwich	755	33	8	1855	67	1	40
Tuna	1 sandwich	843	39	8.5	1954	72	3	44
Ultimate Porker	1 sandwich	760	39	9	1751	67	6	37

PLAIN SLIMS

	SERVING SIZE	CALORIES	TOTAL FAT (G)	SAT FAT (G)	SODIUM (MG)	CARBS (G)	FIBER (G)	PROTEIN (G)
Double Provolone	1 sandwich	545	16	9	991	65	0	29
Ham & Cheese	1 sandwich	505	10	5	1244	66	0	31
Roast Beef	1 sandwich	424	3	1	996	64	0	29
Salami, Capicola & Cheese	1 sandwich	599	20	9	1450	66	0	33
Tuna Salad	1 sandwich	722	31	4	1746	68	1	35
Turkey Breast	1 sandwich	401	1	0	1075	65	0	27

SUBS, 8", ON FRENCH BREAD UNLESS OTHERWISE SPECIFIED

	SERVING SIZE	CALORIES	TOTAL FAT (G)	SAT FAT (G)	SODIUM (MG)	CARBS (G)	FIBER (G)	PROTEIN (G)
Big John	1 sub	533	24	4	1014	49	1	26
J.J.B.L.T.	1 sub	634	35	9	1329	49	1	25
Pepe	1 sub	614	31	8	1262	50	1	28
The J.J. Gargantuan	1 sub	988	54	13	2893	54	1	66
Totally Tuna	1 sub	648	31	4	1592	54	3	33
Turkey Tom	1 sub	515	22	3	1094	50	1	24
Unwich, Hunter's Club, on Lettuce	1 sub	470	35	9.5	1196	4	2	37
Unwich, The J.J. Gargantuan, on Lettuce	1 sub	739	54	13	2469	7	2	56
Vegetarian	1 sub	578	30	8	873	53	2	19

KFC
CHICKEN

	SERVING SIZE	CALORIES	TOTAL FAT (G)	SAT FAT (G)	SODIUM (MG)	CARBS (G)	FIBER (G)	PROTEIN (G)
Extra Crispy, Breast	1 breast	510	33	7	1010	16	0	39

restaurants

	SERVING SIZE	CALORIES	TOTAL FAT (G)	SAT FAT (G)	SODIUM (MG)	CARBS (G)	FIBER (G)	PROTEIN (G)
Extra Crispy, Drumstick	1 drumstick	150	10	2	360	5	0	12
Extra Crispy, Thigh	1 thigh	340	24	5	780	10	0	20
Extra Crispy, Whole Wing	1 wing	190	13	2.5	410	6	0	12
Grilled, Breast	1 breast	220	7	2	730	0	0	40
Grilled, Drumstick	1 drumstick	90	4	1	290	0	0	13
Grilled, Thigh	1 thigh	170	10	3	530	0	0	19
Grilled, Whole Wing	1 wing	80	5	1.5	250	1	0	10
Original Recipe, Breast	1 breast	360	21	5	1080	11	0	34
Original Recipe, Drumstick	1 drumstick	120	7	1.5	310	3	0	11
Original Recipe, Thigh	1 thigh	250	17	4.5	730	7	0	17
Original Recipe, Whole Wing	1 wing	120	7	1.5	380	3	0	11
Spicy Crispy, Breast	1 breast	420	25	5	1250	12	1	38
Spicy Crispy, Drumstick	1 drumstick	160	10	2	440	5	0	11
Spicy Crispy, Thigh	1 thigh	360	27	6	1010	13	1	17
Spicy Crispy, Whole Wing	1 wing	170	12	2.5	470	6	0	11
POT PIE & BOWL								
Chicken Pot Pie	1 pot pie	790	45	37	1970	66	3	29
KFC Famous Bowl, w/Mashed Potatoes & Gravy	1 bowl	680	31	8	2130	74	6	26
SALADS								
Crispy Chicken BLT Salad, w/o Dressing	1 salad	360	19	3.5	1120	18	4	30
Crispy Chicken Caesar Salad, w/o Dressing or Croutons	1 salad	340	18	4.5	930	16	3	28
SANDWICHES								
Crispy Twister	1 sandwich	610	33	6	1380	52	3	28
Double Down w/Filet, Original Recipe	1 sandwich	610	37	11	1880	18	1	52
Doublicious w/Filet, Original Recipe	1 sandwich	520	25	7	1180	40	2	32
Honey BBQ Sandwich	1 sandwich	320	4	1	770	47	3	24
KFC Snacker w/Crispy Strip	1 sandwich	310	15	2.5	600	30	2	15
SIDES, INDIVIDUAL								
Biscuit	as served	180	8	6	530	23	1	4
Cole Slaw	as served	150	6	1	135	21	2	1
Macaroni & Cheese	as served	160	7	2.5	720	19	1	5
Mashed Potatoes w/Gravy	as served	120	4	1	530	19	1	2
Potato Wedges	as served	290	15	2.5	810	35	2	4
STRIPS & FILETS & POPCORN CHICKEN								
Crispy Strips	3 strips	390	21	3	1130	17	0	32

	SERVING SIZE	CALORIES	TOTAL FAT (G)	SAT FAT (G)	SODIUM (MG)	CARBS (G)	FIBER (G)	PROTEIN (G)
Original Filet	1 filet	200	9	1.5	670	8	1	22
Popcorn Chicken, Large	1 serving	560	37	8	1480	26	2	32
WINGS								
Hot Wings	1 wing	70	4	0.5	140	4	0	4
Hot Wings, Firey Buffalo	1 wing	70	4	0.5	270	5	0	4
Hot Wings, Honey BBQ	1 wing	80	4	0.5	240	8	0	4

Kolache Factory

Bacon, Egg & Cheese	as served	400	19	0	520	38	1	17
Egg & Cheese	as served	410	20	0	670	39	1	17
Fruit Varieties	as served	210	5	0	125	37	1	3
Ham & Cheese	as served	190	7	0	770	26	1	7
Italian Chicken	as served	230	9	0	520	25	1	12
Philly Cheese Steak	as served	230	9	0	340	25	1	12
Polish Sausage	as served	500	25	0	950	50	2	18
Potato, Egg & Cheese	as served	350	14	0	840	42	2	12
Ranchero	as served	340	14	0	570	39	2	13
Sausage	as served	160	6	0	109	21	1	4
Sausage, Egg & Cheese	as served	400	19	0	780	38	1	17
Spinach	as served	290	6	0	390	27	1	8
Texas Hot Polish Sausage	as served	470	21	0	970	51	2	17

Krispy Kreme
DOUGHNUTS

Cake, Traditional	1 doughnut	190	12	6	260	19	0	2
Caramel Kreme Crunch	1 doughnut	390	20	10	170	50	< 1	4
Chocolate, Iced, Cake	1 doughnut	280	15	7	320	34	< 1	3
Chocolate, Iced, Custard Filled	1 doughnut	310	17	8	150	36	< 1	4
Chocolate, Iced, Glazed	1 doughnut	240	11	5	95	33	< 1	2
Chocolate, Iced, Kreme Filling	1 doughnut	360	21	10	140	40	< 1	4
Cinnamon, Apple Filled	1 doughnut	290	16	8	150	33	< 1	3
Dulce de Leche	1 doughnut	300	18	9	160	31	< 1	3
Glazed, Blueberry Cake	1 doughnut	300	14	7	230	42	< 1	2
Glazed, Chocolate Cake	1 doughnut	300	15	7	230	41	2	3
Glazed, Cinnamon	1 doughnut	200	11	4.5	90	25	< 1	2
Glazed, Cruller	1 doughnut	220	12	5	260	27	< 1	2
Glazed, Kreme Filling	1 doughnut	340	20	10	140	38	< 1	3
Glazed, Maple Iced	1 doughnut	230	11	5	90	32	< 1	2
Glazed, Original	1 doughnut	190	11	5	90	21	0	2

restaurants

	SERVING SIZE	CALORIES	TOTAL FAT (G)	SAT FAT (G)	SODIUM (MG)	CARBS (G)	FIBER (G)	PROTEIN (G)
Glazed, Raspberry Filled	1 doughnut	290	16	8	125	36	< 1	3
Powdered, Blueberry Filled	1 doughnut	300	17	8	135	34	< 1	4
Powdered, Cake	1 doughnut	220	11	5	240	27	0	2
Powdered, Strawberry Filled	1 doughnut	290	16	8	135	33	< 1	3
Sugar	1 doughnut	190	11	5	85	20	0	2
OTHER								
Cinnamon Bun	1 bun	260	16	8	125	28	< 1	3
Doughnut Hole, Original, Glazed	4 holes	200	11	4.5	90	26	0	2

La Salsa Fresh Mexican Grill

BURRITOS

	SERVING SIZE	CALORIES	TOTAL FAT (G)	SAT FAT (G)	SODIUM (MG)	CARBS (G)	FIBER (G)	PROTEIN (G)
California, Chicken, w/Black Beans	1 burrito	840	33	14	1890	95	7	44
California, Meatless, w/Black Beans	1 burrito	710	29	13	1520	89	7	28
Original Gourmet, Chicken	1 burrito	870	41	13.5	1810	86	10	37
Overstuffed Grilled, Chicken	1 burrito	1260	59	19	3450	110	6	73
FAVORITES								
Fire Roasted Bowl, Chicken, w/Black Beans	1 bowl	730	32	9	1730	74	10	39
Fire Roasted Bowl, Meatless, w/Black Beans	1 bowl	630	29	9	1380	71	10	22
Stuffed Fajita Quesadilla, Chicken	1 quesadilla	863	52	21	1952	56	5	45
PLATTERS								
2 Taquitos & Quesadilla, w/Black Beans	1 entrée	1600	86	36	3020	143	18	70
2 Veggie Tacos, w/Black Beans	1 entrée	780	23	12	1530	117	14	33
Enchilada, Cheese, w/Black Beans	1 entrée	900	47	28	1830	82	10	45
Enchilada, Chicken, w/Black Beans	1 entrée	714	25	11	1821	84	10	47
Fajita, Chicken, w/Black Beans	1 entrée	827	29	11	1959	99	12	52
Mexico City Taco Platter, w/Black Beans	1 entrée	1060	39	13.5	2140	127	11	51
Ranchero Burrito, Chicken, w/Black Beans	1 entrée	936	36	14	2616	113	11	49
Tacos La Salsa, Chicken, w/Black Beans	1 entrée	910	35	10.5	1690	105	13	44
QUESADILLAS								
Classic	1 quesadilla	850	54	30	1440	56	3	38
Classic, Chicken	1 quesadilla	955	57	30	1787	58	3	55
Grande, Chicken, w/Black Beans	1 quesadilla	1133	60	30	2586	92	8	63
SALADS								
Chile Lime	1 salad	634	46	11	1246	45	8	17
Chipotle Shrimp	1 salad	799	56	13	1896	52	14	28

	SERVING SIZE	CALORIES	TOTAL FAT (G)	SAT FAT (G)	SODIUM (MG)	CARBS (G)	FIBER (G)	PROTEIN (G)
Taco, Chicken, w/Black Beans	1 salad	985	42	16	1873	108	10	50
TACOS								
Baja Fish	1 taco	393	22	4.5	367	29	2	20
Baja Shrimp	1 taco	320	19	2	400	30	3	8
Mexico City, Chicken	1 taco	188	3	0	232	27	2	13
Taquitos	3 taquitos	762	42	9	1230	66	15	33
Vegetarian Taco	1 taco	280	10	6	420	37	4	12

Little Caesars
BABY PAN!PAN! PIZZA

	SERVING SIZE	CALORIES	TOTAL FAT (G)	SAT FAT (G)	SODIUM (MG)	CARBS (G)	FIBER (G)	PROTEIN (G)
Just Cheese	1 pizza	320	15	6	520	33	2	14
Pepperoni	1 pizza	360	18	7	650	33	2	16
PIZZA, 14"								
3 Meat Treat	1 slice	340	17	7	730	32	2	16
Deep Dish, Just Cheese	1 slice	320	13	5	510	38	2	14
Deep Dish, Pepperoni	1 slice	360	16	6	640	38	2	16
Round Hot-N-Ready, Just Cheese	1 slice	250	9	4	440	32	1	12
Round Hot-N-Ready, Pepperoni	1 slice	280	11	5	560	32	2	14
Ultimate Supreme	1 slice	310	13	6	640	33	2	15
Veggie	1 slice	270	10	4.5	560	33	2	13
SIDES								
Crazy Bread	1 stick	100	3	0.5	150	15	1	3
Italian Cheese Bread	1 piece	130	6	2.5	240	13	1	6
Pepperoni Cheese Bread	1 piece	150	8	3	280	13	1	6
Wings, Barbecue	1 wing	80	5	1.5	260	3	0	6
Wings, Hot Buffalo	1 wing	70	5	1.5	390	0	0	6
Wings, Mild Buffalo	1 wing	70	5	1.5	290	0	0	6
Wings, Oven-Roasted	1 wing	70	5	1.5	190	0	0	5
Wings, Teriyaki	1 wing	70	5	1.5	240	1	0	6

Lone Star Steakhouse
BURGERS & SANDWICHES

	SERVING SIZE	CALORIES	TOTAL FAT (G)	SAT FAT (G)	SODIUM (MG)	CARBS (G)	FIBER (G)	PROTEIN (G)
Bacon Bleu	1 burger	821	37	16.5	1641	51	3	68
Bubba	1 burger	1087	57	23	4268	67	3	73
Lone Star	1 burger	640	27	10.2	1169	48	3	60
Mesquite Grilled Chicken Sandwich, w/Fries	1 entrée	1047	34	4	4431	135	8	50
Swiss & Mushroom	1 burger	844	38	16.6	1349	53	3	69
Steak Sandwich, w/Bun	1 sandwich	638	22	5	2968	55	3	55

	SERVING SIZE	CALORIES	TOTAL FAT (G)	SAT FAT (G)	SODIUM (MG)	CARBS (G)	FIBER (G)	PROTEIN (G)
CHICKEN & RIBS, W/O SIDES								
Baby Back Ribs	as served	486	40	16.2	126	0	0	29
Bubba BBQ Chicken Breast	as served	167	1	0.4	1394	5	< 1	34
Grilled Chicken	as served	169	4	0.3	1335	0	0	33
Lone Star Chicken, Plain	as served	169	4	0.3	1335	0	0	33
COMBOS, W/O SIDES								
Baby Back Ribs & Chicken	as served	741	30	13.1	9607	46	2	74
Filet & 3 Fried Shrimp	as served	652	23	5.4	3248	50	1	52
Sirloin & Baby Back Ribs	as served	654	33	16	8868	7	1	81
Sirloin Steak & Lobster	as served	334	8	3.2	5971	10	0	56
Texas Trio	as served	1206	55	18.6	8386	64	2	108
SALADS								
Chicken Caesar	1 salad	479	24	5.2	2877	19	5	46
Cobb	1 salad	685	37	13	3357	23	6	67
El Paso	1 salad	351	19	11.4	1087	25	7	24
STARTERS								
Amarillo Cheese Fries	as served	2641	152	38.3	16888	356	15	69
Lone Star Wings, Mild	as served	954	62	8.2	842	15	3	83
Queso	as served	238	15	8.1	1200	13	1	13
Texas Rose	as served	1258	83	37	2704	108	7	20
STEAKS								
Chopped Steak	10 oz	712	52	6.2	364	0	0	62
Delmonico	12 oz	625	43	7.4	529	0	0	58
Five Star Filet	6 oz	333	18	6.8	242	2	0	42
New York Strip	12 oz	525	28	15.6	617	0	0	69
Sirloin	6 oz	244	7	3.3	1933	1	0	43
Texas Ribeye	14 oz	710	40	14.6	1339	6	0	83

Long John Silver's
SANDWICHES & MORE

	SERVING SIZE	CALORIES	TOTAL FAT (G)	SAT FAT (G)	SODIUM (MG)	CARBS (G)	FIBER (G)	PROTEIN (G)
Alaskan Pollock Sandwich	1 sandwich	470	23	5	1180	49	3	18
Baja Chicken Strip Taco	1 taco	370	23	5	890	31	3	11
Baja Fish Taco	1 taco	360	23	4.5	810	30	3	9
Chicken Strip Sandwich	1 sandwich	440	30	6	1350	47	4	22
Chicken Strips	1 piece	140	8	2	480	9	0	8
Freshside Grille Salmon Entrée	1 entrée	280	7	2	1010	27	3	27
Freshside Grille Shrimp Scampi Entrée	1 entrée	330	15	3.5	1230	29	3	20
Freshside Grille Tilapia Entrée	1 entrée	250	5	2	820	27	3	25

	SERVING SIZE	CALORIES	TOTAL FAT (G)	SAT FAT (G)	SODIUM (MG)	CARBS (G)	FIBER (G)	PROTEIN (G)
Ultimate Alaskan Pollock Sandwich	1 sandwich	530	27	8	1500	50	3	21
Zesty Chicken Strip Sandwich	1 sandwich	380	19	4	880	39	3	14
SEAFOOD								
Battered Alaskan Pollock	1 piece	260	16	4	790	17	0	12
Battered Shrimp	3 pieces	130	9	2.5	480	8	0	5
Breaded Clam Strips	1 snack box	320	19	4.5	1190	29	2	9
Buttered Langostino Lobster Bites	1 snack box	230	9	3	520	24	2	13
Grilled Pacific Salmon	2 filets	150	5	1	440	2	0	24
Grilled Tilapia	1 filet	110	3	1	250	1	0	22
Langostino Lobster Stuffed Crab Cake	1 crab cake	170	9	2	390	16	1	6
Popcorn Shrimp	1 snack box	270	16	4	570	23	1	9
Shrimp Scampi	8 pieces	200	13	2.5	650	3	0	17
SIDES								
Breaded Mozzarella Sticks	3 pieces	150	9	3.5	350	13	1	5
Broccoli Cheese Bites	5 pieces	230	12	4.5	550	25	2	5
Broccoli Cheese Soup	1 bowl	220	18	8	650	8	1	5
Cole Slaw	as served	200	15	2.5	340	15	3	1
Corn Cobbette, w/Butter Oil	1 cobbette	150	10	2	30	14	3	3
Fries	as served	310	14	3.5	460	45	4	3
Jalapeño Cheddar Bites	5 pieces	240	14	5	730	23	2	6

Manhattan Bagel
BAGELS

Asiago	1 bagel	370	5	3	840	68	3	17
Everything	1 bagel	350	3	0	980	68	3	12
French Toast	1 bagel	300	6	2	380	54	2	9
Honey Whole Wheat	1 bagel	250	1	0	440	56	3	9
Multigrain	1 bagel	340	2	0	710	70	5	12
Plain	1 bagel	320	1	0	670	68	3	11
BREAKFAST								
Egg & Cheese, Plain Bagel	1 sandwich	520	16	7	1270	69	3	25
Egg, Bacon & Cheese, Plain Bagel	1 sandwich	620	24	10	1660	70	3	32
Egg, Pork Sausage & Cheese, Plain Bagel	1 sandwich	770	39	15	1670	70	3	32
Egg White Benedict, Bagel Thin	1 sandwich	300	8	4.5	1100	33	1	24
Toasted Italian Egg White	1 sandwich	400	11	4	890	49	3	27
Turkey Bacon & Cheddar, Bagel Thin	1 sandwich	290	11	5	730	25	4	23
THE LIGHTER SIDE, LUNCH SANDWICHES								
Avocado BLT, Bagel Thin	1 sandwich	370	24	4	700	30	6	11

restaurants

	SERVING SIZE	CALORIES	TOTAL FAT (G)	SAT FAT (G)	SODIUM (MG)	CARBS (G)	FIBER (G)	PROTEIN (G)
Tuna, Bagel Thin	1 sandwich	370	22	3	560	26	5	19
Turkey, Bagel Thin	1 sandwich	250	7	2.5	980	28	5	25

Maui Tacos
BOWL

Chicken	1 bowl	500	16	5	830	54	9	34
Pork	1 bowl	500	16	5	1140	61	9	27
Steak	1 bowl	520	17	7	830	54	9	36
Vegetarian	1 bowl	340	3	0	700	66	11	13

BURRITO & TACOS

Haiku Burrito	1 burrito	620	22	13	970	83	12	23
Hana Burrito	1 burrito	740	27	12	1430	92	3	30
Honolii Burrito	1 burrito	820	41	21	1020	69	11	42
Hookipa Burrita	1 burrito	760	22	11	1320	96	10	42
Lahaina Burrito, Chicken	1 burrito	740	30	13	1060	77	4	36
Lahaina Burrito, Steak	1 burrito	760	33	15	1040	77	4	37
LaPerouse Burrito	1 burrito	680	21	10	1020	87	12	32
Maui Taco, Fish, Baja Grilled	1 taco	410	22	3	430	34	7	20
Maui Taco, Vegetarian	1 taco	410	15	6	560	57	10	14
Napili Burrito	1 burrito	810	27	12	1250	95	10	43
Puamana Burrito	1 burrito	790	27	15	1330	100	22	38

McDonald's
BREAKFAST

Bacon, Egg & Cheese Bagel	1 sandwich	560	27	9	1300	56	3	24
Bacon, Egg & Cheese Biscuit, Regular	1 item	420	23	12	1160	37	2	15
Bacon, Egg & Cheese McGriddle	1 item	420	18	8	1110	48	2	15
Big Breakfast, w/Hotcakes, Regular	1 platter	1090	56	19	2150	111	6	36
Egg McMuffin	1 item	300	12	5	820	30	2	18
Fruit & Maple Oatmeal	as served	290	5	2	160	57	5	5
Fruit 'n Yogurt Parfait	1 parfait	160	2	1	85	31	1	4
Hash Brown	1 item	150	9	1.5	310	15	2	1
Hotcakes	as served	350	9	2	590	60	3	8
Sausage Burrito	1 burrito	300	16	7	830	26	1	12
Sausage, Egg & Cheese McGriddles	1 item	560	32	12	1360	48	2	20
Sausage McMuffin	1 item	370	22	8	850	29	2	14
Sausage McMuffin, w/Egg	1 item	450	27	10	920	30	2	21

BURGERS & SANDWICHES

Angus Bacon & Cheese	1 burger	790	39	17	2070	63	4	45

	SERVING SIZE	CALORIES	TOTAL FAT (G)	SAT FAT (G)	SODIUM (MG)	CARBS (G)	FIBER (G)	PROTEIN (G)
Angus Chipotle BBQ Bacon	1 burger	800	39	18	2020	66	4	45
Angus Deluxe Snack Wrap	1 wrap	410	25	10	990	27	2	20
Angus Mushroom & Swiss	1 burger	770	40	17	1170	59	4	44
Big Mac	1 burger	540	29	10	1040	45	3	25
Big N' Tasty	1 burger	460	24	8	720	37	3	24
Cheeseburger	1 burger	300	12	6	750	33	2	15
Double Cheeseburger	1 burger	440	23	11	1150	34	2	25
Filet-O-Fish	1 sandwich	380	18	3.5	640	38	2	15
Hamburger	1 burger	250	9	3.5	520	31	2	12
Honey Mustard Snack Wrap, Crispy	1 wrap	330	15	4.5	700	33	1	14
Mac Snack Wrap	1 wrap	330	19	7	690	26	1	15
McChicken	1 sandwich	360	16	3	830	40	2	14
McDouble	1 burger	390	19	8	920	33	2	22
McRib	1 sandwich	500	26	10	980	44	3	22
Premium Crispy Chicken Classic Sandwich	1 sandwich	510	22	3.5	990	56	3	24
Premium Crispy Chicken Club Sandwich	1 sandwich	620	29	7	1200	57	3	31
Quarter Pounder w/Cheese	1 burger	510	26	12	1190	40	3	29
CHICKEN								
Chicken McNuggets	6 pieces	280	18	3	540	18	1	13
Chicken Selects Premium Breast Strips	5 pieces	640	38	6	1240	36	1	38
DESSERTS & SHAKES, MEDIUM								
Baked Hot Apple Pie	1 item	250	13	7	170	32	4	2
Chocolate McCafe Shake	16 fl oz	720	20	12	300	119	1	15
McFlurry, w/M&M's Candies	12 fl oz	640	23	14	190	95	4	13
McFlurry, w/Oreo Cookies	12 fl oz	510	17	9	300	79	3	12
McFlurry, w/Reese's Peanut Butter Cup	12 fl oz	610	25	11	320	85	4	15
Strawberry McCafe Shake	16 fl oz	710	20	12	210	116	0	14
Vanilla McCafe Shake	16 fl oz	680	20	12	220	111	0	14
PREMIUM SALADS, W/O DRESSING								
Bacon Ranch, w/Crispy Chicken	1 salad	390	22	6	870	24	4	26
Bacon Ranch, w/o Chicken	1 salad	140	7	3.5	300	10	3	9
Caesar, w/Crispy Chicken	1 salad	350	18	4.5	740	24	4	23
Caesar, w/Grilled Chicken	1 salad	190	5	3	580	10	4	27
Southwest, w/Crispy Chicken	1 salad	450	21	4.5	820	42	7	23
Southwest, w/Grilled Chicken	1 salad	290	8	2.5	650	28	7	27
SIDES								
Apple Slices	1 package	15	0	0	0	4	0	0

restaurants

	SERVING SIZE	CALORIES	TOTAL FAT (G)	SAT FAT (G)	SODIUM (MG)	CARBS (G)	FIBER (G)	PROTEIN (G)
Large French Fries	as served	500	25	3.5	350	63	6	6
Medium French Fries	as served	380	19	2.5	270	48	5	4
Small French Fries	as served	230	11	1.5	160	29	3	3
Moe's Southwest Grill								
BURRITOS, ON A WHOLE GRAIN TORTILLA, W/BLACK BEANS								
Homewrecker, Chicken	1 burrito	975	37	17	1886	102	21	54
Homewrecker, Steak	1 burrito	956	37	16	2026	102	21	49
Joey Bag of Donuts, Chicken	1 burrito	824	25	11	1643	96	18	51
Joey Bag of Donuts, Steak	1 burrito	805	25	10	1783	96	18	46
Joey Jr.	1 burrito	467	14	6	927	57	10	27
FAJITAS, W/CHICKEN								
Alfredo Garcia	as served	961	45	19	1587	66	7	73
Fat Sam	as served	1021	50	20	1807	70	9	74
NACHOS, W/BLACK BEANS								
Billy Barou	as served	1044	62	28	3470	79	13	49
Ruprict	as served	904	55	26	3090	79	13	30
QUESADILLAS, ON A WHOLE GRAIN TORTILLA								
John Coctostan	as served	814	39	20	1541	58	15	54
Chicken Club	as served	1090	75	29	1898	42	6	56
Super Kingpin	as served	535	32	17	983	39	6	22
RICE BOWLS								
Chicken Rice Bowl	1 bowl	854	42	12	1314	77	12	46
Tofu Rice Bowl	1 bowl	700	23	6	1583	82	14	32
TACOS, ON A SOFT FLOUR TORTILLA, W/GROUND BEEF								
Funkmeister	1 taco	348	13	5	784	39	6	19
Overacheiver	1 taco	423	19	8	906	42	7	20
Unanimous Decision	1 taco	341	15	7	571	39	7	14
SALADS, W/CHICKEN, BLACK BEANS & CHIPOTLE RANCH								
Closetalker	1 salad	1069	69	17	1663	64	13	46
Personal Trainer	1 salad	920	64	14	1874	64	12	22
Mr. Goodcents								
COLD SUBS, ON WHEAT BREAD, 8"								
Censable Sub	1 sub	440	17	7	1500	57	5	23

	SERVING SIZE	CALORIES	TOTAL FAT (G)	SAT FAT (G)	SODIUM (MG)	CARBS (G)	FIBER (G)	PROTEIN (G)
Italian Sub	1 sub	640	37	16	1970	55	5	28
Mr. Goodcents, Original	1 sub	510	25	10	1650	56	5	25
Oven-Roasted Chicken Breast	1 sub	350	6	2	1180	55	5	28
Penny Club	1 sub	350	6	2	1480	57	5	25
Roast Beef	1 sub	350	6	3	1490	55	5	28
Tuna Salad	1 sub	490	21	4	1010	63	6	22
Turkey	1 sub	350	6	1	1340	58	5	23
Veggie Sub	1 sub	290	4	1	840	58	6	13
PASTA								
Chicken Alfredo on Mostaccioli	1 entrée	1370	79	43	2510	112	7	44
Chicken Parmesan on Mostaccioli	1 entrée	660	10	3	1530	100	5	40
Red Sauce on Mostaccioli, w/Meatball	1 entrée	610	20	6	1080	79	4	25
TOASTED SUBS, ON WHEAT BREAD, 8"								
Buffalo Chicken	1 sub	500	13	2	2330	62	5	40
California Turkey Club	1 sub	720	34	11	2230	72	9	43
Chicken Bacon Ranch, w/Cheddar	1 sub	660	27	9	1920	61	5	52
Chipotle Cheesesteak, Steak	1 sub	680	31	10	2280	67	6	39
Meatball, w/Mozzarella	1 sub	680	33	13	1680	67	5	35

Mrs. Fields
BROWNIES

	SERVING SIZE	CALORIES	TOTAL FAT (G)	SAT FAT (G)	SODIUM (MG)	CARBS (G)	FIBER (G)	PROTEIN (G)
Bites, Double Fudge	3 bites	200	10	5	75	27	1	2
Butterscotch Blondie	1 brownie	260	10	6	20	38	0	3
Double Fudge	1 brownie	260	13	8	95	34	1	3
Walnut Fudge	1 brownie	270	15	7	95	32	2	3
COOKIES								
Bite-Size Nibbler Cookies, Semi-Sweet Chocolate	3 cookies	170	8	3.5	140	23	1	2
Butter	1 cookie	200	8	3.5	180	29	< 1	2
Cinnamon Sugar	1 cookie	210	8	3.5	210	31	0	2
Oatmeal, Raisins & Walnuts	1 cookie	200	9	3	180	27	1	3
Peanut Butter	1 cookie	200	12	4	210	24	1	4
Semi-Sweet Chocolate	1 cookie	210	10	5	170	29	1	2
Semi-Sweet Chocolate, w/Walnuts	1 cookie	220	11	4.5	160	28	1	2
Triple Chocolate	1 cookie	210	10	6	170	28	1	2
White Chunk Macadamia	1 cookie	230	12	6	170	28	0	2

restaurants

	SERVING SIZE	CALORIES	TOTAL FAT (G)	SAT FAT (G)	SODIUM (MG)	CARBS (G)	FIBER (G)	PROTEIN (G)
Ninety Nine								
CHICKEN & STEAKS, W/O SIDES								
Broiled Sirloin Tips	1 entrée	910	48	13	2130	5	0	107
Chicken & Sausage Al Forno	1 entrée	1900	89	37	4290	179	14	94
Chicken Broccoli & Ziti Dinner	1 entrée	1920	103	50	3140	169	11	78
Louisiana Sirloin	1 entrée	650	34	12	1750	3	1	81
NY Strip Sirloin	1 entrée	680	28	10	610	1	0	100
Original Crispy Chicken Tenders	1 entrée	1130	75	13	6160	55	2	60
Smothered Sirloin Tips	1 entrée	1010	56	15	2140	12	2	108
St. Louis Ribs	1 entrée	2410	114	41	11850	251	12	75
FIT FOR YOU, W/SIDES								
Grilled Balsamic Chicken & Iceberg Wedge	1 entrée	490	22	6	1510	30	4	43
Herb Salmon & Vegetables	1 entrée	380	22	7	270	10	4	37
Mushroom Bleu Top Sirloin	1 entrée	400	19	6	720	10	5	47
SALADS, W/DRESSING								
Chicken Caesar	1 salad	830	54	9	2190	50	7	47
Crispy Honey Mustard Chicken	1 salad	1150	75	18	1850	66	6	53
Fire Grilled Southwest Cobb	1 salad	890	58	16	1680	30	6	59
SEAFOOD								
Baked Scrod, w/o Sides	1 entrée	560	32	15	520	10	0	53
Captain's Combo Platter, w/o Seafood Chowder	1 entrée	1840	126	21	3750	122	10	62
Fish & Chips	1 entrée	1830	124	21	3550	120	10	66
Panko-Crusted Cod, w/o Sides	1 entrée	1410	63	28	1890	143	8	64
Seasoned Salmon, w/o Sides	1 entrée	550	41	17	340	0	0	44
SOUPS & SIDES								
French Onion Soup	1 crock	300	11	5	2000	39	1	14
Honey Butter Biscuit, w/Honey Butter	1 biscuit	220	9	5	610	29	1	4
Seafood Chowder	1 crock	490	34	18	880	30	2	20
STARTERS								
Boneless Buffalo Wings	as served	1120	75	11	4050	45	2	62
Boneless Wings & Skins Sampler	as served	1660	111	29	4890	72	6	87
Calypso Coconut Shrimp	as served	600	32	12	940	60	4	20
Fried Mozzarella	as served	780	48	19	1780	57	3	32
Gold Fever Wings	as served	1270	77	12	2850	81	4	64
Nachos	as served	1600	103	52	3690	100	12	69

	SERVING SIZE	CALORIES	TOTAL FAT (G)	SAT FAT (G)	SODIUM (MG)	CARBS (G)	FIBER (G)	PROTEIN (G)
Outrageous Potato Skins	as served	1130	84	33	1710	45	6	47
STEAKBURGERS & SANDWICHES, W/O SIDES								
All Star Steakburger	1 burger	1310	96	36	2360	57	2	57
Bacon & Cheese Steakburger	1 burger	1020	67	32	1830	48	2	57
Brewhouse BBQ Steakburger	1 burger	1160	69	31	2310	73	3	58
Grilled Chicken Panini	1 sandwich	970	60	23	1870	53	4	54
Honey BBQ Chicken Wrap	1 wrap	930	40	11	1840	94	4	47
Nacho Burger	1 burger	1020	66	29	1710	59	3	51
Roast Beef & Cheddar Dip Sandwich	1 sandwich	770	37	14	2670	59	2	47
Steakburger	1 burger	860	54	25	1270	46	2	47
Steakburger, w/Cheese	1 burger	940	61	29	1540	48	2	52
Turkey & Havarti on Ciabatta	1 sandwich	600	36	10	1930	42	2	33

Noodles & Company
ADD ONS

Chicken Breast	as served	110	3	0.5	370	0	0	23
Chicken Breast, Parmesan-Crusted	as served	200	10	2.5	820	8	< 1	20
Marinated Steak, Sautéed	as served	170	8	3.5	470	< 1	0	23
Meatballs, Regular	as served	300	23	9	860	6	0	19
Shrimp, Sautéed	as served	80	1	0	360	< 1	0	17
Tofu, Organic	as served	180	11	1.5	310	6	1	16
ENTRÉES, REGULAR								
Bacon, Mac & Cheeseburger	1 entrée	1260	58	31	1830	132	6	53
Bangkok Curry	1 entrée	480	14	9	790	80	7	8
Indonesian Peanut Sauté	1 entrée	830	18	4.5	2030	148	7	18
Japanese Pan Noodles	1 entrée	620	15	1	2200	110	6	13
Mushroom Stroganoff	1 entrée	790	31	17	980	102	6	28
Pad Thai	1 entrée	830	18	3	2050	151	5	15
Pasta Fresca	1 entrée	780	25	7	1030	114	6	26
Pesto Cavatappi	1 entrée	800	31	13	890	102	6	27
Spaghetti & Meatballs	1 entrée	970	39	14	1900	111	6	43
Whole Grain Tuscan Linguine	1 entrée	680	32	13	1220	77	13	22
Wisconsin Mac & Cheese	1 entrée	1030	43	25	1050	122	5	39
SALADS, REGULAR SIZE								
Caesar	1 salad	370	28	7	940	19	2	11
Chinese Chop	1 salad	370	22	1.5	880	39	6	5
Very Berry, Spinach	1 salad	670	42	14	1460	56	9	18

restaurants

	SERVING SIZE	CALORIES	TOTAL FAT (G)	SAT FAT (G)	SODIUM (MG)	CARBS (G)	FIBER (G)	PROTEIN (G)
SANDWICH								
Mmmeatball	1 sandwich	670	32	13	2170	59	3	36
Spicy Chicken Caesar, w/o Dressing	1 sandwich	330	9	2	770	40	1	21
The Med	1 sandwich	330	10	2	970	41	2	20
Wisconsin Cheesesteak, on a Ciabatta Roll	1 sandwich	570	22	10	1820	54	4	39
SIDES								
Flatbread	1 flatbread	200	5	0.5	400	35	1	6
Potstickers, Regular, w/o Sauce	as served	340	10	2	1080	45	3	17

O'Charley's
APPETIZERS

	SERVING SIZE	CALORIES	TOTAL FAT (G)	SAT FAT (G)	SODIUM (MG)	CARBS (G)	FIBER (G)	PROTEIN (G)
Good Time Nach-O's	as served	1030	54	20	2530	114	9	30
Potato Skins, Overloaded	as served	1260	98	43	3380	44	0	56
Spinach & Artichoke Dip	as served	780	44	13	1530	86	6	14
BURGERS								
Better Cheddar, Bacon	1 burger	980	57	23	1710	55	3	59
Classic	1 burger	740	37	12	1180	54	3	44
Turkey, Grilled	1 burger	890	54	14	1710	54	3	47
Wild West	1 burger	1210	79	23	1860	67	4	53
ENTRÉES								
Chicken Tenders, w/Buffalo Sauce	1 entrée	1200	72	12	5650	82	5	61
Chicken Tenders, w/Honey Mustard	1 entrée	1090	61	10	3680	82	4	59
Chicken, Brushetta	1 entrée	470	16	5	1790	25	5	56
Chicken, Italia	1 entrée	1330	75	30	2340	93	6	70
Filet Mignon	1 entrée	450	28	9	910	0	0	47
Fish 'n' Chips, Hand Battered	1 entrée	1190	85	16	2070	43	3	62
Pasta, Cajun Chicken	1 entrée	1730	106	37	4150	131	11	66
Pasta, Prime Rib	1 entrée	1530	101	38	2580	90	5	63
Pasta, Shrimp Scampi	1 entrée	840	33	15	2260	93	5	39
Ribs, Baby Back	1 entrée	1480	96	34	5260	76	3	77
Salmon, Atlantic, Grilled	9 oz	540	33	7	240	2	1	57
Salmon, Cedar-Planked	1 entrée	530	32	6	940	2	1	57
Shrimp Dinner, Fried, Panko-Crusted	1 entrée	570	26	5	1710	53	2	31
Shrimp Dinner, Grilled	1 entrée	290	7	1.5	1220	32	1	22
Sirloin, Louisiana	1 entrée	680	40	14	1220	3	1	74
Steak, Ribeye	1 entrée	810	55	20	960	0	0	72
Tilapia, Cedar Planked	1 entrée	280	11	3	410	2	1	42
Top Sirloin, Grilled	12 oz	590	33	9	2380	1	0	70

	SERVING SIZE	CALORIES	TOTAL FAT (G)	SAT FAT (G)	SODIUM (MG)	CARBS (G)	FIBER (G)	PROTEIN (G)
SALADS								
Caesar, Classic, w/Dressing	1 salad	450	39	8	960	16	3	9
California Chicken, w/o Dressing	1 salad	700	37	9	760	48	8	45
Calypso Spinach, w/Dressing	1 salad	1120	70	17	2530	77	12	45
Pecan Chicken Tender, w/o Dressing	1 salad	1020	60	11	2020	81	10	46
Southern Fried Chicken, w/o Dressing	1 salad	1120	61	19	3670	72	7	75
SANDWICHES								
Grilled Cheese, White Cheddar	1 sandwich	620	30	14	1160	57	2	26
Mediterranean Chicken	1 sandwich	780	36	10	1650	70	11	53
Philly, Prime Rib	1 sandwich	830	46	14	2240	64	4	47
Southern Fried Chicken	1 sandwich	1380	80	21	3790	102	5	66

Old Country Buffet

	SERVING SIZE	CALORIES	TOTAL FAT (G)	SAT FAT (G)	SODIUM (MG)	CARBS (G)	FIBER (G)	PROTEIN (G)
BREADS								
Banana Walnut Muffin	1 muffin	270	13	2	290	35	2	5
Caramel Roll	1 roll	140	5	1	115	22	< 1	3
Corn Bread	1 piece	160	6	1	320	25	< 1	3
French Bread Loaf	1 slice	70	1	0	160	14	< 1	3
Garlic Bread	1 slice	70	3	0.5	110	9	0	2
Garlic Cheese Biscuit	1 biscuit	220	14	6	630	20	< 1	5
DESSERTS								
Apple Crisp	1 spoon	150	3	1	85	32	1	< 1
Frozen Yogurt, Nonfat, Vanilla, Nutrasweet	4 fl oz	80	0	0	80	16	0	4
Fudge Brownie	1 brownie	200	7	2	140	35	1	2
Lemon Bar	1 bar	180	4	2	85	35	0	3
Peach Cobbler	1 spoon	140	2	0	130	32	< 1	1
ENTRÉES								
BBQ Pork Ribs, Country-style	1 rib	140	9	3.5	320	5	0	9
BBQ Smoked Sausage, Grilled	1 spoon	170	13	6	520	8	< 1	6
Beef Brisket, BBQ	3 oz	170	6	2	500	6	0	23
Beef Stroganoff	1 spoon	190	8	2.5	200	19	1	13
Chicken, Country BBQ, Breast	1 breast	310	16	5	780	6	2	40
Chicken, Fried, Hand-Breaded, Thigh	1 thigh	200	13	3.5	230	0	< 1	20
Chicken, Fried, Hand-Breaded, Wing	1 wing	90	6	1.5	115	0	0	10
Chicken, New Orleans Bourbon Street	1 spoon	180	8	1.5	580	9	0	17
Chicken, Rotisserie, Breast	1 breast	310	17	5	680	1	2	40
Chicken, Rotisserie, Drumstick	1 drumstick	90	6	1.5	170	0	0	10
Chicken Strips	1 spoon	170	10	2.5	430	10	0	10

	SERVING SIZE	CALORIES	TOTAL FAT (G)	SAT FAT (G)	SODIUM (MG)	CARBS (G)	FIBER (G)	PROTEIN (G)
Creamy Penne Carbonara	1 spoon	260	17	5	870	17	2	11
Fire Grilled Chicken Alfredo	1 spoon	220	14	4	480	14	2	10
Fish, Baked	1 piece	90	5	1	230	0	0	14
Ham, Carved	3 oz	100	5	3	990	0	0	14
Macaroni & Cheese	1 spoon	110	3	1	500	18	< 1	4
Meatloaf	3 oz	180	11	4.5	440	7	0	12
Perfect Pot Roast	1 spoon	160	7	2.5	780	9	1	15
Pork Loin, Grilled, Carved	3 oz	140	10	3.5	370	0	0	13
Roast Beef, Carved	3 oz	230	15	7	55	0	0	23
Salisbury Steak	1 piece	150	9	3.5	300	8	1	9
Salmon, Wood-Seared	1 piece	220	16	3	280	0	0	19
Shrimp, Fried	11 pieces	120	6	1	590	12	< 1	4
Steak, Country-Fried, w/Gravy	1 piece	230	14	4.5	690	16	< 1	10
Steak, Sirloin, Carved	3 oz	180	9	3.5	170	0	0	25
Turkey, Oven-Roasted, Rotisserie Style	3 oz	100	4	1	450	< 1	0	14
SIDES								
Beans, Baked, BBQ	1 spoon	130	3	1	680	26	4	4
Pasta Salad, Chicken	1 spoon	240	18	3.5	320	13	< 1	6
Potato Salad	1 spoon	120	7	1	300	15	1	2
Potatoes, Grilled, Cowboy	1 spoon	180	9	1.5	640	23	4	3
Potatoes, Red, Ranch	1 spoon	100	5	1	150	16	2	2
Potatoes, Sweet	1 spoon	80	0	0	35	20	3	2
SOUPS								
Chili Bean	4 fl oz ladle	80	4	1.5	340	9	3	7
Clam Chowder, New England	4 fl oz ladle	150	11	8	440	12	< 1	2
Corn Chowder	4 fl oz ladle	80	4	0.5	290	12	1	2
Minestrone	4 fl oz ladle	60	1	0	370	11	1	3
Potato Cheese	4 fl oz ladle	120	9	5	260	9	1	3

Old Spaghetti Factory
APPETIZERS

Olive Tapenade	1/4 plate	800	66	7	1560	46	2	7
Shrimp, Spinach & Artichoke Dip	1/4 plate	590	41	17	1130	39	3	18
Sicilian Garlic Cheese Bread	1/4 plate	1310	76	33	2510	110	6	49
Toasted Cheese Ravioli	1/4 plate	210	6	3.5	810	30	2	8
ENTRÉES								
Baked Lasagna, Dinner	1 entrée	800	43	21	2160	61	7	43
Chicken Marsala	1 entrée	1050	57	26	2260	75	3	56

	SERVING SIZE	CALORIES	TOTAL FAT (G)	SAT FAT (G)	SODIUM (MG)	CARBS (G)	FIBER (G)	PROTEIN (G)
Chicken Parmigiana	1 entrée	810	30	7	1800	80	5	54
Fettuccine Alfredo	1 entrée	1080	70	44	630	91	4	24
Lasagna Vegetariano	1 entrée	830	48	25	1910	68	9	37
Meatloaf, Italian Style	1 entrée	1180	68	32	1590	83	6	56
Spaghetti & Sicilian Meatballs	1 entrée	960	31	10	1940	114	7	53
Spaghetti w/Marinara Sauce	1 entrée	560	5	0.5	870	108	7	19
Spaghetti w/Mizithra Cheese & Brown Butter	1 entrée	1040	59	36	460	99	4	29
Spinach & Cheese Ravioli	1 entrée	480	16	9	1040	63	6	20
Spinach Tortellini, w/Alfredo Sauce	1 entrée	930	55	32	1110	86	5	25

Olive Garden
APPETIZERS

	SERVING SIZE	CALORIES	TOTAL FAT (G)	SAT FAT (G)	SODIUM (MG)	CARBS (G)	FIBER (G)	PROTEIN (G)
Breadstick w/ Garlic-Butter Spread	1 breadstick	140	2	0	370	26	2	5
Calamari	as served	890	54	5	2340	64	2	36
Fried Mozzarella Sampler	as served	370	22	9	800	26	2	17
Hot Spinach-Artichoke Dip	as served	650	31	15	1430	68	6	25

ENTRÉES

	SERVING SIZE	CALORIES	TOTAL FAT (G)	SAT FAT (G)	SODIUM (MG)	CARBS (G)	FIBER (G)	PROTEIN (G)
Braised Beef & Tortellini	1 entrée	1020	53	22	2060	82	10	53
Cheese Ravioli with Marinara Sauce	1 entrée	660	22	11	1440	84	7	32
Chicken Alfredo	1 entrée	1440	82	48	2070	103	5	71
Chicken Parmigiana	1 entrée	1090	49	18	3380	79	27	83
Eggplant Parmigiana	1 entrée	850	35	10	1900	98	19	36
Grilled Sausage & Peppers Rustica	1 entrée	1320	80	30	2860	91	10	59
Lasagna Classico	1 entrée	850	47	25	2830	39	19	68
Parmesan Crusted Tilapia	1 entrée	590	25	10	910	42	6	50
Spaghetti & Meatballs	1 entrée	920	36	14	1770	98	9	50
Steak Toscano	1 entrée	590	20	4.5	1460	62	6	39
Tour di Mare	1 entrée	1050	57	28	2350	88	7	46

SALADS

	SERVING SIZE	CALORIES	TOTAL FAT (G)	SAT FAT (G)	SODIUM (MG)	CARBS (G)	FIBER (G)	PROTEIN (G)
Garden-Fresh Salad w/ Dressing	1 serving	150	10	1.5	760	11	2	2
Grilled Chicken Caesar Salad w/ Dressing	1 serving	610	40	8	1230	19	5	43

SANDWICHES

	SERVING SIZE	CALORIES	TOTAL FAT (G)	SAT FAT (G)	SODIUM (MG)	CARBS (G)	FIBER (G)	PROTEIN (G)
Chicken Parmigiana Sandwich	1 whole sandwich	890	19	4	1270	47	5	26
Italian Meatball	1 whole sandwich	1060	58	27	2050	81	9	54

restaurants

	SERVING SIZE	CALORIES	TOTAL FAT (G)	SAT FAT (G)	SODIUM (MG)	CARBS (G)	FIBER (G)	PROTEIN (G)
Shrimp Scampi Fritta	1 whole sandwich	940	52	13	2590	87	4	31
SOUPS								
Pasta e Fagioli	1 cup	130	2.5	1	680	17	6	9
Zuppa Toscana	1 cup	170	4	2	960	24	2	10

On the Border
APPETIZER

	SERVING SIZE	CALORIES	TOTAL FAT (G)	SAT FAT (G)	SODIUM (MG)	CARBS (G)	FIBER (G)	PROTEIN (G)
Avocado Fries, w/Creamy Red Chile Sauce	as served	1120	83	14	1520	89	11	13
Border Sampler	as served	2060	142	55	4110	101	13	98
Chicken Flautas, w/Original Queso	as served	1250	87	22	2110	65	9	50
Firecracker Stuffed Jalapeños, w/Original Queso	as served	1910	135	38	6050	124	5	61
Grande Fajita Nachos, Steak	as served	1450	89	51	3010	79	16	92
BURRITO & BURRITO ENTRÉES, W/O BEANS								
Big Bordurrito, Chicken, w/Side Salad, w/o Dressing	as served	1690	77	20	4670	173	16	76
Big Bordurrito, Steak, w/Side Salad, w/o Dressing	as served	1750	89	29	3480	171	17	67
Chicken, Classic, w/o Sauce	as served	920	36	16	2340	103	4	46
Chicken, Three Sauce Fajita	as served	1120	40	17	4540	118	6	71
Shredded Beef, Classic, w/o Sauce	as served	1020	41	19	2010	102	3	58
Steak, Three Sauce Fajita	as served	1180	52	27	3330	115	6	62
CHIMICHANGA, CLASSIC								
Chicken, w/o Sauce	1 entrée	1300	79	24	2340	103	4	46
Ground Beef, w/o Sauce	1 entrée	1420	90	29	2440	105	6	47
EMPANADAS, W/RICE, W/O BEANS								
Chicken, w/Chile con Queso	1 entrée	620	46	16	830	32	1	19
Ground Beef, w/Chile con Queso	1 entrée	620	46	16	870	33	2	19
ENCHILADAS, W/RICE, W/O BEANS								
Avocado w/Red Chile Pesto & Rice, Grilled	1 entrée	1080	59	21	1960	111	14	33
Carne Asada	as served	970	38	15	2010	105	5	52
Chicken, Green Chile, w/Rice	1 entrée	850	34	11	2000	103	5	35
Chicken Salsa Fresca	as served	520	9	3	2410	60	12	50
Jalapeño BBQ Salmon	as served	590	21	6	1220	45	24	54

	SERVING SIZE	CALORIES	TOTAL FAT (G)	SAT FAT (G)	SODIUM (MG)	CARBS (G)	FIBER (G)	PROTEIN (G)
Pepper Jack Chicken, w/Rice, Grilled	1 entrée	1050	48	18	2990	106	6	51
Queso Chicken	as served	1030	41	14	2300	110	8	57
Ranchiladas	1 entrée	1260	66	34	3180	96	6	71
Smoky Beef Brisket, w/Rice, Grilled	1 entrée	980	46	20	2510	100	5	47
Suizas	1 entrée	1000	45	20	2220	106	7	45
Fajita, the Ultimate Fajita	as served	1160	96	22	2750	26	7	51
Quesadilla, Chicken	1 quesadilla	560	37	15	1340	25	1	31
SALADS, W/O DRESSING								
Sizzling Fajita, Chicken	1 salad	710	47	22	1770	23	8	52
Taco Grande, Beef	1 taco salad	1280	85	34	2250	80	15	53
Taco Grande, Chicken	1 taco salad	1180	75	29	2180	79	13	52
TACOS, W/RICE, W/O BEANS								
Al Carbon Especiales, Chicken	1 entrée	900	31	14	2190	102	3	52
Al Carbon Especiales, Steak	1 entrée	960	41	21	2270	101	3	50
Chicken, Achiote	1 entrée	650	12	2	1690	98	6	37
Chicken, Southwest, w/Creamy Red Chile Sauce	1 entrée	1280	61	18	2920	129	3	54
Fish, Dos XX, w/Creamy Red Chile Sauce	1 entrée	1950	121	28	3540	158	5	57
Mini, Street Style, Carnitas	1 entrée	930	47	16	2300	89	9	42
Mini, Street Style, Chicken	1 entrée	890	40	13	1990	88	8	47
Soft, Chicken	1 entrée	270	11	5	840	23	1	19
Soft, Ground Beef	1 entrée	340	18	8	880	24	2	20
TRES ENCHILADAS DINNER								
Chicken, w/Sour Cream Sauce	1 entrée	920	39	17	2040	102	5	39
Ground Beef, w/Chile con Carne	1 entrée	1060	48	18	2510	109	10	48

Outback Steakhouse
AUSSIE-TIZERS

	SERVING SIZE	CALORIES	TOTAL FAT (G)	SAT FAT (G)	SODIUM (MG)	CARBS (G)	FIBER (G)	PROTEIN (G)
Aussie Cheese Fries, Regular	1/6 order	327	22	10	463	23	0	9
Blooming Onion	1/6 order	325	27	8	683	19	2	3
Coconut Shrimp	1/2 order	207	11	6	403	20	0	7
Grilled Shrimp on the Barbie	1/2 order	147	8	2	433	12	2	8
Wings	1/4 order	469	38	13	1117	4	0	28
BURGERS & SANDWICHES, W/O SIDES								
Aged Cheddar Bacon Burger	1 burger	1042	75	32	1652	36	2	57
Bloomin' Burger	1 burger	1027	71	31	1766	50	4	47
Filet Focaccia Sandwich	1 sandwich	849	51	16	3977	51	3	44

restaurants

	SERVING SIZE	CALORIES	TOTAL FAT (G)	SAT FAT (G)	SODIUM (MG)	CARBS (G)	FIBER (G)	PROTEIN (G)
Grilled Chicken & Swiss Sandwich	1 sandwich	709	39	13	1352	41	2	50
Outbacker Burger	1 burger	686	40	19	1001	39	3	41
OUTBACK FAVORITES, W/O SIDES								
Alice Springs Chicken	1 entrée	784	49	16	1724	13	1	76
Baby Back Ribs, 1/2 rack	1 entrée	670	43	17	846	19	0	56
Grilled Chicken on the Barbie	1 entrée	305	3	0	893	10	0	57
No Rules Parmesan Pasta	1 entrée	880	51	29	988	73	6	18
SALADS, W/O DRESSING								
Aussie Chicken Cobb Salad, Grilled	1 salad	543	29	13	899	19	3	50
Caesar Salad, w/Chicken	1 salad	725	42	10	1537	21	6	71
California Chicken Salad	1 salad	690	39	9	1472	52	7	45
Filet Wedge Salad	1 salad	736	59	18	1400	16	2	36
SIDES								
Aussie Fries	as served	384	19	9	496	49	0	5
Dressed Baked Potato, Plain	as served	230	1	0	668	49	7	6
Garlic Mashed Potatoes	as served	305	17	7	1142	32	6	7
SIGNATURE STEAKS, W/O SIDES								
Outback Special Steak, 6 oz	1 entrée	254	13	5	226	0	0	37
Ribeye, 10 oz	1 entrée	544	35	15	405	0	0	58
Teriyaki Filet Medallions	1 entrée	694	30	12	3864	65	5	40
Victoria's Filet, 6 oz	1 entrée	218	9	4	206	0	0	36
STRAIGHT FROM THE SEA, W/O SIDES								
Lobster Tails, 4 oz	1 entrée	448	27	15	792	2	1	44
Norwegian Salmon	1 entrée	387	25	4	295	2	1	38
P.F. Chang's								
BEEF & PORK								
Beef w/ Broccoli	1 entrée	670	35	8	3260	33	4	56
Mongolian Beef	1 entrée	720	39	9	2700	31	1	61
Sweet & Sour Pork	1 entrée	710	25	6	1440	94	3	30
CHICKEN								
Almond & Cashew	1 entrée	640	25	4	3780	46	7	61
Kung Pao	1 entrée	1100	66	10	2130	56	7	73
Sesame	1 entrée	790	36	6	1340	50	12	68
Sweet & Sour	1 entrée	840	44	7	940	71	10	40
NOODLES & RICE								
Lo Mein (Combo)	1 entrée	880	31	6	3400	101	6	55

	SERVING SIZE	CALORIES	TOTAL FAT (G)	SAT FAT (G)	SODIUM (MG)	CARBS (G)	FIBER (G)	PROTEIN (G)
P.F. Chang's Fried Rice (Combo)	1 entrée	1210	36	8	2440	157	4	62
SEAFOOD								
Kung Pao Shrimp	1 entrée	830	54	8	2610	46	16	42
Crispy Honey Shrimp	1 entrée	660	38	7	2070	53	2	26
STARTERS & SMALL PLATES								
Chang's Vegetarian Lettuce Wraps	as served	610	36	4.5	2300	39	7	25
Egg Rolls w/o Sauce	2 rolls	280	10	2	1210	37	3	9
Pan Fried Pork Dumplings w/o Sauce	1 dumpling	360	15	4.5	680	33	4	22
Spring Rolls w/o Sauce	2 rolls	110	5	1	230	13	1	3
VEGETARIAN								
Coconut Curry Vegetables	1 entrée	1050	75	24	1360	52	11	43
Fried Rice	1 entrée	1090	19	5	2210	201	11	28
Ma Po Tofu	1 entrée	1030	70	13	3450	44	6	60

Panera Bread
BAKERY, BAGELS & BREADS

	SERVING SIZE	CALORIES	TOTAL FAT (G)	SAT FAT (G)	SODIUM (MG)	CARBS (G)	FIBER (G)	PROTEIN (G)
Cinnamon Sweet Roll	1 roll	630	24	14	490	91	4	13
French Baguette	as served	150	1	0	370	30	1	5
French Toast Bagel	1 bagel	340	4	2	620	67	2	9
Plain Bagel	1 bagel	290	1.5	0	460	49	2	10
Sourdough Soup Bowl	as served	660	3	0	1340	131	4	23
Whole Grain Bagel	1 bagel	340	2.5	0	400	67	6	13
Wild Blueberry Muffin	1 muffin	440	17	3	330	66	2	6
HOT PANINIS								
Half Chipotle Chicken on Artisan French	1/2 panini	420	19	6	1070	35	2	27
Half Italian Combo on Ciabatta	1/2 panini	490	21	8	1310	47	2	29
Half Smokehouse Turkey on Three Cheese	1/2 panini	360	13	6	1230	34	3	26
Half Tomato & Mozzarella on Ciabatta	1/2 panini	370	13	5	780	47	3	15
SANDWICHES								
Egg & Cheese on Ciabatta	1 sandwich	390	15	7	710	43	2	19
Half Smoked Ham & Swiss on Rye	1/2 sandwich	290	8	4	930	32	2	22
Half Smoked Turkey Breast on Country	1/2 sandwich	210	1.5	0	820	33	2	16
Half Tuna Salad on Honey Wheat	1/2 sandwich	250	8	2	580	31	3	14
SOUPS & SALADS								
Broccoli Cheddar	as served	300	19	13	1250	21	7	12
Chicken Caesar Salad	1 salad	440	26	7	660	19	3	34
Chopped Chicken Cobb w/Avocado Salad	1 salad	580	42	9	970	16	6	38
New England Clam Chowder	as served	630	54	35	890	27	3	8

restaurants

	SERVING SIZE	CALORIES	TOTAL FAT (G)	SAT FAT (G)	SODIUM (MG)	CARBS (G)	FIBER (G)	PROTEIN (G)
Papa John's								
PIZZA								
12" BBQ Chicken Bacon	1 slice	250	8	3.5	740	32	1	11
12" Cheese	1 slice	210	8	3.5	530	26	1	8
12" Garden Fresh	1 slice	200	7	3	500	27	2	8
12" Hawaiian BBQ Chicken	1 slice	250	8	3.5	740	33	1	11
12" Pepperoni	1 slice	230	10	4	610	26	1	9
12" Spicy Italian	1 slice	270	13	5	690	27	1	10
12" Spinach Alfredo	1 slice	200	8	3.5	500	26	1	8
12" The Meats	1 slice	250	12	5	710	26	1	11
12" The Works	1 slice	230	9	4	650	27	1	9
12" Tuscan Six Cheese	1 slice	230	9	4.5	580	26	1	10
SIDES								
Breadsticks	2 sticks	290	4.5	0.5	540	54	2	8
Spicy Buffalo Wings	2 wings	170	13	3	1070	3	0	12
Papa Murphy's								
CALZONES, LARGE								
Combination	1 slice	436	19	9.6	1016	45	<1	20
Italian	1 slice	433	18	9	1072	46	<1	21
Vegetarian	1 slice	384	15	7.7	899	45	1	17
deLITE THIN CRUST PIZZAS, LARGE								
Cheese	1 slice	143	7	4	202	13	<1	7
Chicken Bacon Artichoke	1 slice	179	9	3.8	389	13	<1	11
Gourmet Vegetarian	1 slice	160	8	3.9	306	13	<1	8
Herb Chicken Mediterranean	1 slice	180	9	3.9	344	15	1	10
Meat	1 slice	190	11	5.5	393	14	<1	11
Pepperoni	1 slice	171	9	4.9	300	13	<1	8
ORIGINAL CRUST PIZZAS, LARGE								
Cheese	1 slice	237	10	5	565	26	<1	11
Cowboy	1 slice	305	15	6.9	851	27	<1	15
Gourmet Vegetarian	1 slice	271	12	5.5	613	28	<1	12
Murphy's Combo	1 slice	317	16	7.1	891	28	<1	16
Pepperoni	1 slice	279	13	6.5	706	26	<1	13
SALADS								
Caesar, w/Chicken	1 salad	220	7	3.2	774	9	5	30
Club	1 salad	280	16	7.7	963	12	6	23
Italian	1 salad	263	19	8.6	738	13	6	14

	SERVING SIZE	CALORIES	TOTAL FAT (G)	SAT FAT (G)	SODIUM (MG)	CARBS (G)	FIBER (G)	PROTEIN (G)
Mediterranean	1 salad	381	16	9.2	1367	40	17	20
SIDE ITEMS								
Apple Dessert Pizza	1 slice	243	5	2	338	45	1	4
Cheesy Bread, w/o Sauce	2 slices	219	7	2.8	484	31	< 1	7
Cherry Dessert Pizza	1 slice	235	5	1	331	43	1	4
Cinnamon Wheel, w/o Frosting	2 slices	250	7	2.2	415	42	< 1	5
S'mores Dessert Pizza	2 slices	258	8	3.6	291	44	1	5
STUFFED PIZZAS, LARGE								
5-Meat	1 slice	362	16	7.5	906	38	< 1	17
Chicago Style	1 slice	360	16	7.6	857	39	< 1	16
Chicken Bacon	1 slice	365	15	6.8	830	38	< 1	19

Peet's Coffee & Tea

	SERVING SIZE	CALORIES	TOTAL FAT (G)	SAT FAT (G)	SODIUM (MG)	CARBS (G)	FIBER (G)	PROTEIN (G)
BAKERY								
Almond Biscotti	1 cookie	184	10	1.3	25	20	2	4
Banana Nut Bread	as served	470	20	9	450	65	2	7
Blueberry Muffin	1 muffin	480	21	9	530	65	2	8
Chocolate Chip Cookie	1 cookie	410	20	9	280	50	4	5
Cinnamon Twist Croissant	1 croissant	460	27	17	480	45	2	7
Classic Coffee Cake	as served	590	27	14	400	75	2	8
Cranberry Walnut Scone	1 scone	320	13	4	130	46	3	3
Low-Fat Banana Blueberry Muffin	1 muffin	290	3	1	240	54	2	7
Peanut Butter Cookie	1 cookie	470	24	9	260	52	2	9
Reduced-Fat Pumpkin Ginger Muffin	1 muffin	460	14	1.5	530	75	3	8
Sugar Cookie	1 cookie	290	12	7	180	54	3	4
BLENDED FREDDOS, W/REDUCED-FAT MILK, W/O WHIPPED CREAM, MEDIUM								
Caffe Freddo	16 fl oz	210	3	2	200	48	1	5
Chai Freddo	16 fl oz	330	4	2	231	67	0	8
Chocolate & Caramel Swirl	16 fl oz	370	3	2	245	84	2	8
Dark Chocolate Caramel Mocha Freddo	16 fl oz	410	5	3	203	83	2	8
Mocha Freddo	16 fl oz	250	3	2	196	51	1	6
Vanilla Caffe Freddo	16 fl oz	310	3	2	186	67	0	5
BREWED COFFEE, W/REDUCED-FAT MILK								
Caffe au Lait	16 fl oz	70	3	2	70	7	0	7
ESPRESSO BEVERAGES, W/REDUCED-FAT MILK, W/O WHIPPED CREAM, MEDIUM								
Caffe Latte	16 fl oz	211	8	5	228	21	0	21

restaurants

	SERVING SIZE	CALORIES	TOTAL FAT (G)	SAT FAT (G)	SODIUM (MG)	CARBS (G)	FIBER (G)	PROTEIN (G)
Caffe Mocha	16 fl oz	300	8	5	230	40	2	17
Caffe Vanilla Latte	16 fl oz	310	8	5	210	46	0	15
Cappuccino	16 fl oz	130	5	3	140	13	0	10
Caramel Caffe Latte	16 fl oz	381	8	4	254	61	0	17
Latte Macchiato	16 fl oz	211	8	5	228	21	0	16
ICED COFFEES, W/REDUCED-FAT MILK								
Caffe Latte	16 fl oz	175	6	4	175	18	0	3
Caffe Latte, w/Vanilla	16 fl oz	275	6	4	175	43	0	13
Caffe Mocha	16 fl oz	248	6	3	178	35	2	13
Cappuccino	16 fl oz	158	6	3	158	16	0	11
Caramel Latte	16 fl oz	338	6	3	210	56	0	14
TEAS, W/REDUCED-FAT MILK								
Masala Chai Latte, Hot or Iced	16 fl oz	213	4	3	133	34	0	9

Pepe's Mexican Restaurant
BURRITOS, SUIZA

	SERVING SIZE	CALORIES	TOTAL FAT (G)	SAT FAT (G)	SODIUM (MG)	CARBS (G)	FIBER (G)	PROTEIN (G)
Beef	1 burrito	640	34	14	1170	55	10	30
Chicken	1 burrito	610	31	13	1140	54	9	30
Pork	1 burrito	600	29	12	1150	54	10	32
FLAUTAS, W/CHEESE & SAUCE								
Beef	1 flauta	190	12	3	300	11	2	10
Chicken	1 flauta	230	13	2	250	17	2	11
TACO SALAD, W/SHELL								
Beef	1 salad	550	26	10	1570	52	8	27
Chicken	1 salad	520	23	8	1540	51	7	27
Pork	1 salad	500	20	7	1560	52	8	29
TACOS								
Crisp, Chicken	1 taco	190	9	3	380	15	2	12
Crisp, Pork	1 taco	170	6	2.5	390	16	3	13
Soft, Corn, Beef	1 taco	250	10	4	440	28	4	13
Soft, Corn, Chicken	1 taco	230	8	3.5	420	27	4	13
Soft, Corn, Pork	1 taco	220	6	2.5	430	27	4	14
TOSTADAS, SUIZA								
Beef	1 tostada	440	29	11	750	26	4	19
Chicken	1 tostada	410	26	10	740	25	4	19
Pork	1 tostada	410	25	9	740	26	4	20

Perkins Restaurant & Bakery

	SERVING SIZE	CALORIES	TOTAL FAT (G)	SAT FAT (G)	SODIUM (MG)	CARBS (G)	FIBER (G)	PROTEIN (G)
APPETIZERS								
Buffalo Dippers	1 entrée	1090	74	13	6010	64	2	46
Chick'n Cheese Quesadilla	1 entrée	920	48	25	2490	67	4	56
Perkins Sampler Platter	1 entrée	1990	124	27	4010	157	5	64
BREAKFAST								
Belgian Waffle	1 entrée	700	33	14	1020	92	2	9
Cheesy Bacon Scramber	1 entrée	1450	76	28	2880	139	6	52
Classic Eggs, w/Bacon	1 entrée	1420	58	16	3920	181	7	44
Country Sausage Biscuit Platter	1 entrée	1770	99	49	5080	163	9	54
Ooh-la-la French Toast	1 entrée	1000	42	12	1220	121	3	36
Pancakes, Short Stack	1 entrée	730	35	11	1500	92	0	12
Smoked Bacon & Ham Omelette	1 entrée	1690	79	26	4350	185	7	60
Southern Fried Chicken Scrambler	1 entrée	1440	69	20	3120	158	6	47
Steak & Eggs	1 entrée	1490	54	15	3460	181	7	71
ENTRÉES								
Cavatappi Marinara Pasta	1 entrée	960	54	16	1610	96	8	23
Down Home Meatloaf	1 entrée	1040	65	26	2530	72	6	41
Grilled Pork Chops	1 entrée	1110	58	20	2050	75	9	69
Island Tilapia Dinner	1 entrée	450	6	1.5	1060	50	5	50
Jumbo Shrimp Dinner	1 entrée	1030	50	14	1970	117	10	30
Mushroom 'n Swiss Chicken Dinner	1 entrée	1130	45	15	2320	123	8	58
Roast Beef Dinner	1 entrée	780	42	17	2210	57	6	41
Top Sirloin Steak Dinner	1 entrée	770	34	12	470	67	8	50
SALADS								
Chef Deluxe	1 salad	880	58	22	2120	30	6	59
Chicken & Spinach	1 salad	960	65	14	2210	37	5	56
Honey Mustard Chicken Crunch	1 salad	1220	83	21	2510	72	6	52
SANDWICHES & BURGERS								
Buffalo Wrap	1 wrap	1460	98	25	5270	105	6	42
Chef Wrap	1 wrap	1160	74	18	3000	90	6	38
Chicken Crisp Melt	1 sandwich	1710	111	28	3750	119	5	61
Country Club Melt	1 sandwich	1380	84	29	3630	95	5	62
French Dip	1 sandwich	930	51	13	2580	77	4	43
Ham & Turkey BLT Wrap	1 wrap	1080	69	14	3090	89	6	31
Hamburger	1 burger	1060	62	18	1220	71	6	56

restaurants

	SERVING SIZE	CALORIES	TOTAL FAT (G)	SAT FAT (G)	SODIUM (MG)	CARBS (G)	FIBER (G)	PROTEIN (G)
Kickin Chicken Sandwich	1 sandwich	1350	75	20	3450	118	8	54
SOUP, BOWL								
Broccoli & Cheddar Cheese	1 bowl	280	18	8	1480	20	2	10
Homestyle Chicken Noodle	1 bowl	150	5	1	340	16	2	11
New England Clam Chowder	1 bowl	260	14	8	1130	19	2	14
Vegetable Beef	1 bowl	150	5	1	1190	19	5	10

Peter Piper Pizza
APPETIZERS & DESSERTS

	SERVING SIZE	CALORIES	TOTAL FAT (G)	SAT FAT (G)	SODIUM (MG)	CARBS (G)	FIBER (G)	PROTEIN (G)
Breadsticks	1/2 order	250	10	1.5	760	36	0	7
Cinnamon Crunch Dessert	1/2 order	220	2	0	220	49	2	5
Garlic Cheese Bread	1/2 order	310	14	4	610	37	2	10
Regular Boneless Wings, Buffalo	1/2 order	397	19	3	2203	22	2	28
Wings	1/2 order	110	8	2	190	0	0	9
PIZZA, 5 MEAT SUPREME, LARGE								
Hand-Tossed	1 slice	350	13	6	970	38	2	19
Original	1 slice	350	13	6	850	38	2	21
Pan	1 slice	380	13	6	1010	46	2	20
Thin	1 slice	180	8	4	540	14	1	12
PIZZA, CALIFORNIA VEGGIE, LARGE								
Hand-Tossed	1 slice	270	7	3	560	39	2	13
Original	1 slice	200	6	3	430	23	2	12
Pan	1 slice	300	7	3	610	47	3	14
Thin	1 slice	130	5	2	290	15	1	8
PIZZA, CHEESE, LARGE								
Hand-Tossed	1 slice	290	9	4.5	590	38	2	17
Original	1 slice	300	9	4.5	470	37	2	18
Pan	1 slice	290	9	4.5	590	38	2	17
Thin	1 slice	150	5	3	290	14	1	10
PIZZA, PEPPERONI, LARGE								
Hand-Tossed	1 slice	290	10	4.5	670	37	2	14
Original	1 slice	300	10	4.5	550	36	2	16
Pan	1 slice	330	10	4.5	710	44	2	15
Thin	1 slice	150	6	3	340	13	1	9
SALADS								
Chicken Caesar	1 salad	200	8	1	900	10	4	21
Garden	1 salad	50	0	0	45	10	2	3
Italian Chef	1 salad	290	16	4	1910	14	2	24

	SERVING SIZE	CALORIES	TOTAL FAT (G)	SAT FAT (G)	SODIUM (MG)	CARBS (G)	FIBER (G)	PROTEIN (G)
Side	1 salad	20	0	0	30	4	1	2

Piccadilly
DESSERTS

Bread Pudding, w/Rum Sauce	1 slice	807	23	13	569	107	2	50
Cupcakes	1 each	171	8	2	141	24	0	2
Lemon Icebox Pie	1 slice	589	31	21	305	71	1	10
Mississippi Mud Pie	1 slice	439	29	15	251	43	2	6
Old Fashion Brownie	1 slice	1005	35	6	691	176	0	9
Peach Cobbler	1 slice	545	22	9	515	82	6	6
Pumpkin Pie	1 slice	310	11	5	581	48	2	5
Red Velvet Cake	1 slice	833	54	10	382	83	1	6

ENTRÉES

Baked Cajun Boneless Chicken Breast	1 entrée	379	19	9	1766	9	1	41
Blackened Boneless Chicken Breast	1 entrée	297	14	8	194	3	1	40
Blackened Pork Chop, w/Fettuccine Alfredo	1 entrée	658	30	13	480	35	3	60
Blackened Shrimp, w/Fettuccine	1 entrée	827	40	6	256	73	5	44
Cajun Baked Tilapia	1 entrée	332	20	12	1095	4	1	37
Chicken Teriyaki, w/Polynesian Rice	1 entrée	659	16	6	2341	79	3	48
Crawfish Etouffee	1 entrée	555	14	3	2605	84	3	20
Large Angus Chop Steak	1 entrée	884	65	23	473	5	1	67
Salmon Pattie	1 entrée	231	9	3	390	24	1	13
Shrimp Diablo	1 entrée	443	10	3	1894	54	3	32
Shrimp Scampi & Fettuccini	1 entrée	648	42	25	1090	35	2	34
Sliced Roast Beef	1 entrée	640	53	21	1487	0	0	39
Smothered Pork Chop	1 entrée	732	34	9	1184	46	4	56

SENSATIONAL SALADS & SAVORY SIDES

Breaded Okra	1 side	242	13	3	473	26	4	4
Carrot Souffle	1 side	392	17	10	205	58	3	4
Greens, Turnip, w/Diced Turnips	1 side	62	2	1	633	11	4	2
Mashed Potatoes	1 serving	117	4	2	173	19	2	2
Neptune Salad	1 salad	244	14	2	944	25	2	7
Pea Salad	1 salad	291	17	7	719	20	5	15
Piccadilly Fruit Salad	1 salad	72	0	0	11	18	2	1
Southwest Fiesta Chicken Salad	1 salad	698	37	19	1979	35	7	58

restaurants

	SERVING SIZE	CALORIES	TOTAL FAT (G)	SAT FAT (G)	SODIUM (MG)	CARBS (G)	FIBER (G)	PROTEIN (G)
SPECIALTY SOUPS								
Chicken-Rice	1 cup	100	0	0	933	20	0	4
Seafood Gumbo Over Rice	1 bowl	227	6	2	1236	32	2	11
Vegetable	1 cup	45	0	0	556	9	2	2

Pita Pit
BREAKFAST PITAS, WHITE PITA, INCLUDES EGGS, HASHBROWNS, GREEN PEPPERS & ONIONS

	SERVING SIZE	CALORIES	TOTAL FAT (G)	SAT FAT (G)	SODIUM (MG)	CARBS (G)	FIBER (G)	PROTEIN (G)
Awakin' w/Bacon	1 pita	610	27	9	1610	57	4	31
Chicken Classic	1 pita	555	18	6	1270	59	4	34
Ham n' Eggs	1 pita	510	17	6	1610	58	4	28
Morning Glory	1 pita	505	19	5.5	970	61	7	20
Sausage Scramble	1 pita	530	21	7	1220	59	5	23
PITAS, WHITE PITA								
Black Forest Ham	1 pita	320	5	2	1610	43	2	25
BLT	1 pita	455	19	6	1290	44	4	26
Chicken Breast	1 pita	300	4	1	630	43	2	22
Chicken Caesar	1 pita	385	10	3	950	44	3	29
Chicken Crave	1 pita	360	6	2	1270	44	2	31
Chicken Souvlaki	1 pita	357	10	1.4	829	42	2	21
Club	1 pita	385	9	3	1800	42	2	31
Dagwood	1 pita	410	9	3.3	1795	44	2	37
Falafel	1 pita	456	14	1.5	1092	65	6	16
Feta	1 pita	320	9	5	1070	43	2	17
Garden	1 pita	200	1	0	330	41	2	7
Gyro	1 pita	560	29	12	1110	49	2	23
Hummus	1 pita	300	8	0	590	49	4	11
Philly Steak	1 pita	320	6	2	1160	44	3	24
Prime Rib	1 pita	410	12	4.5	960	44	2	31
Spicy Black Bean	1 pita	310	3	0	1100	57	9	18
Turkey	1 pita	290	2	0	1350	41	2	25
SAUCES								
Ancho Chipotle	as served	90	7	1	250	7	0	0
Caribbean Jerk	as served	40	0	0	760	10	0	0
Chipotle BBQ Sauce	as served	45	1	0	200	9	0	0
Jalapeño Ranch Dressing	as served	110	12	1	230	2	0	1
Mango Habeñero	as served	20	0	0	100	5	0	0

	SERVING SIZE	CALORIES	TOTAL FAT (G)	SAT FAT (G)	SODIUM (MG)	CARBS (G)	FIBER (G)	PROTEIN (G)
Red Thai Curry Sauce	as served	30	3	2	80	3	0	0
Salsa Roja	as served	15	0	0	20	2	0	0
Salsa Verde	as served	10	0	0	170	2	0	0
Secret Sauce	as served	190	21	1.5	65	0	0	0
Sundried Tomato Pesto Vinaigrette	as served	100	11	2	270	2	0	0
Sweet Chili Sauce	as served	60	0	0	220	14	0	0
Tzatziki	as served	45	4	3.5	75	2	0	0

Pizza Hut
BONE OUT WINGS
All American	2 pieces	150	8	1.5	490	11	1	10
Average for Buffalo Flavors	2 pieces	190	9	1.5	1003	18	1	10

CRISPY BONE-IN WINGS
All American	2 pieces	200	14	2.5	500	8	1	9
Average for All Buffalo Flavors	2 pieces	230	15	3	1023	16	1	9

PIZZA, FIT 'N DELICIOUS, 12"
Chicken, Red Onion & Green Pepper	1 slice	180	5	1.5	510	23	1	11
Ham, Red Onion & Mushroom	1 slice	160	5	1.5	550	23	1	8

PIZZA, HAND-TOSSED, LARGE
Cheese Only	1 slice	320	12	6	800	38	2	15
Meat Lover's	1 slice	440	23	9	1250	38	2	20
Pepperoni	1 slice	330	14	6	910	38	2	15
Veggie Lover's	1 slice	290	9	4.5	760	39	2	13

PIZZA, PAN, LARGE
Cheese Only	1 slice	360	17	7	740	37	2	15
Meat Lover's	1 slice	480	28	10	1180	37	2	20
Pepperoni	1 slice	380	19	7	840	36	2	15
Veggie Lover's	1 slice	330	15	5	690	38	2	13

PIZZA, PERSONAL PAN, 6"
Cheese Only	whole pizza	590	24	10	1290	69	3	26
Meat Lover's	whole pizza	830	46	17	2110	68	3	36
Pepperoni	whole pizza	610	26	10	1410	67	3	26
Veggie Lover's	whole pizza	550	20	8	1190	70	4	22

PIZZA, P'ZONE
Classic	1/2 order	470	16	7	1070	61	2	20
Meaty	1/2 order	550	23	10	1370	61	2	24
Pepperoni	1/2 order	450	15	7	1120	60	2	19

restaurants

	SERVING SIZE	CALORIES	TOTAL FAT (G)	SAT FAT (G)	SODIUM (MG)	CARBS (G)	FIBER (G)	PROTEIN (G)
PIZZA, STUFFED CRUST, LARGE								
Cheese Only	1 slice	340	14	7	900	39	2	16
Meat Lover's	1 slice	480	26	11	1380	39	2	22
Pepperoni	1 slice	370	17	8	1040	39	2	17
Veggie Lover's	1 slice	330	12	6	880	41	2	15
PIZZA, THIN 'N CRISPY, LARGE								
Cheese Only	1 slice	260	11	6	740	29	1	12
Meat Lover's	1 slice	390	23	9	1210	28	1	18
Pepperoni	1 slice	280	13	6	850	28	1	13
Veggie Lover's	1 slice	240	9	4	710	30	2	10
SIDES								
Breadsticks	1 each	140	5	1	260	19	1	5
Cheese Breadsticks	1 each	170	6	2.5	390	20	1	8

Pizza Ranch
PIZZAS, SKILLET CRUST, MEDIUM

	SERVING SIZE	CALORIES	TOTAL FAT (G)	SAT FAT (G)	SODIUM (MG)	CARBS (G)	FIBER (G)	PROTEIN (G)
Bacon Cheeseburger	1 slice	200	9	3	390	23	1	7
Beef	1 slice	170	6	2	270	23	1	6
Cheese	1 slice	190	8	3	250	23	1	7
Garlic Cheese	1 slice	190	9	2	200	21	1	4
Italian Sausage	1 slice	180	7	2	260	23	1	5
Pepperoni	1 slice	190	8	3	300	22	1	6
STARTERS & SIDES								
Cactus Bread, Large	1 slice	320	11	2	248	50	1	5
Chicken, Breast, Broasted	1 breast	440	23	7	370	4	0	52
Chicken, Leg, Broasted	1 leg	190	12	3.5	180	2	0	18
Chicken, Thigh, Broasted	1 thigh	370	26	7	340	4	0	30
Chicken, Wing, Broasted	1 wing	190	13	3.5	170	2	0	15
Garlic Bread, w/Cheese	1 piece	288	18	8	456	12	1	8
Hot Wings	1 wing	111	10	3	283	1	0	5
Ranch Stix, w/Cheese	1 piece	218	11	4	270	25	0	7

Planet Smoothie
SMOOTHIES

	SERVING SIZE	CALORIES	TOTAL FAT (G)	SAT FAT (G)	SODIUM (MG)	CARBS (G)	FIBER (G)	PROTEIN (G)
Acai	1 smoothie	410	7	1.5	15	85	8	3
Acai Bowl	1 smoothie	370	10	2	50	66	6	4
Berry Bada-Bing	1 smoothie	410	0	0	110	101	11	8
Big Bang, Protein Blast	1 smoothie	300	0	0	20	61	5	13
Big Bang, Workout Blast	1 smoothie	280	0	0	20	68	5	1

	SERVING SIZE	CALORIES	TOTAL FAT (G)	SAT FAT (G)	SODIUM (MG)	CARBS (G)	FIBER (G)	PROTEIN (G)
Billy Bob Banana	1 smoothie	360	1	0	130	87	12	9
Chocolate Chimp, Protein Blast	1 smoothie	320	1	0	0	69	3	14
Chocolate Elvis	1 smoothie	490	17	3.5	280	79	12	15
Hangover Over	1 smoothie	350	0	0	100	90	11	6
Leapin' Lizard	1 smoothie	260	0	0	0	67	3	1
Lunar Lemonade, Raspberry	1 smoothie	310	0	0	20	77	6	2
Mediterranean Monster	1 smoothie	300	0	0	20	78	5	1
Mr. Mongo, Chocolate, Protein Blast	1 smoothie	330	1	0	140	63	10	22
Mr. Mongo, Chocolate, Workout Blast	1 smoothie	300	1	0	150	70	10	10
Mr. Mongo, Strawberry, Protein Blast	1 smoothie	430	0	0	140	90	12	21
Mr. Mongo, Strawberry, Workout Blast	1 smoothie	400	0	0	150	97	12	9
Rasmanian Devil	1 smoothie	340	0	0	50	78	7	3
Road Runner	1 smoothie	310	0	0	30	77	6	1
Screamsicle	1 smoothie	320	1	0	100	77	4	5
Shag-a-delic	1 smoothie	380	0	0	150	91	13	9
The Last Mango	1 smoothie	330	2	0	60	80	4	2
Thelma & Louise	1 smoothie	250	0	0	30	63	6	1
Twig & Berries	1 smoothie	340	0	0	100	87	12	6
Two Piece Bikini, Strawberry	1 smoothie	310	0	0	75	75	5	4
Werewolf	1 smoothie	270	0	0	50	66	5	2
Yo' Adriane	1 smoothie	330	0	0	110	83	11	6

Pollo Tropical
DESSERTS

	SERVING SIZE	CALORIES	TOTAL FAT (G)	SAT FAT (G)	SODIUM (MG)	CARBS (G)	FIBER (G)	PROTEIN (G)
Cream Smoothies, Average of All Flavors	17 oz	330	8	6	80	64	0	3
Flan	1 flan	210	9	5	550	26	0	8
Guava Cheesecake	1 slice	310	17	10	230	36	1	5
Tres Leches	1 item	380	9	5	210	76	0	9
TropiChiller, Average of All Flavors	16 oz	297	1	1	30	73	1	1

ENTRÉES

	SERVING SIZE	CALORIES	TOTAL FAT (G)	SAT FAT (G)	SODIUM (MG)	CARBS (G)	FIBER (G)	PROTEIN (G)
1/4 Chicken, Dark Meat	as served	290	22	6	430	0	0	24
1/4 Chicken, White Meat	as served	360	20	6	730	0	0	43
Caribbean Ribs	1/2 rack	400	31	13	680	2	0	29
Chicken Breasts, Grilled	1 breast	150	3	1	440	0	0	30
Fajitas, Chicken, w/o Rice or Beans	1 fajita	710	26	11	1680	61	6	59
Grilled Tropical Wings	1 wing	50	3	1	190	1	0	5
Mojo Roast Pork, w/Grilled Onions	as served	370	22	8	620	3	1	39

restaurants

	SERVING SIZE	CALORIES	TOTAL FAT (G)	SAT FAT (G)	SODIUM (MG)	CARBS (G)	FIBER (G)	PROTEIN (G)
SALADS & SANDWICHES								
Chicken Chipotle, Sandwich	1 sandwich	510	20	3	960	44	3	38
Chicken Quesadilla Salad	1 salad	1110	67	16	2070	71	9	51
Guava Pork BBQ, Sandwich	1 sandwich	430	13	4	650	52	3	27
SIDES								
Fried Yuca	6 pieces	360	16	2	640	54	3	1
Waffle Fries, Regular	as served	390	27	2	730	34	3	3
Yellow Rice w/Vegetables, Regular	as served	240	4	1	620	48	3	5
TROPICAL TRIOS, W/BREAD ROLL								
Chicken (White), Mojo Roast Pork & Carribean Ribs	1 entrée	1010	59	20	1830	20	2	100
Wings (White) & Caribbean Ribs	1 entrée	800	46	15	1780	21	1	77
Wings (White) & Mojo Roast Pork	1 entrée	970	53	16	2060	23	2	102

Popeye's Lousiana Kitchen

	SERVING SIZE	CALORIES	TOTAL FAT (G)	SAT FAT (G)	SODIUM (MG)	CARBS (G)	FIBER (G)	PROTEIN (G)
BIG EASYS								
Chicken & Sausage Jambalaya	1 item	220	11	3	760	20	1	10
Chicken Po' Boy	1 item	660	34	9	2120	61	3	31
Loaded Chicken Wrap	1 wrap	310	13	6	890	33	3	14
BREAKFAST								
Bacon Biscuit	1 item	400	25	12	780	37	3	8
Egg Biscuit	1 item	510	29	15	1155	41	1	13
Hashbrowns	1 item	360	20	9	450	41	4	3
Sausage Biscuit	1 item	540	36	18	1100	41	1	13
LOUISIANA TRAVELERS								
Mild Tenders	3 pieces	340	14	6	1350	26	1	27
Naked Tenders	3 pieces	170	2	0	550	2	0	26
Nuggets	6 pieces	230	14	6	350	14	1	11
MILD CHICKEN								
Breast	1 breast	440	27	11	1330	16	2	35
Leg	1 leg	160	9	4	460	5	1	14
Thigh	1 thigh	280	21	8	640	7	1	14
Wing	1 wing	210	14	4	610	8	1	13
SHRIMP								
Butterfly	8 shrimp	290	17	8	820	21	3	12
Popcorn	as served	330	9	9	1290	28	3	11

	SERVING SIZE	CALORIES	TOTAL FAT (G)	SAT FAT (G)	SODIUM (MG)	CARBS (G)	FIBER (G)	PROTEIN (G)
SIDES								
Cajun Fries, Large	1 item	770	41	16	1700	89	7	10
Macaroni & Cheese, Regular	1 item	600	21	11	1470	78	3	24
Mashed Potatoes, Regular	1 item	330	12	6	1770	54	3	9
Onion Rings	12 rings	560	38	17	920	50	5	6

Port of Subs
GRILLERS, 8", ON CIABATTA, W/PROVOLONE CHEESE

	SERVING SIZE	CALORIES	TOTAL FAT (G)	SAT FAT (G)	SODIUM (MG)	CARBS (G)	FIBER (G)	PROTEIN (G)
BBQ Pulled Pork	1 sandwich	461	11	5	1872	59	2	32
Grilled Chicken	1 sandwich	594	15	6	1827	62	3	55
Meatball	1 sandwich	883	50	21	2423	65	5	46
SALADS								
Antipasto, w/Capicola, Salami, Pepperoni & Provolone	1 salad	333	23	10	1137	9	3	22
Chef, w/Ham, Turkey, Provolone & American Cheese	1 salad	300	18	11	1290	10	3	23
Grilled Chicken	1 salad	188	3	1	720	10	3	29
Tuna	1 salad	249	18	3	395	9	3	12
SANDWICHES, 8", W/CHEESE, LETTUCE, TOMATO & ONION								
Bacon, Lettuce, Tomato	1 sandwich	754	41	14	1424	61	5	34
Ham, American	1 sandwich	634	23	10	2347	68	5	38
Ham, Turkey, Provolone	1 sandwich	577	17	8	1907	66	5	39
Peppered Pastrami, Swiss	1 sandwich	581	19	9	964	66	5	36
Roast Beef, Provolone	1 sandwich	590	19	8	1290	66	5	41
Roasted Chicken, Provolone	1 sandwich	563	16	7	1539	66	5	40
Salami, Provolone	1 sandwich	667	30	11	1753	66	5	35
Smoked Ham, Swiss	1 sandwich	632	23	10	1749	67	5	42
Tuna, Provolone	1 sandwich	885	50	12	1364	69	5	40
Turkey, Provolone	1 sandwich	584	17	7	1940	69	5	41

Pret A Manger
BAGUETTES

	SERVING SIZE	CALORIES	TOTAL FAT (G)	SAT FAT (G)	SODIUM (MG)	CARBS (G)	FIBER (G)	PROTEIN (G)
Chicken Mozzarella	1 baguette	620	22	6	1060	92	6	37
Pret's Famous Ham & Cheese	1 baguette	600	20	6	1540	77	3	26
Pret's Vietnamese	1 baguette	550	16	2	1070	92	4	30
Roasted Turkey & Cheddar	1 baguette	630	21	8	1690	77	3	38
Slow-Roasted Beef, Arugula & Parmesan	1 baguette	580	17	5	910	55	2	38

restaurants

	SERVING SIZE	CALORIES	TOTAL FAT (G)	SAT FAT (G)	SODIUM (MG)	CARBS (G)	FIBER (G)	PROTEIN (G)
HOT FOOD								
BBQ Pulled Pork Hot Wrap	1 wrap	470	16	9	1290	60	1	15
Falafel & Red Peppers Hot Wrap	1 wrap	490	23	9	1100	55	6	7
Ham, Cheese & Mustard Toastie	1 toastie	540	26	10	1350	44	4	30
Mozzarella & Pesto Toastie	1 toastie	400	16	7	510	48	6	17
SALAD & SUSHI								
Chicken & Avocado Salad	1 salad	440	28	3	140	43	12	22
Farmer's Market Salad	1 salad	260	12	1	430	34	12	8
Harvest Salad	1 salad	260	15	3	160	30	5	7
Pret's Cobb & Greens Salad	1 salad	440	23	8	880	32	6	27
Tuna Quinoa Salad Pot	1 salad	200	9	1.5	250	16	3	15
SANDWICHES								
Balsamic Chicken & Avocado	1 sandwich	530	23	2	940	58	12	23
Chicken & Bacon	1 sandwich	470	18	3	810	59	9	26
Mozzarella, Roasted Tomato & Pesto	1 sandwich	450	19	8	720	52	8	18
Pret's Classic Cheddar & Tomato	1 sandwich	490	23	10	830	51	7	19
Pret's Egg Salad & Arugula	1 sandwich	460	22	4	910	47	6	17
Pret's Perfect Ham & Cheddar	1 sandwich	490	20	6	1400	47	6	24
SOUPS								
Hungarian Mushroom	12 oz	285	20	9	1380	20	3	5
Moroccan Lentil	12 oz	435	19	2.3	960	54	14	17
Pret's Hearty Turkey Chili	12 oz	300	6	2	915	33	11	29
Pretzel Roll	1 roll	100	2	0	260	18	1	3
Shrimp & Roasted Corn Chowder	12 oz	360	20	11	840	32	3	17
Steak & Ale	12 oz	525	35	21	1125	30	3	23
WRAPS								
Avocado Pine Nut	1 wrap	440	26	5	470	41	9	9
Spicy Shrimp & Cilantro	1 wrap	290	7	2	640	34	3	22

Qdoba

3-CHEESE NACHOS, ALL W/CHIPS, 3-CHEESE QUESO, LETTUCE, BLACK BEANS, GUACAMOLE, SOUR CREAM & SALSA ROJA

	SERVING SIZE	CALORIES	TOTAL FAT (G)	SAT FAT (G)	SODIUM (MG)	CARBS (G)	FIBER (G)	PROTEIN (G)
As Is	as served	1095	58	20	1850	119	28	26
Grilled Chicken	as served	1285	68	22.5	2190	120	28	51
Ground Beef	as served	1335	75	27	2380	120	29	46

	SERVING SIZE	CALORIES	TOTAL FAT (G)	SAT FAT (G)	SODIUM (MG)	CARBS (G)	FIBER (G)	PROTEIN (G)
BURRITOS, ALL W/12.5" FLOUR TORTILLA, CLIANTRO-LIME RICE, BLACK BEANS, SALSA VERDE & SOUR CREAM								
Grilled Chicken	1 burrito	925	27	9	2190	120	18	47
Grilled Steak	1 burrito	925	26	10	2090	122	18	47
Grilled Vegetables	1 burrito	795	21	7	1950	124	21	23
Pulled Pork	1 burrito	880	19	7.5	2100	130	18	43
GRILLED QUESADILLA, ALL W/12.5" TORTILLA & SOUR CREAM								
Cheese	as served	800	47	28.5	1450	54	3	39
Grilled Chicken	as served	990	57	31	1790	55	3	64
Grilled Steak	as served	990	56	32	1690	57	3	64
SIGNATURE BURRITOS, ALL 12.5" FLOUR TORTILLA, W/GRILLED CHICKEN, CILANTRO-LIME RICE & SALSA ROJA								
Ancho Chile BBQ	1 burrito	815	25	7	2640	111	6	38
Fajita Ranchera	1 burrito	770	24	6	2380	101	8	38
Grilled Veggie	1 burrito	725	22	6	2090	95	5	37
Mexican Gumbo	1 burrito	815	27	7	3070	104	6	40
Queso Burrito	1 burrito	825	30	12	2390	98	6	40
TACO SALADS, ALL W/CRUNCHY TORTILLA BOWL, CORN & BLACK BEAN SALSA, CHEESE & SOUR CREAM, W/O DRESSING								
Grilled Chicken	1 salad	795	44	15	815	56	9	43
Grilled Steak	1 salad	795	43	16	715	58	9	43
TACOS, ALL W/CRISPY TACO TORTILLA, LETTUCE, CHEESE, SOUR CREAM & PICO DE GALLO								
Grilled Chicken	1 taco	200	13	5	310	10	1	12
Grilled Vegetables	1 taco	160	10	4	230	12	2	5
Ground Beef	1 taco	220	15	6.5	375	10	1	11

Quiznos
CLASSIC SUBS, REGULAR SIZE, ALL BREADS

	SERVING SIZE	CALORIES	TOTAL FAT (G)	SAT FAT (G)	SODIUM (MG)	CARBS (G)	FIBER (G)	PROTEIN (G)
Classic Club	1 sub	870	50	14	2300	66	5	40
Classic Italian	1 sub	810	46	17	2420	67	6	34
Pork Cuban	1 sub	760	37	10	1960	61	5	43

restaurants

	SERVING SIZE	CALORIES	TOTAL FAT (G)	SAT FAT (G)	SODIUM (MG)	CARBS (G)	FIBER (G)	PROTEIN (G)
The Traditional	1 sub	680	31	11	1950	68	6	32
Tuna Melt	1 sub	1060	74	17	1300	63	5	43
Turkey Ranch & Swiss	1 sub	660	29	7	1770	69	6	31
Ultimate Turkey Club	1 sub	880	54	16	2080	65	5	37
Veggie	1 sub	790	45	14	1860	68	10	27
FLATBREAD SAMMIES								
Bistro Steak Melt	1 sandwich	410	23	5.5	1100	31	1	17
Chicken Bacon Ranch	1 sandwich	380	19	4.5	780	28	1	20
Italiano	1 sandwich	420	25	8	1175	28	1	20
Roadhouse Steak	1 sandwich	270	6	1	1060	39	1	14
Smoky Chipotle Turkey	1 sandwich	390	23	6	1210	29	1	17
Veggie	1 sandwich	340	20	4.5	740	29	3	9
SALADS, REGULAR, W/DRESSING								
Chicken Caesar w/Caesar Dressing	1 salad	610	55	11.5	1620	11	2	22
Cobb w/Ranch Dressing	1 salad	610	48	11	1320	10	2	21
Harvest Chicken w/Acai Vinaigrette	1 salad	450	23	4.5	840	48	4	12
Mediterranean Chicken w/Tzatziki	1 salad	630	53	11.5	1580	16	4	28
SIGNATURE SUBS, REGULAR, ALL BREADS								
Black Angus on Rosemary Parmesan	1 sub	790	26	13	2130	83	5	57
Buffalo Chicken	1 sub	750	35	13	2710	72	5	40
Double Cheese Cheesesteak	1 sub	1100	68	16	2010	68	5	54
Harvest Chicken Sub	1 sub	590	17	5	1360	85	6	26
Mesquite Chicken	1 sub	810	40	15	1740	65	5	40
Prime Rib & Peppercorn	1 sub	980	57	16	1920	68	5	48
Southern BBQ Pulled Pork	1 sub	800	32	15	2700	73	5	53
TOASTY BULLETS, SERVED ON BAGUETTES								
Beef, Bacon & Cheddar	1 bullet	450	18	5.5	1325	48	2	21
Italian	1 bullet	500	25	8	1480	47	3	20
Pesto Turkey	1 bullet	380	13	3	1250	48	3	18
Tuna Melt	1 bullet	510	31	6	660	39	2	17
Turkey Club	1 bullet	460	21	5	1330	48	3	20
TOASTY FAVORITES, REGULAR, ALL BREADS								
Honey-Cured Ham	1 sandwich	740	42	11	1628	60	5	32
Meatball	1 sandwich	630	26	9	1905	71	9	29
Oven-Roasted Turkey	1 sandwich	750	42	11	1755	63	5	30

	SERVING SIZE	CALORIES	TOTAL FAT (G)	SAT FAT (G)	SODIUM (MG)	CARBS (G)	FIBER (G)	PROTEIN (G)
Veggie Caprese	1 sandwich	600	32	23	1410	62	6	24

Ranch 1
FRIES

	SERVING SIZE	CALORIES	TOTAL FAT (G)	SAT FAT (G)	SODIUM (MG)	CARBS (G)	FIBER (G)	PROTEIN (G)
Cheese Fries, Medium	as served	490	27	9	1050	46	6	11
Fries, Medium	as served	380	19	3.5	480	43	6	6

OTHER FAVORITES

Chicken Platter w/Rice	1 entrée	270	6	0.5	660	28	3	28
Chicken Tenders	1 entrée	360	14	1.5	430	28	1	31
Chicken Teriyaki Bowl	1 entrée	500	7	0.5	2160	86	1	34
Grilled Chicken Caesar Wrap	1 entrée	750	41	9	1460	55	4	44

SALADS

Grilled Chicken Caesar, w/Dressing	1 salad	430	30	4	580	14	5	29
Mandarin Chicken, w/Dressing	1 salad	820	43	7	840	78	14	39
Mixed Greens, w/Chicken, w/o Dressing	1 salad	317	19	2.4	793	14	6	28
Southwest Chicken, w/Dressing	1 salad	680	43	6	1170	44	7	33

SANDWICHES

Chicken Philly	1 sandwich	410	13	4.5	780	40	2	36
Grilled Classic	1 sandwich	680	47	8	750	37	2	29
Grilled Spicy Chicken	1 sandwich	360	7	1.5	950	46	2	31
Original Crispy Chicken	1 sandwich	640	31	5	950	60	3	33
Original Spicy Crispy Chicken	1 sandwich	470	9	2	1070	68	3	34

Red Hot & Blue
ENTRÉES

BBQ Surf & Turf, w/Catfish	1 entrée	1231	84	4	2254	37	< 1	n/a
Beef Brisket Platter	1 entrée	358	20	7	1330	6	0	n/a
Blues Baker Combo	1 entrée	947	34	11	2350	135	16	n/a
Delta Double, w/Pulled Pork	1 entrée	1122	85	8	587	15	0	n/a
Delta Double, w/RHB Sausage	1 entrée	1264	97	12	1735	23	< 1	n/a
Five Meat Treat	1 entrée	1163	84	18	1530	14	< 1	n/a
Full Slab of Ribs, Half & Half	1 entrée	2555	196	1	4072	44	8	n/a
Idaho Pig, w/Chili	1 entrée	932	31	10	2632	134	17	n/a
Memphis Half Chicken Platter	1 entrée	1511	103	29	1875	11	< 1	n/a
Mississippi Delta Catfish	1 entrée	852	42	9	3743	57	2	n/a
Pig & Link Combo	1 entrée	931	57	20	1855	52	2	n/a
Pig Squealin Combo	1 entrée	718	33	10	550	74	4	n/a
Pulled Pork Platter	1 entrée	483	33	12	244	6	< 1	n/a
Rib & Catfish Platter	1 entrée	1231	84	4	2254	37	< 1	n/a

restaurants

	SERVING SIZE	CALORIES	TOTAL FAT (G)	SAT FAT (G)	SODIUM (MG)	CARBS (G)	FIBER (G)	PROTEIN (G)
Rib & Crisper Platter	1 entrée	1059	69	5	2026	36	0	n/a
Smoked Sausage Platter	1 entrée	947	67	24	2845	36	2	n/a
Tennessee Triple w/Memphis Chicken, Sausage & Pulled Chicken	1 entrée	2104	151	27	1662	23	<1	n/a
SANDWICHES								
Cheeseburger, w/Cheddar	1 sandwich	1028	68	23	666	46	4	n/a
Delta Catfish	1 sandwich	712	25	5	2864	81	5	n/a
Have Your Cake & Eat It Too	1 sandwich	1256	86	31	898	46	1	n/a
Hickory Burger	1 sandwich	1248	83	29	1407	60	2	n/a
Hoochie Coochie Cajun Burger	1 sandwich	991	73	26	748	26	1	n/a
Pulled Chicken, Jumbo	1 sandwich	593	28	7	637	47	3	n/a
Smoked Sausage	1 sandwich	695	37	13	1773	4	60	n/a

Red Lobster
LOBSTER & CRAB

	SERVING SIZE	CALORIES	TOTAL FAT (G)	SAT FAT (G)	SODIUM (MG)	CARBS (G)	FIBER (G)	PROTEIN (G)
Bar Harbor Lobster Bake	1 entrée	670	28	7	3090	57	n/a	48
Chef's Signature Lobster & Shrimp Pasta, Full	as served	1020	50	21	2170	86	n/a	56
Crab Linguini Alfredo, Full	as served	1120	50	24	3650	95	n/a	74
Harborside Lobster & Shrimp	1 entrée	470	13	2.5	2650	35	n/a	53
Live Maine Lobster, w/Stuffing	as served	310	5	1.5	1120	8	n/a	58
New England Lobster Rolls	as served	590	34	4	1530	47	n/a	24
SEASIDE STARTERS								
Crispy Calamari & Vegetables	as served	1520	97	11	3050	115	n/a	47
Lobster Artichoke and Seafood Dip	as served	1200	74	20	1950	101	n/a	0
Lobster Crab and Seafood Stuffed Mushrooms	as served	330	18	9	1110	18	n/a	0
Lobster Pizza	as served	720	30	13	1390	69	n/a	42
New England Seafood Sampler	as served	750	42	10	2160	45	n/a	33
Pan-Seared Crab Cakes	as served	280	14	2.5	1110	13	n/a	26
Parrot Isle Jumbo Coconut Shrimp	as served	530	36	9	1110	34	n/a	18
SHRIMP								
Crunchy Popcorn Shrimp	as served	560	27	2.5	2100	51	n/a	27
Shrimp Linguini Alfredo, Full	as served	1100	58	21	3200	84	n/a	62
Walt's Favorite Shrimp	as served	550	30	2.5	2270	39	n/a	32
SIGNATURE COMBINATIONS								
Admiral's Feast	as served	1280	73	6	4300	92	n/a	63
Seaside Shrimp Trio	as served	1010	55	13	3940	65	n/a	64

	SERVING SIZE	CALORIES	TOTAL FAT (G)	SAT FAT (G)	SODIUM (MG)	CARBS (G)	FIBER (G)	PROTEIN (G)
Ultimate Feast	as served	600	28	3.5	3660	25	n/a	63
SOUPS & SALADS								
Lobster Bisque	1 cup	210	14	8	830	12	n/a	8
New England Clam Chowder	1 cup	230	17	10	680	13	n/a	9
TRADITIONAL FAVORITES								
Broiled Seafood Platter	as served	300	10	3	1880	9	n/a	43
Cajun Chicken Linguini Alfredo, Full	as served	1260	53	19	3110	91	n/a	103
Hand-Battered Fish & Chips	as served	730	33	3	1980	64	n/a	44
Parmesan-Crusted Tilapia, Full	as served	810	41	17	2590	25	n/a	84
Seafood-Stuffed Flounder	as served	320	11	3.5	1520	13	n/a	43
WOOD–FIRE GRILLED SELECTIONS								
Garlic-Grilled Jumbo Shrimp	as served	370	9	2	2160	40	n/a	35
Grilled Lobster, Shrimp & Scallops	as served	500	11	2.5	3220	42	n/a	60
Grilled Peppercorn Sirloin & Shrimp	as served	590	22	10	2230	30	n/a	67
Grilled Scallops, Shrimp & Chicken	as served	600	13	3	3190	42	n/a	77
Maple-Glazed Chicken	as served	570	9	2.5	1950	62	n/a	59
Maple-Glazed Shrimp & Salmon	as served	670	17	3.5	2690	57	n/a	71
NY Strip & Rock Lobster Tail	as served	590	29	12	1700	0	n/a	82
Peach-Bourbon BBQ Shrimp & Scallops	as served	490	22	4	1680	34	n/a	38
Pecan-Crusted Jumbo Shrimp	as served	730	25	4	3780	60	n/a	67
Steak Lobster-and-Shrimp Oscar	as served	1120	72	31	2670	20	n/a	97

Red Robin
BURGERS & SANDWICHES

	SERVING SIZE	CALORIES	TOTAL FAT (G)	SAT FAT (G)	SODIUM (MG)	CARBS (G)	FIBER (G)	PROTEIN (G)
Bacon Cheeseburger	1 burger	1033	69	n/a	1937	51	2	51
Bleu Ribbon Burger	1 burger	1001	55	n/a	1793	71	3	48
California Chicken Sandwich	1 sandwich	824	43	n/a	1923	52	3	53
Crispy Arctic Cod Sandwich	1 sandwich	606	28	n/a	1938	61	3	27
Crispy Chicken Sandwich	1 sandwich	909	54	n/a	1864	70	3	36
Garden Burger	1 burger	478	13	n/a	1754	74	5	9
Gourmet Cheeseburger	1 burger	959	60	n/a	1979	61	2	45
Grilled Turkey Burger	1 burger	578	29	n/a	898	51	2	29
Guacamole Bacon Burger	1 burger	1046	64	n/a	1404	55	3	61
Lettuce-Wrap Your Burger	1 burger	423	27	n/a	397	7	2	35
Sautéed 'Shroom Burger	1 burger	961	56	n/a	1352	58	6	60
Simply Grilled Chicken Sandwich	1 sandwich	409	7	n/a	993	51	2	37
Whiskey River BBQ Burger	1 burger	1182	74	n/a	1516	73	4	50

restaurants

	SERVING SIZE	CALORIES	TOTAL FAT (G)	SAT FAT (G)	SODIUM (MG)	CARBS (G)	FIBER (G)	PROTEIN (G)
ENTRÉES & COMBOS								
Artic Cod Fish & Chips	1 entrée	1118	67	n/a	2833	84	6	44
Classic Creamy Mac 'N' Cheese	1 entrée	1230	73	n/a	2604	91	6	49
Clucks & Fries	1 entrée	1026	75	n/a	2172	40	3	48
Red's Nantucket Seafood Scatter	1 entrée	1246	75	n/a	4543	97	7	48
Southwest Chicken Pasta	1 entrée	1169	46	n/a	2336	127	10	62
Triple S Riblet Basket	1 entrée	1426	85	n/a	3227	60	3	107
SALADS								
Apple Harvest Chicken	1 salad	804	43	n/a	1750	64	8	44
Avo-Cobb-O	1 salad	734	37	n/a	1500	42	10	54
Crispy Chicken Tender	1 salad	1450	96	n/a	2512	87	8	61
Mighty Caesar	1 salad	648	44	n/a	1122	43	6	18
Southwest Grilled Chicken	1 salad	856	52	n/a	1922	42	8	47
SIDES								
Steak Fries	as served	1290	70	n/a	2366	103	12	53
Robeks								
SHAKES & FREEZES								
800 lb. Gorilla Shake	12 fl oz	434	9	n/a	276	58	2	30
Banana Split Shake	12 fl oz	274	0	n/a	92	56	2	3
Orange Freeze	12 fl oz	290	1	n/a	115	63	0	8
P-Nut Power Shake	12 fl oz	362	16	n/a	230	39	4	11
SMOOTHIES								
Acai Energizer	12 fl oz	161	1	n/a	23	33	2	5
Awesome Acai	12 fl oz	146	1	n/a	23	32	1	2
Big Wednesday	12 fl oz	201	1	n/a	0	49	2	1
Cardio Cooler	12 fl oz	244	1	n/a	46	45	3	9
Citrus Stinger	12 fl oz	198	1	n/a	23	44	2	5
Dr. Robeks	12 fl oz	186	1	n/a	0	42	2	2
Green Tea Sensation	12 fl oz	199	2	n/a	207	37	0	8
Infinite Orange	12 fl oz	182	1	n/a	23	42	2	4
Mahalo Mango	12 fl oz	201	1	n/a	23	50	2	1
Outrageous Raspberry	12 fl oz	182	1	n/a	23	44	1	0
Robeks Rejuvenator	12 fl oz	221	1	n/a	23	51	2	4
Strawnana Berry	12 fl oz	188	0	n/a	46	44	1	3
Roly Poly Sandwich								
SANDWICHES								
Classic Tuna Melt	1 sandwich	338	17	6	740	26	2	25

	SERVING SIZE	CALORIES	TOTAL FAT (G)	SAT FAT (G)	SODIUM (MG)	CARBS (G)	FIBER (G)	PROTEIN (G)
Italian Classic	1 sandwich	334	12	4	910	32	5	20
Pesto Turkey Club	1 sandwich	376	19	6	1049	28	3	22
Philly Melt	1 sandwich	278	11	5	715	25	2	20
Popeye's Tuna, on Wheat	1 sandwich	303	4	2	778	31	4	21
Thanksgiving	1 sandwich	285	7	1	850	36	3	14
Tuscan Turkey	1 sandwich	219	2	1	764	31	5	18
Ultimate Veggie	1 sandwich	180	1	1	223	33	6	8
SALADS, W/O DRESSING								
Cobb	1 salad	517	27	11	1481	12	4	50
Frisco Chicken	1 salad	527	25	12	1250	20	7	47
Just Veggies	1 salad	95	0	0	64	19	8	6
Roly Chef	1 salad	340	19	6	1385	12	2	31
Spa	1 salad	255	15	2	30	26	7	9
SIGNATURE SOUPS								
Broccoli Cheddar	1 cup	160	11	6	710	10	1	6
Classic Chili	1 cup	160	5	2	730	18	6	9
Garden Vegetable	1 cup	60	0	0	610	12	2	3
Old Fashioned Chicken Noodle	1 cup	70	2	0	800	11	1	4
Seafood Bisque	1 cup	217	14	9	735	12	0	8

Romano's Macaroni Grill

ENTREES

	SERVING SIZE	CALORIES	TOTAL FAT (G)	SAT FAT (G)	SODIUM (MG)	CARBS (G)	FIBER (G)	PROTEIN (G)
Grilled Chicken Speidini	1 entrée	410	11	2	990	38	10	39
Mediterranean Sea Bass	1 entrée	570	36	3	920	29	5	37
Pan-Roasted Pork Chop	1 entrée	1370	91	39	1900	58	7	76
Pollo Caprese	1 entrée	560	22	7	1530	31	5	60
NEAPOLITAN PIZZA								
Margherita	as served	840	31	14	1310	101	7	39
Primo Pepperoni	as served	980	41	19	1960	97	6	53
PASTA								
Carmela's Chicken	1 entrée	930	31	11	1540	111	8	45
Chicken & Mushroom Canneloni	1 entrée	780	68	19	2100	39	4	51
Chicken Parmesan	1 entrée	940	57	12	1330	74	7	30
Eggplant Parmesan	1 entrée	950	56	12	1250	76	12	32
Fettuccine Alfredo	1 entrée	1180	73	41	2000	91	6	46
Lasagna Bolognese	1 entrée	630	40	16	1810	27	4	36
Mushroom Ravioli	1 entrée	900	62	31	1020	52	5	21

restaurants	SERVING SIZE	CALORIES	TOTAL FAT (G)	SAT FAT (G)	SODIUM (MG)	CARBS (G)	FIBER (G)	PROTEIN (G)
Pasta Milano	1 entrée	1010	42	15	1660	111	7	47
Penne Rustica	1 entrée	1160	49	18	2490	110	7	72
SALADS								
Caesar, w/ Dressing	1 salad	420	39	8	740	11	4	7
Market Chop, w/ Dressing	1 salad	1010	71	19	2300	33	10	56
Parmesan-Crusted Chicken, w/ Dressing	1 salad	930	58	15	1720	53	5	51

Round Table Pizza
ORIGINAL CRUST, MEDIUM

	SERVING SIZE	CALORIES	TOTAL FAT (G)	SAT FAT (G)	SODIUM (MG)	CARBS (G)	FIBER (G)	PROTEIN (G)
Chicken & Garlic Gourmet	1 slice	270	12	5	670	27	1	13
Guinevere's Garden Delight	1 slice	240	9	4	540	28	2	10
King Arthur Supreme	1 slice	300	15	6	720	28	2	14
Maui Zaui, w/Zesty Red Sauce	1 slice	270	11	5	720	29	2	13
Montague's All Meat Marvel	1 slice	330	17	7	820	27	2	15
Ulti-Meat	1 slice	330	17	7	830	27	2	15
Wombo Combo	1 slice	300	14	7	840	29	2	14

PAN CRUST, MEDIUM

	SERVING SIZE	CALORIES	TOTAL FAT (G)	SAT FAT (G)	SODIUM (MG)	CARBS (G)	FIBER (G)	PROTEIN (G)
Chicken & Garlic Gourmet	1 slice	360	14	6	870	42	2	17
Guinevere's Garden Delight	1 slice	320	11	5	720	42	2	13
King Arthur Supreme	1 slice	360	15	7	850	42	2	16
Maui Zaui, w/Zesty Red Sauce	1 slice	360	13	6	920	44	2	16
Montague's All Meat Marvel	1 slice	380	16	7	920	41	2	17
Ulti-Meat	1 slice	410	19	8	1020	41	2	18
Wombo Combo	1 slice	390	16	7	1030	43	3	17

SKINNY CRUST, MEDIUM

	SERVING SIZE	CALORIES	TOTAL FAT (G)	SAT FAT (G)	SODIUM (MG)	CARBS (G)	FIBER (G)	PROTEIN (G)
Chicken & Garlic Gourmet	1 slice	230	12	5	580	20	1	12
Guinevere's Garden Delight	1 slice	200	9	4	450	21	2	9
King Arthur Supreme	1 slice	260	14	6	640	21	2	13
Maui Zaui, w/Zesty Red Sauce	1 slice	230	11	5	640	22	1	12
Montague's All Meat Marvel	1 slice	290	17	7	730	20	1	14
Ulti-Meat	1 slice	290	17	7	750	20	1	14
Wombo Combo	1 slice	270	14	6	750	21	2	13

Roy Rogers
BURGERS & SANDWICHES

	SERVING SIZE	CALORIES	TOTAL FAT (G)	SAT FAT (G)	SODIUM (MG)	CARBS (G)	FIBER (G)	PROTEIN (G)
Chicken Griller	1 sandwich	350	10	2	980	39	2	28
Double Double R Burger	1 burger	876	49	20	1997	37	2	64
Double R Burger	1 burger	549	27	11	1349	36	2	35
Gold Rush Chicken	1 sandwich	641	32	11	1531	61	3	31

	SERVING SIZE	CALORIES	TOTAL FAT (G)	SAT FAT (G)	SODIUM (MG)	CARBS (G)	FIBER (G)	PROTEIN (G)
Hamburger	1 burger	462	21	8	757	36	2	33
Large Roast Beef	1 sandwich	467	10	3	944	36	2	57
Roast Beef Sliders	6 sliders	999	18	3	1873	126	0	79
CHICKEN								
Chicken & Biscuit	3 pieces	1375	91	31	2660	83	2	59
Chicken Strips	5 pieces	439	15	6	1103	20	1	52
SIDES								
Baked Apples	as served	140	0	0	0	37	2	0
Baked Beans, Large	as served	434	4	1	1637	90	11	14
Holster Fries	as served	546	29	10	535	63	5	8
Mashed Potatoes & Gravy, Large	as served	255	5	0	1488	51	3	8

Rubio's
BURRITOS, SERVED W/O CHIPS

	SERVING SIZE	CALORIES	TOTAL FAT (G)	SAT FAT (G)	SODIUM (MG)	CARBS (G)	FIBER (G)	PROTEIN (G)
Baja Grill, Grilled Chicken	1 burrito	630	28	11	1800	55	5	40
Big Especial Grilled Chicken	1 burrito	820	31	9	1980	102	7	33
Chile-Lime Wild Salmon	1 burrito	680	33	8	1180	59	5	38
Grilled Mesquite Shrimp	1 burrito	730	34	12	2200	75	4	31
Grilled Ono	1 burrito	670	31	7	1330	60	5	38
Grilled Veggie	1 burrito	770	35	12	1520	83	7	22
HealthMex Grilled Ono Burrito	as served	560	12	3	1550	74	9	40
HealthMex Grilled Veggie Burrito	as served	490	9	3	1260	80	11	13
OTHER FAVORITES								
Nachos Grande Chicken	as served	1340	78	27	2260	114	22	54
Three Cheese Quesadilla	as served	1120	70	30	1940	87	7	39
TACO PLATES, W/CORN TORTILLA, PINTO BEANS & CHIPS								
Chile-Lime Wild Salmon	1 plate	840	33	5	1050	106	20	31
Classic Grilled Chicken	1 plate	860	38	9	1390	101	20	31
Fish Especial, 2 Tacos	1 plate	1090	59	10	1710	113	21	32
Grilled Gourmet Chicken	1 plate	1010	49	15	1830	102	20	44
Grilled Gourmet Chicken & Grilled Gourmet Steak	1 plate	1020	51	15	1830	102	19	44
Grilled Gourmet Garlic Herb Shrimp	1 plate	1040	53	16	1760	102	19	42
Grilled Gourmet Portobello & Poblano & Grilled Gourmet Chicken	1 plate	980	49	14	1560	105	20	36
Grilled Ono	1 plate	840	32	5	1150	106	19	32
HealthMex Grilled Chicken Taco	as served	130	1	0	340	22	3	10

restaurants

	SERVING SIZE	CALORIES	TOTAL FAT (G)	SAT FAT (G)	SODIUM (MG)	CARBS (G)	FIBER (G)	PROTEIN (G)
The Original Fish, 2 Tacos	1 plate	960	48	5	1540	110	19	25

Ruby Tuesday's
BURGERS & SANDWICHES

	SERVING SIZE	CALORIES	TOTAL FAT (G)	SAT FAT (G)	SODIUM (MG)	CARBS (G)	FIBER (G)	PROTEIN (G)
Alpine Swiss Burger	1 burger	1017	65	n/a	1246	60	6	50
Bacon Cheeseburger	1 burger	1007	67	n/a	1426	58	4	49
Boston Blue Burger	1 burger	1165	72	n/a	1913	82	6	51
Buffalo Chicken Burger	1 burger	888	49	n/a	2159	70	4	45
Chicken BLT	1 sandwich	898	48	n/a	1909	70	4	48
Classic Cheeseburger	1 burger	947	61	n/a	1216	58	4	46
Ruby's Classic Burger	1 burger	877	55	n/a	976	57	4	42
Triple Prime Bacon Cheddar Burger	1 burger	1136	82	n/a	1247	47	4	54
Triple Prime Burger	1 burger	916	63	n/a	757	47	4	41
Turkey Burger	1 burger	801	48	n/a	1349	56	4	41

FIT & TRIM ENTRÉES

Chicken Fresco, Petite	as served	397	21	n/a	1108	25	4	30
Grilled Salmon	as served	386	22	n/a	553	9	3	36
Parmesan Shrimp Pasta, Petite	as served	678	36	n/a	1559	54	3	54
Sirloin, Petite	as served	476	27	n/a	967	12	3	45

FORK TENDER RIBS

Classic Barbecue	half rack	500	24	n/a	500	29	0	44

FRESH ALL NATURAL CHICKEN

Chicken Bella	1 entrée	405	18	n/a	1304	8	3	54
Chicken Fresco	1 entrée	397	19	n/a	1268	10	1	49

FRESH COMBINATIONS

Buffalo Chicken Minis	as served	763	36	n/a	1869	89	6	24
Chicken Vegetable Harvest Soup	as served	200	8	n/a	1177	22	4	14
Ruby Minis	as served	915	53	n/a	1519	78	6	31
White Bean Chicken Chili	as served	300	10	n/a	1902	37	10	24
Zucchini Cake Minis	as served	824	36	n/a	2240	112	9	15

GARDEN FRESH SALAD

Carolina Chicken Salad	1 salad	1101	46	n/a	1057	52	11	33
Grilled Chicken Salad	1 salad	795	28	n/a	1057	48	7	24

PASTA CLASSICS

Chicken & Broccoli Pasta	1 entrée	1521	92	n/a	3340	96	8	78
Chicken & Mushroom Alfredo	1 entrée	1253	64	n/a	3031	88	9	83
Lobster Carbonara	1 entrée	1406	95	n/a	3796	80	7	61
Parmesan Shrimp Pasta	1 entrée	1065	54	n/a	2400	88	5	100

	SERVING SIZE	CALORIES	TOTAL FAT (G)	SAT FAT (G)	SODIUM (MG)	CARBS (G)	FIBER (G)	PROTEIN (G)
Spaghetti Squash Marinara	1 entrée	257	12	n/a	836	29	9	7
PREMIUM SEAFOOD								
Asian Glazed Salmon	1 entrée	417	25	n/a	650	14	1	34
Herb-Crusted Tilapia	1 entrée	401	24	n/a	944	11	2	39
Louisiana Fried Shrimp	1 entrée	560	29	n/a	3040	47	4	28
SHAREABLES								
Asian Dumplings	1/4 order	115	5	n/a	306	12	1	5
Fire Wings	1/4 order	178	11	n/a	603	4	1	16
Four Way Sampler	1/4 order	288	14	n/a	769	18	2	21
Southwestern Spring Rolls	1/4 order	158	8	n/a	305	18	1	4
Spinach Artichoke Dip	1/4 order	310	19	n/a	470	27	3	8
STEAKHOUSE STEAKS								
Rib Eye	1 entrée	912	71	n/a	1040	7	0	61
Top Sirloin	1 entrée	468	25	n/a	720	4	0	55

Runza
BURGERS

	SERVING SIZE	CALORIES	TOTAL FAT (G)	SAT FAT (G)	SODIUM (MG)	CARBS (G)	FIBER (G)	PROTEIN (G)
Bacon Cheeseburger, 1/4 lb	1 burger	510	31	10	1200	26	1	32
BBQ, Bacon & Swiss, 1/4 lb	1 burger	540	32	13	1090	26	1	33
Cheeseburger, 1/4 lb, The Runza Way	1 burger	410	22	7	1030	27	2	28
Double Cheeseburger, 1/2 lb, The Runza Way	1 burger	670	39	13	1450	29	2	49
Double Hamburger, 1/2 lb, The Runza Way	1 burger	570	31	11	850	25	2	43
Hamburger, 1/4 lb, The Runza Way	1 burger	360	18	6	730	25	2	25
Swiss Cheese Mushroom, 1/4 lb	1 burger	480	29	10	1110	24	2	29
CHICKEN								
Buffalo Grilled Chicken Sandwich	1 sandwich	350	10	1	1800	36	1	30
Buffalo Mini Chicken Wrap	1 wrap	310	16	4	1110	31	1	13
Chicken Strips	4 pieces	440	24	4	1200	28	0	32
Deluxe Grilled Chicken Sandwich	1 sandwich	360	11	0.5	1420	37	1	30
Ranch Mini Chicken Wrap	1 wrap	310	16	4	750	30	1	13
Smothered Grilled Chicken Sandwich	1 sandwich	430	17	4.5	1730	36	2	35
RUNZA SANDWICHES								
Cheese	1 sandwich	580	24	7	1660	69	4	23
Jalapeño	1 sandwich	650	31	10	2300	69	4	23
Mini Cheese	1 sandwich	290	12	4	850	35	2	12
Mini Original	1 sandwich	270	10	3.5	700	34	2	10
Mini Swiss Cheese Mushroom	1 sandwich	320	14	5	2070	35	3	13

restaurants

	SERVING SIZE	CALORIES	TOTAL FAT (G)	SAT FAT (G)	SODIUM (MG)	CARBS (G)	FIBER (G)	PROTEIN (G)
Original	1 sandwich	530	20	6	1360	67	4	20
Swiss Cheese Mushroom	1 sandwich	630	28	10	2040	68	5	25
SALADS								
Asian Grilled Chicken Salad, w/Dressing	1 salad	400	6	0.5	2110	58	3	25
Side Salad, w/o Dressing	1 salad	20	0	0	10	4	2	1
Southwest Chicken Salad, w/o Dressing	1 salad	320	15	3.5	1220	29	3	20
Sweet Berry Chicken Salad, w/o Dressing	1 salad	360	19	5	1180	18	4	31
SHAKES								
Chocolate Shake, Regular	16 fl oz	480	12	8	280	81	0	12
Strawberry Shake, Regular	16 fl oz	490	12	8	250	84	0	12
Vanilla Shake, Regular	16 fl oz	430	12	8	250	66	0	12
SIDES, MEDIUM								
French Fries	as served	390	15	2.5	430	41	5	4
Frings!	as served	370	18	3	350	39	4	5
Onion Rings	as served	320	19	3	260	35	3	5
Saladworks								
PANINIS								
Buffalo Chicken	1 sandwich	657	29	9.9	1690	56	2	43
Caprese	1 sandwich	586	27	9.4	1208	59	2	26
Chicken Mozzarella	1 sandwich	620	25	9.0	1687	63	2	44
Turkey Melt	1 sandwich	797	40	14.4	1932	60	2	47
SALADS								
Autumn Harvest	1 salad	301	12	1.5	232	40	15	13
Bently	1 salad	245	10	5.9	653	11	3	29
Buffalo Bleu	1 salad	250	7	1.9	713	24	6	22
Chicken Caesar	1 salad	286	4	0.2	789	19	3	42
Cobb	1 salad	269	16	3.9	824	13	6	23
Fire Roasted Cabo Jack	1 salad	389	19	8.5	553	31	6	25
Garden Deluxe	1 salad	239	2	0.2	642	50	10	12
Greek	1 salad	185	10	4.9	488	18	7	8
Mandarin Chicken	1 salad	228	7	0.1	191	37	11	12
Sophie's Salad	1 salad	312	14	2.8	385	35	12	12
Tivoli	1 salad	430	19	9	934	32	4	33
Turkey Club	1 salad	217	5	0.9	471	29	4	18
SANDWICHES								
BLT	1 sandwich	343	13	4	1084	32	1	17

	SERVING SIZE	CALORIES	TOTAL FAT (G)	SAT FAT (G)	SODIUM (MG)	CARBS (G)	FIBER (G)	PROTEIN (G)
Chicken Monterey	1 sandwich	383	12	5	897	35	1	34
Ham Continental	1 sandwich	395	11	7.0	1296	38	1	32
Turkey Continental	1 sandwich	375	10	5.0	937	36	1	32
SOUPS, LARGE								
Asparagus & Pea	1 bowl	263	20	12	732	14	2	7
Butternut Squash	1 bowl	160	5	3	820	22	0	2
Chicken Noodle	1 bowl	100	4	2	1120	10	0	6
Chicken Orzo	1 bowl	160	3	2	1120	14	2	6
Chicken Pot Pie	1 bowl	180	9	5	1200	18	2	8
Cream of Broccoli	1 bowl	180	6	4	1120	20	4	8
Fiesta Tortilla	1 bowl	120	4	0	1260	18	4	4
Garden Fresh Pea	1 bowl	100	2	0	960	14	4	6
Italian Wedding	1 bowl	100	6	3	1220	8	0	6
Lasagna	1 bowl	175	7	3	1064	18	2	9
Loaded Baked Potato	1 bowl	312	23	12	730	21	1	6
Maryland Crab	1 bowl	144	0	0	2036	25	2	8
Roasted Corn Tomato w/Smoked Cheddar	1 bowl	428	33	19	1490	18	2	17
Tomato Bisque	1 bowl	140	7	4	640	12	0	2
Vegetarian Chili	1 bowl	140	4	0	940	22	4	4
Vegetarian Veggie	1 bowl	60	1	0	620	10	0	2

Samurai Sam's Teriyaki Grill

SIGNATURE BOWLS, LARGE								
Orange Peel White Chicken, White Rice	1 bowl	810	6	1.5	730	132	4	53
"Riceless" White Chicken, No Sauce	1 bowl	310	5	1.5	300	20	6	46
Spicy Steak & Broccoli, White Rice	1 bowl	830	11	4.0	1360	130	4	36
Sweet & Sour White Chicken, White Rice	1 bowl	790	6	1.5	320	128	2	51
TERIYAKI RICE BOWLS, W/VEGETABLES								
Salmon, Brown Rice	1 bowl	590	5	0.5	1240	105	8	33
Shrimp, White Rice, Large	1 bowl	650	2	0.5	940	121	3	32
Spicy White Chicken, White Rice, Large	1 bowl	810	6	1.5	910	132	3	53
Steak, White Rice, Large	1 bowl	800	11	4.0	1350	122	3	35
Sumo Bowl, Brown Rice	1 bowl	1020	23	7.0	1520	111	9	81
Sumo Bowl, White Rice	1 bowl	1080	21	6.0	1520	128	3	81
Veggie, Brown Rice, Large	1 bowl	500	3	0.5	790	108	10	12
White Chicken, Brown Rice, Large	1 bowl	720	8	2	940	107	8	53

restaurants

	SERVING SIZE	CALORIES	TOTAL FAT (G)	SAT FAT (G)	SODIUM (MG)	CARBS (G)	FIBER (G)	PROTEIN (G)
White Chicken, White Rice, Large	1 bowl	790	6	1.5	940	124	3	53
White Chicken & Steak, Brown Rice, Large	1 bowl	730	10	3	1150	106	8	44
White Chicken & Steak, White Rice, Large	1 bowl	790	8	3	1140	123	3	44
TERIYAKI YAKISOBA NOODLE BOWLS, LARGE, W/VEGETABLES								
Salmon	1 bowl	630	8	0	1440	121	6	43
Shrimp	1 bowl	620	6	0	1140	120	6	42
Steak	1 bowl	780	16	4	1550	121	6	45
Veggie	1 bowl	550	6	0	930	124	8	22
White Chicken	1 bowl	770	11	1.5	1140	123	6	63
White Chicken & Steak	1 bowl	770	13	2.5	1350	122	6	54

Sandella's Flatbread Café

GRILLED FLATBREADS

Brazilian Chicken	1 flatbread	510	10	6	1170	73	3	33
Buffalo Chicken	1 flatbread	420	10	6	2150	47	3	33
Cheese	1 flatbread	370	9	6	790	49	4	20
Hawaiian	1 flatbread	610	17	8	1580	89	5	31
Margherita	1 flatbread	360	9	5	480	51	5	21
Perfecto Pepperoni	1 flatbread	530	23	11	1310	49	4	28
Spinach & Bacon	1 flatbread	660	39	14	1590	52	6	30
PANINIS								
Buffalo	1 sandwich	600	25	12	1430	48	4	35
Chicken Delicato	1 sandwich	490	18	7	990	51	3	33
Provolone & Veggie	1 sandwich	450	17	8	780	56	6	20
Tuscan Chicken	1 sandwich	540	21	7	1050	55	5	34
QUESADILLAS								
Cheese	1 serving	450	19	12	960	49	3	21
Chicken Fajita	1 serving	510	19	11	1190	52	4	34
Southwestern	1 serving	550	23	12	1160	62	8	26
RICE BOWLS								
Black Beans & Rice	1 bowl	840	20	11	1270	130	18	38
Chicken Fajita	1 bowl	750	20	11	1200	104	8	40
SALADS, W/DRESSING								
Chicken Caesar	1 salad	320	5	1.5	1160	36	7	22
Fiesta	1 salad	360	8	1	870	54	11	24
Greek	1 salad	310	15	5	850	37	7	11

	SERVING SIZE	CALORIES	TOTAL FAT (G)	SAT FAT (G)	SODIUM (MG)	CARBS (G)	FIBER (G)	PROTEIN (G)
Santa Fe	1 salad	420	24	11	950	35	7	20
WRAPS								
Buffalo Chicken	1 wrap	400	7	1	1100	51	5	22
Chicken Caesar	1 wrap	390	5	1.5	1260	54	6	24
Chicken Verona	1 wrap	510	18	7	990	54	4	34
Chipotle Chicken	1 wrap	350	7	1	650	55	5	22
Classic BLT	1 wrap	480	23	6	1270	59	5	26
Classic Ham & Swiss	1 wrap	590	25	11	1610	59	6	34
Georgetown Turkey	1 wrap	540	3	0.5	1750	96	5	34
Hummus	1 wrap	320	6	1	460	59	8	13
Pacific Chicken	1 wrap	460	16	2.5	1030	59	6	28
Pesto Turkey	1 wrap	460	15	6	1390	54	6	32
Roast Beef Club	1 wrap	490	16	3.5	1390	60	5	35
Sweet & Spicy Chicken	1 wrap	400	7	2	920	64	5	27
Turkey & Bacon	1 wrap	440	12	3	1360	55	5	34

Schlotzsky's
PIZZA, 8"

	SERVING SIZE	CALORIES	TOTAL FAT (G)	SAT FAT (G)	SODIUM (MG)	CARBS (G)	FIBER (G)	PROTEIN (G)
Combination Special	1 pizza	649	26	10	1716	77	4	27
Fresh Veggie	1 pizza	568	20	7	1480	75	4	23
Pepperoni & Double Cheese	1 pizza	727	33	15	1830	74	3	34
SALADS								
Cranberry, Apple, Pecan & Chicken	1 salad	655	28	7	924	63	6	38
Hearts of Romaine Chicken Caesar	1 salad	490	18	6	1360	39	2	47
Turkey Avocado Cobb	1 salad	659	35	9	1899	44	11	41
SANDWICHES, MEDIUM								
Angus Beef & Provolone	1 sandwich	814	33	11	2116	84	5	42
Angus Corned Beef Reuben	1 sandwich	911	40	19	2200	79	5	59
Angus Pastrami & Swiss	1 sandwich	905	36	18	2480	83	6	64
Angus Roast Beef & Cheese	1 sandwich	786	33	15	2188	75	4	47
BLT	1 sandwich	669	30	9	1855	73	4	29
Chicken & Pesto	1 sandwich	568	13	2	1853	75	4	34
Chipotle Chicken	1 sandwich	544	11	1	1729	75	4	32
Deluxe Original-Style	1 sandwich	957	46	18	4084	80	5	55
Dijon Chicken	1 sandwich	589	11	1	2541	82	8	37
Fresh Veggie	1 sandwich	512	14	7	1203	76	6	21
Ham & Cheese, Original-Style	1 sandwich	734	27	12	2980	79	5	44
Smoked Turkey Reuben	1 sandwich	896	38	17	2163	84	5	51

	SERVING SIZE	CALORIES	TOTAL FAT (G)	SAT FAT (G)	SODIUM (MG)	CARBS (G)	FIBER (G)	PROTEIN (G)
The Original	1 sandwich	772	34	15	2634	77	5	40
Turkey & Guacamole	1 sandwich	575	14	2	1692	80	9	32
Turkey Bacon Club	1 sandwich	828	35	14	2561	77	5	50
SOUPS								
Timberline Chile	1 cup	275	9	4	890	31	7	18
Wisconsin Cheese	1 cup	263	20	4	1154	20	0	4
WRAPS								
Grilled Chicken & Guacamole	1 wrap	700	36	9	1541	62	8	37
Homestyle Tuna	1 wrap	479	18	4	1389	55	4	26
Parmesan Chicken Caesar	1 wrap	602	23	7	2035	62	5	38

Shakey's Pizza Parlor

SHAKEY'S FAMOUS FRIED CHICKEN

	SERVING SIZE	CALORIES	TOTAL FAT (G)	SAT FAT (G)	SODIUM (MG)	CARBS (G)	FIBER (G)	PROTEIN (G)
Breast	1 breast	477	26	6.6	1383	16	<1	43
Leg	1 leg	172	9	2.3	542	6	<1	15
Thigh	1 thigh	352	24	6.3	900	10	<1	23
Wing	1 wing	129	9	2.3	317	4	<1	8
SHAREABLES								
Chicken Strips	5 strips	621	31	4.4	1725	48	3	38
Mojo Potatoes	as served	216	11	2.2	547	25	3	3
Mojo Supreme	as served	1949	120	40.3	4984	160	17	53
Shakey's Spicy Wings	6 pieces	494	29	7.1	2768	27	1	30
PAN PIZZA, LARGE								
Firehouse	1 slice	257	12	5.2	585	27	2	10
Garden Veggie	1 slice	184	6	2.3	380	27	2	7
Plain Cheese	1 slice	185	6	3	382	26	3	8
Rustic Garlic Chicken	1 slice	191	6	2.5	415	26	1	10
Shakey's Special	1 slice	209	7	1.9	545	31	3	7
Texas BBQ Chicken	1 slice	204	5	2.4	504	29	1	10
Ultimate Meat	1 slice	281	14	5.5	706	26	2	14
THIN CRUST PIZZA, LARGE								
Firehouse	1 slice	221	12	5.3	505	19	2	9
Garden Veggie	1 slice	148	5	2.4	299	19	2	6
Plain Cheese	1 slice	149	6	3.1	301	18	1	7
Rustic Garlic Chicken	1 slice	155	6	2.6	335	18	1	9
Shakey's Special	1 slice	195	10	4.1	442	18	1	8
Texas BBQ Chicken	1 slice	168	5	2.5	424	21	1	9

	SERVING SIZE	CALORIES	TOTAL FAT (G)	SAT FAT (G)	SODIUM (MG)	CARBS (G)	FIBER (G)	PROTEIN (G)
Ultimate Meat	1 slice	245	13	5.6	626	18	1	12

Sheetz

BREAKFAST

	SERVING SIZE	CALORIES	TOTAL FAT (G)	SAT FAT (G)	SODIUM (MG)	CARBS (G)	FIBER (G)	PROTEIN (G)
Hashbrownz	as served	130	8	4	250	14	3	1
Pretzel Meltz, Ham, Egg & Cheese	1 sandwich	520	23	10	1554	50	1	29
Pretzel Meltz, Steak, Egg & Cheese	1 sandwich	605	28	11	1208	47	1	33
Shmagelz, Bacon, Egg & Cheese	1 sandwich	642	36	15	1800	53	2	32
Shmagelz, Ham, Egg & Cheese	1 sandwich	533	22	9	1754	54	2	32
Shmiscuitz, Egg & Cheese	1 sandwich	450	27	10	1517	36	1	16
Shmiscuitz, Sausage & Egg	1 sandwich	515	35	10	1453	36	1	16
Shmuffin, Bacon, Egg & Cheese	1 sandwich	521	34	15	1549	29	2	27
Shmuffin, Egg & Cheese	1 sandwich	320	17	8	858	26	2	15
Shmuffin, Sausage, Egg & Cheese	1 sandwich	495	34	14	1251	26	2	20

BURGERZ ON A TOASTED CORN-DUSTED ROLL, W/O CHEESE OR TOPPINGS UNLESS INDICATED

	SERVING SIZE	CALORIES	TOTAL FAT (G)	SAT FAT (G)	SODIUM (MG)	CARBS (G)	FIBER (G)	PROTEIN (G)
Double JR Burger	1 burger	230	11	3	359	22	1	10
JR Burger	1 burger	340	20	6	488	22	1	16
Made to Order Burgerz	1 burger	579	31	11	495	45	1	26
Made to Order Cheeseburgerz	1 burger	689	40	17	952	45	1	31

BURRITOS, W/O TOPPINGS

	SERVING SIZE	CALORIES	TOTAL FAT (G)	SAT FAT (G)	SODIUM (MG)	CARBS (G)	FIBER (G)	PROTEIN (G)
Cheese	1 burrito	522	16	6	1254	77	4	17
Grilled Chicken & Cheese	1 burrito	639	20	8	1890	77	4	39
Steak & Cheese	1 burrito	705	24	9	1601	78	4	34
Chicken Strips (5)	as served	404	13	2	1722	38	0	34

CLASSIC HOT SUBZ, 12", W/O CHEESE OR TOPPINGS UNLESS INDICATED

	SERVING SIZE	CALORIES	TOTAL FAT (G)	SAT FAT (G)	SODIUM (MG)	CARBS (G)	FIBER (G)	PROTEIN (G)
Made-to-Order Grilled Chicken on Wheat	1 sub	820	15	4	2431	116	7	65
Made-to-Order Steak on White	1 sub	851	21	6	1631	93	3	51
Meatball Parmesan on White	1 sub	768	26	10	1632	99	5	29
Pepperoni Pizza on White	1 sub	1098	59	26	3153	90	3	45

CLASSIC SUBZ, 12", W/O CHEESE OR TOPPINGS UNLESS INDICATED

	SERVING SIZE	CALORIES	TOTAL FAT (G)	SAT FAT (G)	SODIUM (MG)	CARBS (G)	FIBER (G)	PROTEIN (G)
BLT on Wheat	1 sub	988	42	15	2541	122	7	45
Chicken Salad on Wheat	1 sub	1084	50	8	2051	134	7	36
Classic Italian on White	1 sub	727	21	7	2167	94	3	37
Club Combo on Wheat	1 sub	686	11	1	2111	120	7	40

restaurants

	SERVING SIZE	CALORIES	TOTAL FAT (G)	SAT FAT (G)	SODIUM (MG)	CARBS (G)	FIBER (G)	PROTEIN (G)
Deli on White	1 sub	767	27	9	1843	94	3	31
Ham & Cheese on White	1 sub	845	27	15	2839	96	3	45
Roast Beef & Cheese on White	1 sub	784	26	15	2272	92	3	39
Roasted Turkey & Cheese on Wheat	1 sub	905	29	14	3026	120	7	50
Tuna Salad on Wheat	1 sub	1013	39	6	1908	134	7	43
FLATBREAD SANDWICHEZ, W/O CHEESE OR TOPPINGS UNLESS INDICATED								
California Turkey	1 sandwich	697	37	9	1789	65	2	32
Cuban	1 sandwich	478	15	7	1769	60	2	26
Grilled Cheese, American	1 sandwich	516	22	14	1595	55	2	21
Italian	1 sandwich	621	29	10	1752	62	1	31
Mozzarella & Tomato	1 sandwich	622	30	12	987	59	1	37
Grilled Chicken Breast Sandwich, Corn-Dusted Bun	1 sandwich	368	6	1	1000	46	2	30
HOT DOGZ & PRETZELZ								
Gourmet Pretzels, Cinnamon Sugar	1 pretzel	570	12	2	720	102	3	15
Gourmet Pretzels, Jalapeño-Filled	1 pretzel	480	12	6	1380	75	3	18
Gourmet Pretzels, Salted	1 pretzel	540	12	2	2250	93	3	15
Hot Dog	1 hot dog	260	15	5	670	24	1	9
Nachoz, Bueno or Grande	as served	513	23	4	636	65	6	7
PERFECT SANDWICHEZ, W/O CHEESE OR TOPPINGS UNLESS INDICATED								
Chicken Salad on Wheat	1 sandwich	363	23	4	732	30	1	11
Deli on White	1 sandwich	285	17	5	823	21	5	14
Ham & Cheese on White	1 sandwich	300	14	7	1334	22	5	22
Italian on White	1 sandwich	258	13	4	1038	21	5	18
Roast Beef & Cheese on Wheat	1 sandwich	277	13	7	1026	222	1	17
Roasted Turkey on White	1 sandwich	147	4	0	693	20	5	14
Tuna Salad on White	1 sandwich	310	18	3	592	27	5	7
PIZZA								
Cheese	1 slice	350	15	9	821	37	4	16
Mushroom	1 slice	364	16	9	881	38	4	16
Pepperoni	1 slice	416	21	12	953	38	4	19
Vegetable	1 slice	397	18	9	1010	41	5	16
PRETZEL MELTS, W/O CHEESE OR TOPPINGS UNLESS INDICATED								
Bacon	1 sandwich	552	22	9	1052	70	2	21

	SERVING SIZE	CALORIES	TOTAL FAT (G)	SAT FAT (G)	SODIUM (MG)	CARBS (G)	FIBER (G)	PROTEIN (G)
Club	1 sandwich	402	7	2	837	69	2	18
Ham	1 sandwich	422	7	3	857	70	2	18
Roast Beef	1 sandwich	351	5	2	361	67	2	9
Roasted Turkey	1 sandwich	402	7	2	837	69	2	18
QUESADILLAZ, W/O TOPPINGS								
Cheese	as served	731	40	22	1448	57	2	36
Chicken & Cheese	as served	848	44	23	2080	57	2	57
Steak & Cheese	as served	915	48	24	1797	58	2	53
SALADZ, W/O TOPPINGS OR DRESSING UNLESS INDICATED								
Classic Chef's Salad	1 salad	149	4	1	999	12	2	20
Garden Salad	1 salad	27	0	0	27	7	2	2
Grilled Chicken Caesar	1 salad	365	29	6	1361	4	0	26
Made-to-Order Crispy Chicken Salad	1 salad	269	8	1	1060	30	2	22
Made-to-Order Grilled Chicken Salad	1 salad	144	4	1	663	7	2	24
Made-to-Order Steak Salad	1 salad	211	8	2	376	8	2	19
Taco Salad	1 salad	254	10	2	173	38	5	5
SIDEZ								
Fryz, Cup	as served	258	10	3	568	36	3	3
Garlic Fryz, Side	as served	554	49	33	1186	102	35	35
Mac & Cheese	1 entrée	129	6	3	934	14	0	5
Nacho Cheese Fryz, Side	as served	672	32	8	2018	81	7	9
Three Cheese Mac & Cheese	1 entrée	180	10	6	1020	15	0	9
WRAPZ, W/O CHEESE OR TOPPINGS UNLESS INDICATED								
Grilled Chicken Caesar	1 wrap	470	25	5	1842	32	9	37
Made-to-Order Grilled Chicken	1 wrap	259	7	1	1118	23	9	34
Made-to-Order Steak	1 wrap	326	11	2	831	24	9	29
Roasted Turkey & Cheese	1 wrap	323	15	6	1575	27	9	29

Sizzler
BURGERS & SANDWICHES

	SERVING SIZE	CALORIES	TOTAL FAT (G)	SAT FAT (G)	SODIUM (MG)	CARBS (G)	FIBER (G)	PROTEIN (G)
Grilled Chicken Club	1 sandwich	667	31	12	1339	48	3	45
Mega Bacon Cheeseburger	1 burger	1009	61	27	2475	48	3	64
Sizzler Burger, 1/2 lb	1 burger	619	30	12	1344	47	3	36
Vegetable Medley	1 sandwich	82	4.1	2.4	41	8.4	2.8	2.9

CHICKEN & RIBS

Grilled Chicken Fettuccine Alfredo	1 entrée	1018	59	36	2219	62	2	50

restaurants

	SERVING SIZE	CALORIES	TOTAL FAT (G)	SAT FAT (G)	SODIUM (MG)	CARBS (G)	FIBER (G)	PROTEIN (G)
Lemon Herb Chicken, Double	1 entrée	440	23	6	1249	3	0	52
Malibu Chicken, Double	1 entrée	725	50	16	1367	23	0	43
Ribs, Full Rack	1 entrée	1157	79	30	1609	51	0	57
SEAFOOD								
Dozen Fried Shrimp	1 entrée	433	12	1	2263	48	2	29
Grilled Salmon, w/Rice Pilaf	1 entrée	532	20	6	921	40	1	47
Grilled Shrimp Fettuccine Alfredo	1 entrée	986	55	35	2082	64	2	53
Unlimited Shrimp	1 entrée	720	19	3	3749	80	3	48
SIDES								
Cheese Toast	1 slice	238	19	9	395	13	1	5
Rice Pilaf	1 side	224	5	2	738	39	1	5
Sweet Potato, w/Maple Topping	1 whole	442	16	7	244	69	8	5
STEAKS & STEAK COMBOS								
Bacon Wrapped Sirloin Filets	1 entrée	554	35	12	2318	5	1	49
Big Appetite Trio	1 entrée	1098	50	15	3855	67	2	85
Chopped Steak	1 entrée	519	30	11	1402	17	1	42
Classic, 8 oz	1 entrée	318	14	3	1578	2	1	41
Classic Trio	1 entrée	836	40	12	2893	37	2	76
Rib Eye, 12 oz	1 entrée	949	62	23	1278	1	0	91
Steak & Colossal Shrimp, w/Rice Pilaf	1 entrée	625	19	5	2507	43	2	66
Steak & Grilled Shrimp Skewers, w/Rice Pilaf	1 entrée	641	27	10	2495	43	2	51
Steak & Hibachi Chicken	1 entrée	457	19	4	2179	9	0	58
Steak & Lemon Herb Chicken	1 entrée	476	24	6	2100	4	0	58
Steak & Lobster Tail	1 entrée	369	13	2	1939	4	1	56
Steak & Malibu Chicken	1 entrée	619	37	11	2159	14	1	53
Steak & Unlimited Shrimp	1 entrée	976	31	5	5224	82	3	80

Skyline Chili
BOWLS

	SERVING SIZE	CALORIES	TOTAL FAT (G)	SAT FAT (G)	SODIUM (MG)	CARBS (G)	FIBER (G)	PROTEIN (G)
Coney	1 bowl	780	61	33	2120	8	1	48
Loaded Chili	1 bowl	510	31	17	1530	23	5	34
Vegetarian Black Beans & Rice	1 bowl	370	14	4.5	710	47	8	13
BURRITOS & CHILITO								
Chili Bean Mix Burrito Deluxe	1 burrito	650	29	15	1220	64	10	33
Chili Burrito Deluxe	1 burrito	640	33	17	1480	44	5	36
Chilito	1 chilito	370	17	8	450	36	3	17

	SERVING SIZE	CALORIES	TOTAL FAT (G)	SAT FAT (G)	SODIUM (MG)	CARBS (G)	FIBER (G)	PROTEIN (G)
Vegetarian Black Bean Burrito Deluxe	1 burrito	700	32	14	920	73	9	27
CHILI, REGULAR								
3-Way	1 serving	780	41	23	1550	52	4	47
4-Way Bean	1 serving	850	42	23	1780	65	8	52
4-Way Onion	1 serving	800	41	23	1550	58	5	48
5-Way	1 serving	870	42	23	1790	70	8	52
Chili Spaghetti	1 serving	440	13	5	1020	51	4	26
Vegetarian Black Bean & Rice 3-Way	1 serving	820	36	19	1290	83	9	38
CONEYS & SANDWICHES								
Cheese Coney	as served	290	23	12	940	6	1	15
Chili Cheese Sandwich	as served	290	17	9	800	24	2	21
Regular Chili Sandwich, w/o Cheese	as served	120	7	2.5	840	5	1	9
Regular Coney, w/o Cheese	as served	170	13	6	760	5	1	8
FRIES								
Chili Cheese Fries	as served	750	40	18	1820	66	6	32
French Fries	as served	390	13	2.5	790	63	6	6
POTATOES								
3-Way Potato	as served	600	25	14	1100	63	7	33
Cheddar Potato	as served	700	42	16	650	61	6	21
Sour Cream Potato	as served	520	28	8	310	61	6	8
SALADS								
Buffalo Chicken, w/o Dressing	1 salad	190	8	3	1820	10	1	19
Regular Greek, w/Dressing	1 salad	380	37	9	1990	7	5	6
WRAPS								
Buffalo Chicken, w/Ranch Dressing	1 wrap	700	37	10	2970	17	3	34
Classic Chicken, w/Chili Ranch Dressing	1 wrap	660	34	10	2030	23	3	34
Greek Chicken, w/Greek Dressing	1 wrap	740	38	10	5230	67	8	31

Snappy Tomato Pizza
PIZZA, LARGE

	SERVING SIZE	CALORIES	TOTAL FAT (G)	SAT FAT (G)	SODIUM (MG)	CARBS (G)	FIBER (G)	PROTEIN (G)
Cheese	1 slice	220	7	3.5	360	30	1	9
Pepperoni	1 slice	340	17	8	760	31	1	15
Snapperoni	1 slice	390	22	10	990	31	1	17
Snappy Meat Topper	1 slice	430	23	10	1000	31	1	23
Snappy Ultimate	1 slice	460	26	10	1230	33	2	22
Supreme	1 slice	340	17	7	730	32	2	14
Veggie	1 slice	240	8	3.5	420	33	2	10

SONIC Drive-In

	SERVING SIZE	CALORIES	TOTAL FAT (G)	SAT FAT (G)	SODIUM (MG)	CARBS (G)	FIBER (G)	PROTEIN (G)
BREAKFAST								
CroisSONIC, Bacon, Egg & Cheese	1 sandwich	510	39	15	1480	28	0	24
CroisSONIC, Sausage, Egg & Cheese	1 sandwich	600	49	18	1420	28	0	24
SuperSONIC, Breakfast Burrito	1 burrito	540	33	12	1910	46	3	23
Toaster, Bacon, Egg & Cheese	1 sandwich	540	29	10	1570	52	2	27
Toaster, Sausage, Egg & Cheese	1 sandwich	630	39	13	1510	52	2	27
BURGERS & CHICKEN								
Jr. Deluxe Cheeseburger	1 burger	450	28	9	800	33	1	19
Jr. Double Cheeseburger	1 burger	600	38	16	1350	35	1	31
Jumbo Popcorn Chicken, Large	1 sandwich	560	32	6	1890	41	5	27
SONIC Cheeseburger, w/Ketchup	1 burger	720	43	17	1190	47	2	35
SONIC, w/Ketchup	1 burger	650	37	14	860	46	2	32
SuperSONIC Bacon Double Cheeseburger, w/Mayo	1 burger	1280	92	36	1630	44	2	67
SuperSONIC Double Cheeseburger, w/Ketchup	1 burger	1130	76	32	1620	47	2	63
Veggie, w/Ketchup	1 burger	450	14	3.5	1410	67	5	15
CONEYS, 6" UNLESS INDICATED								
All Beef, All American Style Dog	1 hot dog	370	18	7	1180	40	1	12
All Beef, Chili Cheese Coney	1 hot dog	410	26	11	1140	30	2	17
All Beef, Regular Hot Dog	1 hot dog	320	18	7	870	27	1	11
Corn Dog	1 corn dog	210	11	3.5	530	23	2	6
Footlong Quarter Pound Coney	1 hot dog	830	54	22	1940	54	3	30
CREAMSLUSH TREATS, LARGE								
Cherry	20 fl oz	610	28	21	280	86	0	7
Lemon	20 fl oz	610	28	21	270	86	0	7
Strawberry	20 fl oz	640	28	21	280	93	1	7
MALTS, LARGE								
Chocolate	20 fl oz	870	40	29	450	115	0	11
Vanilla	20 fl oz	720	41	29	410	79	0	11
REAL FRUIT SLUSHES, MEDIUM								
Average of All Flavors	20 fl oz	285	0	0	45	75	1	0
SANDWICHES & WRAPS								
Chicken Strips Sandwich	1 sandwich	450	24	4	740	43	1	19
Country Fried Steak Sandwich	1 sandwich	670	37	10	1410	71	2	14
Crab Sandwich	1 sandwich	460	20	2.5	380	57	2	14

	SERVING SIZE	CALORIES	TOTAL FAT (G)	SAT FAT (G)	SODIUM (MG)	CARBS (G)	FIBER (G)	PROTEIN (G)
Crispy Chicken Sandwich on Wheat	1 sandwich	570	33	5	1060	47	4	23
Crispy Chicken Wrap	1 wrap	490	23	5	1280	49	3	21
Grilled Chicken Wrap	1 wrap	390	14	3.5	1420	39	2	28
Philly Cheesesteak Sandwich	1 sandwich	540	23	10	1240	48	3	36
SHAKES, LARGE								
Chocolate	20 fl oz	850	40	29	440	113	0	10
Vanilla	20 fl oz	690	40	29	380	75	0	10
SNACKS & SIDES								
French Fries, Medium	as served	330	13	2.5	440	48	4	4
French Fries, w/Cheese, Medium	as served	460	23	7	990	55	4	9
Onion Rings, Large	as served	640	31	5	630	80	4	9
Tater Tots, Medium	as served	200	13	2.5	440	20	2	2
Tater Tots, w/Chili & Cheese, Medium	as served	390	27	9	1100	25	3	11
SONIC BLAST, LARGE								
M&M'S	20 fl oz	1250	68	47	580	146	2	18
Oreo	20 fl oz	1230	65	42	880	146	2	17
Reese's Peanut Butter Cups	20 fl oz	1200	57	40	690	153	2	22

Souper Salad
HANDCRAFTED SOUPS

	SERVING SIZE	CALORIES	TOTAL FAT (G)	SAT FAT (G)	SODIUM (MG)	CARBS (G)	FIBER (G)	PROTEIN (G)
Beef Noodle	1 bowl	70	2	1	410	8	1	4
Beef Stroganoff	1 bowl	120	5	3	680	9	1	4
Broccoli Cheese	1 bowl	70	3	1	780	10	1	2
Chicken Enchilada	1 bowl	170	11	5	630	10	1	6
Chicken Tortilla	1 bowl	60	2	0	530	7	1	5
Cream of Mushroom	1 bowl	80	4	1.5	480	10	1	2
French Onion	1 bowl	40	1	0	750	6	1	1
Italian Wedding	1 bowl	90	4	1.5	710	10	1	4
Mexican Corn Cheddar	1 bowl	80	3	1.5	680	14	1	2
Minestrone	1 bowl	70	1	0	420	13	2	2
Pasta e Fagioli	1 bowl	80	2	0.5	430	14	4	5
Potato Corn Chowder	1 bowl	120	5	2.5	610	16	1	3
Potato Leek	1 bowl	100	3	1.5	810	16	1	2
Red Beans & Rice, w/Sausage	1 bowl	90	2	1	530	19	9	7
Santa Fe Chicken	1 bowl	90	3	1.5	690	10	1	5
Seafood Gumbo	1 bowl	110	5	2.5	530	13	1	5
Tuscan Tomato Basil	1 bowl	70	3	1.5	460	9	1	1
Vegetarian Black Bean	1 bowl	80	2	1	370	20	11	8

restaurants

	SERVING SIZE	CALORIES	TOTAL FAT (G)	SAT FAT (G)	SODIUM (MG)	CARBS (G)	FIBER (G)	PROTEIN (G)
SALADS								
Caesar Salad	1 cup	50	4	1	220	4	1	2
Fettuccine Pasta Salad	1/3 cup	170	10	1.5	440	16	3	3
Ham & Macaroni Salad	1/3 cup	190	13	2	470	15	1	4

Souplantation & Sweet Tomatoes

	SERVING SIZE	CALORIES	TOTAL FAT (G)	SAT FAT (G)	SODIUM (MG)	CARBS (G)	FIBER (G)	PROTEIN (G)
DESSERTS								
Apple Medley, Fat-Free	1/2 cup	70	0	0	5	18	1	1
Banana Royale, Fat-Free	1/2 cup	80	0	0	5	20	1	1
Carrot & Cream Cheese Lava Cake	1 piece	320	15	5	250	40	1	3
Chocolate Chip Cookie, Small	1 cookie	75	3	2	100	10	0	1
Chocolate Lava Cake	1/2 cup	330	8	4	290	62	0	2
Gooey Caramel Pumpkin Cake	1/2 cup	280	9	5	270	45	2	5
Orchard Apple Cobbler	3/4 cup	390	7	3	170	77	2	2
MUFFINS								
Chocolate Brownie	1 muffin	180	8	2	190	26	1	3
Chocolate Peanut Butter Chip	1 muffin	220	10	2	230	31	1	2
Fruit Medley Bran, 96% Fat-Free	1 muffin	130	1	0	290	29	3	2
Georgia Peach Poppyseed	1 muffin	150	6	1	210	20	1	2
Spiced Pumpkin w/Cranberries	1 muffin	180	7	1	170	29	1	2
Tangy Lemon	1 muffin	140	4	1	190	24	1	2
Wildly Blue Blueberry	1 muffin	140	5	1	180	22	1	2
Zucchini Nut	1 muffin	150	7	1	190	22	1	2
PREPARED SALADS								
German Potato	1/2 cup	150	6	1	290	23	2	2
Red, White & Blue Potato, w/Bacon	1/2 cup	190	13	4	360	15	1	3
Smoky Ham & Cheddar Broccoli Slaw	1/2 cup	260	18	5	540	21	3	5
Tuna Tarragon	1/2 cup	250	15	3	480	21	1	6
Vegan, 100% Whole Wheat Arugula Citrus	1/2 cup	210	10	1	250	29	3	4
Vegan, 100% Whole Wheat Sicilian Penne w/Feta & Pepperoni	1/2 cup	250	14	3	450	30	5	6
Vegan, 100% Whole Wheat Spicy Asian Peanut	1/2 cup	260	14	2	460	32	4	6
Vegan, Cuban Rice & Bean	1/2 cup	210	12	1	280	24	2	2
Vegan, Dijon Potato w/Garlic Dill Vinaigrette	1/2 cup	150	12	1	40	9	3	1

	SERVING SIZE	CALORIES	TOTAL FAT (G)	SAT FAT (G)	SODIUM (MG)	CARBS (G)	FIBER (G)	PROTEIN (G)
Vegan & Fat-Free, Sweet Marinated Vegetables	1/2 cup	80	0	0	210	19	4	1
Vegan & Low-Fat, Baja Bean & Cilantro	1/2 cup	180	3	0	190	29	5	9
Vegan, Roasted Potato w/Chipotle Chile Vinaigrette	1/2 cup	140	6	1	250	18	4	3
Vegan, Three Bean Marinade	1/2 cup	170	6	1	320	27	3	4
Vegetarian, BBQ Potato	1/2 cup	170	9	2	370	21	2	2
Vegetarian, Bistro Potato	1/2 cup	290	19	2	490	27	3	5
Vegetarian, Buffalo Blue Potato	1/2 cup	190	13	3	370	16	2	3
Vegetarian & Low-Fat, Carrot Raisin	1/2 cup	90	3	0	80	17	2	1
Vegetarian, Greek Couscous w/Feta Cheese & Pine Nuts	1/2 cup	210	10	1	480	25	4	5
Vegetarian, Red Potato & Tomato	1/2 cup	170	11	2	520	17	3	2
Vegetarian, Sweet Tomato, Basil & Mozzarella	1/2 cup	170	6	2	220	25	4	5
Vegetarian, Whole Grain Fiesta Couscous	1/2 cup	280	11	1	520	39	8	8
SOUPS								
Beef & Barley Stew	1 cup	240	10	4	930	19	3	12
Better Than Mom's Beef Stew	1 cup	270	17	8	1150	19	2	9
Buffalo Chicken	1 cup	180	6	3	740	21	1	9
Chesapeake Corn Chowder	1 cup	290	17	9	890	30	2	6
Low-Fat, Chicken Tortilla w/Jalapeño Chiles & Tomatoes	1 cup	100	3	1	870	11	1	6
Loaded Baked Potato & Cheese w/Bacon	1 cup	290	18	10	690	24	2	9
Marvelous Minestrone w/Bacon	1 cup	220	8	2	950	31	4	7
Minestrone w/Italian Sausage	1 cup	220	12	5	890	17	4	9
Three Cheese Tortellini	1 cup	180	6	2	900	28	2	7
Tomato Chipotle Bisque	1 cup	250	17	10	1150	20	2	5
Vegetarian, Broccoli Cheese	1 cup	270	19	10	810	17	1	7
Vegetarian, Creamy Vegetable Chowder	1 cup	270	14	8	810	26	2	8
Vegetarian, Irish Potato Leek	1 cup	260	16	9	850	23	2	5
Vegetarian & Low-Fat, Garden Fresh Vegetable	1 cup	150	2	0	890	27	4	4
Vegetarian & Low-Fat, Vegetable Medley	1 cup	90	1	0	520	14	3	2
TOSSED SALADS								
Azteca Taco w/Turkey	1 cup	130	9	3	230	7	4	6

restaurants

	SERVING SIZE	CALORIES	TOTAL FAT (G)	SAT FAT (G)	SODIUM (MG)	CARBS (G)	FIBER (G)	PROTEIN (G)
Buffalo Chicken	1 cup	180	14	2	440	10	1	4
Caesar Salad Asiago	1 cup	270	22	8	590	10	2	5
California Cobb w/Bacon	1 cup	190	15	5	370	7	2	5
Chicken Tortilla	1 cup	180	10	3	300	16	2	6
Club Blue BLT w/Bacon	1 cup	270	17	5	620	20	3	6
Mediterranean Bistro Potato	1 cup	230	11	1	420	26	2	6
Ranch House BLT w/Turkey & Bacon	1 cup	190	13	5	390	11	6	6
Smoked Turkey & Spinach w/Almonds	1 cup	190	10	2	480	20	3	6
Spinach Gorgonzola w/Spiced Pecans & Bacon	1 cup	230	19	5	460	9	3	5
Traditional Spinach w/Bacon	1 cup	190	13	4	370	11	3	5
Vegan, Field of Greens, Citrus Vinaigrette	1 cup	150	12	1	110	10	2	1
Vegan, Mandarin Spinach w/Caramelized Walnuts	1 cup	160	10	1	110	14	2	2
Vegetarian, Roasted Vegetables w/Feta & Olives	1 cup	180	14	2	310	13	2	2
Wonton Chicken Happiness	1 cup	150	7	1	290	17	2	4

Spaghetti Warehouse
APPETIZERS

	SERVING SIZE	CALORIES	TOTAL FAT (G)	SAT FAT (G)	SODIUM (MG)	CARBS (G)	FIBER (G)	PROTEIN (G)
Calamari, w/Marinara Sauce & Garlic Aioli	1 serving	1050	81	16	2496	45	n/a	35
Garlic Cheese Bread	1 serving	1330	90	36	3276	81	n/a	53
Stuffed Mushrooms	1 serving	310	19	8	657	14	n/a	21
LASAGNE								
Incredible 15-Layer Lasagne	as served	1051	52	25	1908	80	n/a	65
Vegetable Garden Lasagne	as served	770	23	11	862	100	n/a	34
ORIGINAL RECIPE SPAGHETTI								
Chicken Tettrazini	as served	690	19	9	1344	85	n/a	41
Spaghetti & Meatballs	as served	770	27	10	1322	91	n/a	40
Spaghetti & Mushrooms in Garlic Butter Sauce	as served	970	63	37	1017	80	n/a	23
Spaghetti, w/Marinara Sauce	as served	400	4	1	302	76	n/a	14
PASTA FAVORITES								
Baked Penne	as served	780	37	20	776	81	n/a	31
Cheese Ravioli, w/Tomato Sauce	as served	500	17	8	828	67	n/a	24
Chicken Florentine	as served	990	47	26	1195	91	n/a	49
Fettuccini Alfredo	as served	600	24	8	556	76	n/a	20

	SERVING SIZE	CALORIES	TOTAL FAT (G)	SAT FAT (G)	SODIUM (MG)	CARBS (G)	FIBER (G)	PROTEIN (G)
Four Cheese Manicotti	as served	810	41	22	1780	70	n/a	43
Roasted Garlic Shrimp Sauté	as served	1060	60	37	1789	91	n/a	39
SALAD								
Chopped Salad "Warehouse Style," w/Dressing	1 salad	800	59	19	3113	19	n/a	47
Classic Caesar Salad, w/Croutons, Dressing & Romano Cheese	1 salad	460	38	8	1200	17	n/a	10
House Salad, w/o Dressing	1 salad	50	2	0	80	8	n/a	1
Tuscan Tender Salad, w/o Dressing	1 salad	1070	63	17	1930	71	n/a	56
WAREHOUSE SPECIALTIES								
Chicken Parmigiana	as served	750	27	10	1010	73	n/a	53
Eggplant Parmigiana	as served	1370	74	21	1273	130	n/a	44
Trolley Stop Sirloin & Spaghetti	as served	900	27	11	1785	85	n/a	77
Warehouse Scampi	as served	1030	71	33	1281	56	n/a	39

Starbucks
BAKED GOODS

	SERVING SIZE	CALORIES	TOTAL FAT (G)	SAT FAT (G)	SODIUM (MG)	CARBS (G)	FIBER (G)	PROTEIN (G)
Banana Nut Loaf	1 slice	490	19	2.5	210	75	4	7
Blueberry Scone	1 scone	460	22	12	420	61	2	7
Blueberry Streusel Muffin	1 muffin	360	11	6	390	59	2	7
Chocolate Chunk Cookie	1 cookie	380	17	10	230	51	2	4
Iced Lemon Pound Cake	1 slice	490	23	13	370	67	< 1	5
Reduced-Fat Cinnamon Swirl Coffee Cake	1 slice	340	9	5	390	62	2	4
BEVERAGES, ICED								
Caffe Latte, Nonfat Milk	16 fl oz	90	0	0	105	13	0	8
Caffe Latte, Whole Milk	16 fl oz	150	7	4.5	105	13	0	8
Caramel Macchiato, Nonfat Milk	16 fl oz	190	1	1	125	34	0	10
Caramel Macchiato, Whole Milk	16 fl oz	260	10	6	125	34	0	9
Flavored Latte, Nonfat Milk	16 fl oz	160	0	0	90	31	0	7
Flavored Latte, Whole Milk	16 fl oz	210	6	3.5	90	30	0	7
CAPPUCCINOS, HOT								
Cappuccino, Nonfat Milk	16 fl oz	80	0	0	90	12	0	8
Cappuccino, Whole Milk	16 fl oz	140	7	4	90	12	0	7
FRAPPUCCINO BLENDED BEVERAGES, W/O WHIPPED CREAM								
Caffe Vanilla Frappuccino Light Blended Beverage, Nonfat Milk	16 fl oz	180	0	0	200	40	0	3

restaurants

	SERVING SIZE	CALORIES	TOTAL FAT (G)	SAT FAT (G)	SODIUM (MG)	CARBS (G)	FIBER (G)	PROTEIN (G)
Caffe Vanilla, Nonfat Milk	16 fl oz	290	0	0	220	69	0	4
Caffe Vanilla, Whole Milk	16 fl oz	310	3	2	220	68	0	3
Caramel, Whole Milk	16 fl oz	410	15	9	240	66	0	4
Java Chip Frappuccino Light Blended Beverage, Nonfat Milk	16 fl oz	200	4	3	230	40	2	5
Java Chip, Nonfat Milk	16 fl oz	430	15	10	260	72	2	6
Java Chip, Whole Milk	16 fl oz	460	18	12	260	72	2	6
Mocha, Nonfat Milk	16 fl oz	370	12	7	230	64	< 1	5
Mocha, Whole Milk	16 fl oz	400	15	9	230	64	< 1	5
Tazo Chai Crème, Whole Milk	16 fl oz	250	4	2.5	210	49	0	4
Tazo Chai Crème, Nonfat Milk	16 fl oz	210	0	0	210	49	0	5
HOT CHOCOLATE, W/WHIPPED CREAM								
Made w/Nonfat Milk	16 fl oz	320	10	6	150	51	2	14
Made w/Whole Milk	16 fl oz	410	20	12	150	50	2	14
LATTES, HOT								
Caffe Nonfat Milk	16 fl oz	130	0	0	150	19	0	13
Caffe Whole Milk	16 fl oz	220	11	7	140	18	0	12
MACCHIATOS, HOT								
Caramel Nonfat Milk	16 fl oz	190	1	1	130	35	0	11
Caramel Whole Milk	16 fl oz	270	11	6	135	34	0	10
MOCHAS, HOT, W/WHIPPED CREAM								
Caffe, Nonfat Milk	16 fl oz	290	10	6	130	45	2	13
Caffe, Whole Milk	16 fl oz	370	19	11	135	44	2	13
Steak Escape								
BURGERS								
Bacon Cheddar Char-Burger	1 burger	660	34	n/a	1060	46	2	43
Char-Burger	1 burger	610	32	n/a	780	48	3	31
Double Bacon Cheddar Char-Burger	1 burger	870	48	n/a	1120	46	2	63
Double Char-Burger	1 burger	870	50	n/a	1100	49	3	53
Double Philly Char-Burger	1 burger	770	37	n/a	660	56	6	55
Philly Burger	1 burger	490	21	n/a	680	43	2	32
Single Burger	1 burger	590	32	n/a	1570	48	2	30
FRESH-CUT FRIES								
Cheddar, Bacon & Ranch, Regular	as served	1240	87	n/a	2090	93	11	20
SANDWICHES, 9"								
BBQ Chicken	1 sandwich	670	20	n/a	2310	77	2	48

	SERVING SIZE	CALORIES	TOTAL FAT (G)	SAT FAT (G)	SODIUM (MG)	CARBS (G)	FIBER (G)	PROTEIN (G)
Cheesesteak, Mexicano	1 sandwich	680	20	n/a	1690	70	3	55
Cheesesteak, Mignon	1 sandwich	970	40	n/a	4030	83	2	69
Chicken Club	1 sandwich	630	20	n/a	2460	65	1	52
Chicken Parmesan	1 sandwich	940	37	n/a	2760	104	4	44
Classic Italian	1 sandwich	910	50	n/a	3460	70	2	42
Fire Escape	1 sandwich	710	23	n/a	2010	70	3	56
Grand Chicken	1 sandwich	620	19	n/a	2110	68	2	49
Honey Ham	1 sandwich	730	31	n/a	3140	82	2	32
Teriyaki Chicken	1 sandwich	660	19	n/a	3940	74	2	52
Turkey Club	1 sandwich	550	14	n/a	2490	65	2	41
Vegetarian	1 sandwich	550	20	n/a	1830	71	4	27
Wild West BBQ	1 sandwich	700	20	n/a	1540	75	2	55
WRAPS								
BBQ Chicken	1 wrap	530	19	n/a	1780	57	1	33
Cheesesteak, Mexicano	1 wrap	540	19	n/a	1360	52	2	37
Cheesesteak, Mignon	1 wrap	730	32	n/a	2930	61	2	46
Cheesesteak, Triple	1 wrap	700	34	n/a	1810	52	2	47
Chicken Club	1 wrap	500	19	n/a	1820	49	1	34
Chicken Parmesan	1 wrap	700	30	n/a	2080	75	3	30
Classic Italian	1 wrap	690	39	n/a	2550	52	1	28
Fire Escape	1 wrap	560	21	n/a	1590	52	2	38
Honey Ham	1 wrap	570	27	n/a	2390	61	1	22
Turkey Club	1 wrap	440	15	n/a	1900	49	1	28
Vegetarian	1 wrap	430	17	n/a	1450	52	3	17
Wild West BBQ	1 wrap	550	19	n/a	1270	56	2	37

Subway
EGG MUFFIN MELTS, W/REGULAR EGG & LIGHT WHEAT ENGLISH MUFFIN

	SERVING SIZE	CALORIES	TOTAL FAT (G)	SAT FAT (G)	SODIUM (MG)	CARBS (G)	FIBER (G)	PROTEIN (G)
Bacon, Egg & Cheese	1 sandwich	200	7	3	550	24	6	13
Egg & Cheese	1 sandwich	170	6	2	460	24	6	12
Egg & Cheese, w/Ham	1 sandwich	190	6	2	590	24	6	14
Sunrise Subway Melt	1 sandwich	230	8	3	810	26	6	18
OMELET SANDWICHES, 6", W/REGULAR EGG & 9-GRAIN WHEAT BREAD								
Bacon, Egg & Cheese	1 sandwich	410	16	6	1080	45	5	23
Breakfast B.M.T. Melt	1 sandwich	490	22	8	1690	46	5	28
Steak, Egg & Cheese	1 sandwich	430	15	5	1220	47	5	28

restaurants

	SERVING SIZE	CALORIES	TOTAL FAT (G)	SAT FAT (G)	SODIUM (MG)	CARBS (G)	FIBER (G)	PROTEIN (G)
SALADS, INCLUDES LETTUCE, TOMATOES, ONIONS, GREEN PEPPERS, CUCUMBERS & OLIVES, W/O DRESSING								
Grilled Chicken & Baby Spinach	1 salad	130	3	0.5	330	10	3	20
Oven-Roasted Chicken Breast	1 salad	130	3	0.5	270	9	4	19
Subway Club	1 salad	140	4	1	640	11	4	17
Sweet Onion Chicken Teriyaki	1 salad	200	3	1	660	24	4	20
Turkey Breast	1 salad	110	2	0.5	570	11	4	12
Veggie Delite	1 salad	50	1	0	65	9	4	3
SUBS, 6", INCLUDES 9-GRAIN WHEAT BREAD, LETTUCE, TOMATO, ONION, GREEN PEPPER & CUCUMBER								
Black Forest Ham	1 sub	290	5	1	830	46	5	18
BLT	1 sub	320	9	4	680	43	5	15
Big Philly Cheesesteak	1 sub	500	17	9	1310	51	6	38
Buffalo Chicken, w/Ranch dressing	1 sub	420	15	3	1130	46	5	25
Cold Cut Combo	1 sub	370	13	4	1140	46	5	18
Meatball Marinara	1 sub	480	18	7	950	59	8	21
Oven-Roasted Chicken	1 sub	320	5	1.5	640	47	5	23
Roast Beef	1 sub	320	5	1.5	700	45	5	24
Spicy Italian	1 sub	480	24	9	1520	46	5	20
Steak & Cheese	1 sub	380	10	4.5	1060	48	5	26
Subway Club	1 sub	310	5	1.5	880	46	5	23
Tuna	1 sub	470	24	4	620	44	5	20
Turkey Breast	1 sub	280	4	1	810	46	5	18
Veggie Delite	1 sub	230	3	0.5	310	44	5	8
Swiss Chalet **DESSERTS & BEVERAGES**								
Fudge Cake	as served	490	28	9	240	55	3	3
Super Sundae, Chocolate	as served	360	16	9	110	58	3	3
Super Sundae, Strawberry	as served	270	12	7	65	42	2	2
ENTRÉE SALADS, STIR-FRYS & FISH								
Chicken Stir-Fry, w/Rice	as served	900	36	6	2260	103	8	46
Fish & Chips, 2 Pieces of Fish, w/Fries, Tartar Sauce & Coleslaw	as served	1460	92	10	1630	122	10	34
Rotisserie Chicken Caesar Salad, w/o Dressing	1 salad	420	11	3.5	910	38	4	45

	SERVING SIZE	CALORIES	TOTAL FAT (G)	SAT FAT (G)	SODIUM (MG)	CARBS (G)	FIBER (G)	PROTEIN (G)
Spinach Chicken Salad, w/o Dressing	1 salad	410	16	3	530	28	6	41
Vegetable Stir-Fry, w/Rice	as served	690	28	3	1980	103	7	11
West Coast Salad, w/Chicken, w/o Dressing	1 salad	460	21	7	970	21	5	47
FROM THE GRILL								
Classic Bacon Cheese Burger, w/Bun	as served	890	54	24	2240	46	2	56
Classic Hamburger, w/Bun	as served	710	39	17	1630	43	2	44
Full Rack BBQ Ribs	as served	1300	85	32	900	11	6	120
Striploin Steak	as served	580	38	6	410	0	0	55
Veggie Burger, w/Bun	as served	330	12	2.5	1050	52	8	32
ROTISSERIE CHICKEN								
Chicken Pot Pie	as served	560	32	9	1190	39	4	29
Double Leg, w/Skin	as served	490	31	10	440	0	1	53
Double Leg, w/o Skin	as served	320	16	5	370	0	1	45
Half Chicken, w/Skin	as served	530	27	8	550	0	1	74
Half Chicken, w/o Skin	as served	380	14	4.5	520	0	1	67
Quarter Chicken, Dark Meat, w/Skin	as served	240	16	5	220	0	1	27
Quarter Chicken, Dark Meat, w/o Skin	as served	160	8	2.5	180	0	1	22
Quarter Chicken, White Meat, w/Skin	as served	290	11	3.5	330	0	1	48
Quarter Chicken, White Meat w/o Skin	as served	220	6	2	340	0	0	44
SIDE SERVINGS								
Creamy Coleslaw	as served	200	14	0	460	15	3	2
Fresh-Cut Fries	as served	530	27	2	95	64	6	7
STARTERS								
Chalet Chicken Noodle Soup	1 bowl	200	5	1.5	1050	18	2	20
Chalet Chicken Wings, w/Mild Sauce	8 pieces	550	34	7	790	23	2	39
Cheese Perogies	7 pieces	420	10	2	790	69	4	12
Chicken Spring Rolls	4 pieces	510	27	3.5	490	47	1	20
Garlic Cheese Loaf	as served	910	58	19	1200	73	5	26
Poutine	as served	910	50	11	930	94	9	21
Seasoned Dry Ribs	as served	920	64	24	1880	4	0	76
WRAPS & SANDWICHES								
Chicken on a Kaiser, White Meat	1 sandwich	480	8	2.5	910	47	2	58
Classic Hot Chicken Sandwich, White Meat	1 sandwich	520	11	3.5	1850	51	3	58
Hickory Chicken Flatbread Sandwich	1 sandwich	700	32	10	2020	70	3	36
Rotisserie Chicken Club Wrap	1 wrap	710	32	11	1450	57	3	49
Rotisserie Chicken Quesadilla, w/o Salsa or Sour Cream	1 quesadilla	640	29	13	1310	66	5	31

restaurants

	SERVING SIZE	CALORIES	TOTAL FAT (G)	SAT FAT (G)	SODIUM (MG)	CARBS (G)	FIBER (G)	PROTEIN (G)
Southwest Chicken Flatbread Sandwich	1 sandwich	710	37	11	1810	64	2	33
T.J. Cinnamons								
Cinnamon Twist	1 pastry	260	14	5	190	33	1	3
Mocha Chill, w/o Whipped Cream	12 fl oz	264	4	2.4	214	46	1	11
Original Gourmet Cinnamon Roll	1 pastry	507	10	4	373	73	4	10
Pecan Sticky Bun	1 pastry	688	22	5	420	91	5	12
Sticky Bun Smear, w/Pecans	1 pastry	181	12	1.6	47	18	1	1
TJ Icing	1 oz	117	5	2	50	18	0	1
Taco Bell								
BURRITOS								
7-Layer	1 burrito	510	19	7	1070	69	11	16
Bean	1 burrito	370	11	4	960	56	9	13
Beefy 5-Layer	1 burrito	550	22	8	1270	68	8	19
Cheesy Bean & Rice	1 burrito	480	21	5	1030	60	7	12
Chili Cheese	1 burrito	380	17	8	930	41	5	16
Fresco Bean	1 burrito	350	8	2.5	990	57	11	12
Fresco Supreme, Chicken	1 burrito	350	8	2.5	1060	50	7	18
Grilled Chicken	1 burrito	430	18	5	870	48	3	18
Supreme, Beef	1 burrito	420	16	6	1100	53	9	17
Volcano	1 burrito	780	41	11	1590	80	8	24
XXL Grilled Stuft, Beef	1 burrito	880	42	14	2050	95	14	32
CHALUPAS								
Supreme, Beef	1 item	370	21	5	570	31	4	13
Supreme, Chicken	1 item	350	18	4	520	29	3	17
GORDITAS								
Cheesy Crunch	1 item	490	29	10	810	39	5	20
Supreme, Beef	1 item	300	14	5	550	31	4	13
Supreme, Chicken	1 item	270	10	3.5	510	29	2	17
NACHOS								
BellGrande	as served	770	42	7	1020	79	13	19
Supreme	as served	440	25	5	640	42	8	12
Volcano	as served	980	60	9	1590	89	15	20
SPECIALTIES								
Cheese Quesadilla	1 item	480	27	11	1000	40	4	19
Chicken Quesadilla	1 item	530	28	12	1210	41	4	28
Crunchwrap Supreme	1 item	540	21	6	1110	71	7	16

	Serving Size	Calories	Total Fat (g)	Sat Fat (g)	Sodium (mg)	Carbs (g)	Fiber (g)	Protein (g)
Mexican Pizza	1 item	540	30	8	870	47	7	20
TACO SALADS								
Express Taco, w/Chips	1 salad	580	29	9	1280	59	9	23
Fiesta Taco, Beef	1 salad	770	42	10	1350	74	11	26
Fiesta Taco, Chicken	1 salad	730	35	7	1270	70	9	34
TACOS								
Crunchy Supreme	1 taco	200	12	4.5	320	15	3	9
Double Decker Supreme	1 taco	350	15	6	680	40	8	14
Fresco Chicken Soft	1 taco	150	4	1	480	18	2	12
Fresco Crunchy	1 taco	150	8	2	310	13	3	6
Fresco Soft	1 taco	180	7	2.5	520	20	3	8
Grilled Steak Soft	1 taco	250	14	4	550	19	2	11
Soft, Beef	1 taco	200	9	4	510	19	3	10
Soft, Chicken	1 taco	180	6	2.5	460	18	1	14
Volcano	1 taco	230	16	4.5	410	14	3	8

Taco Cabana
CHALUPAS

	Serving Size	Calories	Total Fat (g)	Sat Fat (g)	Sodium (mg)	Carbs (g)	Fiber (g)	Protein (g)
Bean & Cheese	as served	290	17	7	350	23	5	11
Ground Beef	as served	310	16	6	640	24	5	16
Guacamole	as served	340	21	6	610	30	9	9
Stewed Chicken	as served	290	14	5	640	26	5	16
NACHOS, SHREDDED CHEESE, REGULAR								
Average of Fajita Nachos	as served	1465	97	40.5	1730	84	14	64
Bean & Cheese	as served	1420	90	38	1340	100	17	54
Brisket Nachos	as served	1650	114	47	1750	85	15	72
Ground Beef	as served	1330	84	35	1680	78	11	62
Stewed Chicken	as served	1280	79	33	1690	81	12	61
Super Ground Beef	as served	1770	114	48	2360	109	20	74
Super Stewed Chicken	as served	1720	109	45	2370	112	21	73
PLATES								
Beef Street Taco	1 entrée	910	27	10	2280	135	13	36
Brisket Taco	1 entrée	1270	48	19	3140	157	12	47
Chicken Fajita Taco	1 entrée	950	25	9	3160	132	15	45
Chicken Street Taco	1 entrée	1080	43	12	2480	134	13	37
Enchilada	1 entrée	1270	66	31	2800	115	12	52
Mexican	1 entrée	1130	53	23	2600	114	12	47
Steak Fajita Taco	1 entrée	980	29	10	3160	132	15	41

	SERVING SIZE	CALORIES	TOTAL FAT (G)	SAT FAT (G)	SODIUM (MG)	CARBS (G)	FIBER (G)	PROTEIN (G)
Super Tex-Mex	1 entrée	1490	76	31	3190	141	20	59
Taco	1 entrée	990	40	16	2400	112	12	41
QUESADILLAS								
Brisket	1 personal	860	50	24	1910	62	5	40
Cheese	1 personal	710	39	21	1630	61	5	29
Steak Fajita	1 personal	770	42	21	1900	62	5	36
SOFT TACOS								
Bean & Cheese	1 taco	300	14	7	590	32	4	11
Black Bean	1 taco	200	4	2	630	34	2	6
Brisket	1 taco	270	14	5	570	21	2	15
Carne Guisada	1 taco	190	6	2	330	21	1	12
Ground Beef	1 taco	230	9	5	720	22	1	13
Stewed Chicken	1 taco	210	7	3	720	23	2	13

Taco John's
BURRITOS

	SERVING SIZE	CALORIES	TOTAL FAT (G)	SAT FAT (G)	SODIUM (MG)	CARBS (G)	FIBER (G)	PROTEIN (G)
Bean Burrito	1 burrito	370	11	5	1090	53	7	14
Grilled Burrito, Average of Beef & Chicken	1 burrito	595	31	13	1840	52	4	27
Meat & Potato, Beef	1 burrito	520	25	8	1490	57	5	15
Meat & Potato, Chicken	1 burrito	480	21	7	1590	56	4	18
Super Burrito	1 burrito	450	20	9	1190	50	6	19
DESSERTS								
Churro	as served	200	9	2.5	170	29	4	3
Cini-Sopapilla Bites	as served	200	8	1.5	180	34	4	4
SIDES								
Chili, w/Cheese	1 bowl	200	11	5	1130	16	4	12
Chips & Queso	as served	430	25	6	1130	43	2	9
Nachos	as served	380	23	5	940	39	1	6
Potato Olés, Medium	as served	670	38	8	1930	73	8	7
SPECIALTIES								
Crunchy Chicken, w/o Sauce	as served	370	18	3	920	29	0	22
Quesadilla Melt, Average of Beef & Chicken	1 quesadilla	535	27	13	1640	46	3	27
Quesadilla Melt, Cheesy	1 quesadilla	450	24	12	1400	40	1	19
Super Nachos, Regular	as served	790	47	15	1650	72	7	22
Super Potato Olés, Regular	as served	1090	67	21	3300	98	14	24
Taco Salad, w/o Dressing	1 salad	540	33	13	820	40	6	22

	SERVING SIZE	CALORIES	TOTAL FAT (G)	SAT FAT (G)	SODIUM (MG)	CARBS (G)	FIBER (G)	PROTEIN (G)
TACOS								
Crispy	1 taco	170	10	4	290	11	2	9
Beef, Soft	1 taco	220	10	4.5	580	23	2	11
Chicken, Soft	1 taco	190	6	3	680	21	2	14
Stuffed Grilled	1 wrap	540	27	10	1320	58	3	18
Taco Bravo	1 taco	330	13	5	750	38	6	14
Taco Burger	1 burger	280	12	4.5	570	29	2	14

Taco Mayo
BURRITOS

	SERVING SIZE	CALORIES	TOTAL FAT (G)	SAT FAT (G)	SODIUM (MG)	CARBS (G)	FIBER (G)	PROTEIN (G)
Bean Burrito	1 burrito	496	16	n/a	1504	71	12	21
Fajita Grilled, Chicken	1 burrito	492	23	n/a	1373	42	3	27
Fajita Grilled, Steak	1 burrito	519	25	n/a	1353	42	3	29
Mexicali Grilled, Chicken	1 burrito	607	30	n/a	1730	54	2	28
Mexicali Grilled, Steak	1 burrito	633	32	n/a	1710	54	2	30
SalsaLITA Beef, Grilled	1 burrito	411	13	n/a	1442	55	4	18
SalsaLITA Chicken, Grilled	1 burrito	387	8	n/a	1553	54	3	23
SalsaLITA Steak, Grilled	1 burrito	413	10	n/a	1553	54	3	25
Super, Chicken	1 burrito	407	16	n/a	1089	39	2	25
Super, Steak	1 burrito	434	18	n/a	1069	39	2	27
NACHOS								
Classic Nachos, Beef Supreme	as served	719	37	n/a	1755	70	12	28
Classic Nachos, Cheese	as served	377	19	n/a	834	45	4	6
Classic Nachos, Chicken Supreme	as served	643	29	n/a	1716	69	11	28
Ultimate Grandé Nacho	as served	1040	55	n/a	2580	98	18	40
OTHER ITEMS								
Guac-N-Chips	as served	399	22	n/a	4	45	371	7
Loco Melt	as served	814	57	n/a	1538	56	7	20
Queso-N-Chips	as served	449	22	n/a	14	49	1296	3
QUESADILLAS								
Cheese	1 quesadilla	596	35	n/a	1174	45	4	25
Fajita Chicken	1 quesadilla	698	39	n/a	1679	47	5	40
Fajita Steak	1 quesadilla	725	40	n/a	1659	47	5	42
SALADS								
Taco Salad, Beef	1 salad	705	38	n/a	1766	57	13	37
Taco Salad, Chicken	1 salad	438	23	n/a	1169	30	3	27
TACOS								
Crispy Beef	1 taco	161	9	n/a	243	10	1	9

restaurants

	SERVING SIZE	CALORIES	TOTAL FAT (G)	SAT FAT (G)	SODIUM (MG)	CARBS (G)	FIBER (G)	PROTEIN (G)
SalsaLITA Chicken, Soft	1 taco	167	4	n/a	693	18	1	14
SalsaLITA Steak, Soft	1 taco	187	5	n/a	678	18	1	16
Soft Beef	1 taco	228	11	n/a	584	17	2	14
Soft Chicken	1 taco	184	6	n/a	592	16	1	15

Taco Time
BURRITOS

Beef, Bean & Cheese	1 burrito	490	17	7	2310	55	11	26
Big Juan, Average of Beef & Pork	1 burrito	640	25	10	2545	72	13	31
Big Juan, Chicken	1 burrito	580	16	8	2550	70	11	34
Casita, Average of Beef & Pork	1 burrito	545	26	11.5	2235	44	6	30
Casita, Chicken	1 burrito	490	17	10	2350	42	5	34
Chicken & Black Bean	1 burrito	490	16	6	1270	54	9	30
Chicken BLT	1 burrito	690	39	10	1600	43	8	39
Crisp Chicken	1 burrito	380	17	6	540	33	2	22
Crispy Chicken Ranchero	1 burrito	600	31	7	1250	51	7	29
Ground Beef, Average of Soft & Crisp	1 burrito	430	19	6.5	960	40	6	23
Pinto Bean, Average of Soft & Crisp	1 burrito	365	12	4	2005	51	8	14

DESSERTS

Churro, w/Cinnamon & Sugar	1 churro	250	16	5	160	27	0	2
Crustos	1 crustos	290	6	1	270	58	3	6
Empanada, Average of All	1 empanada	243	8	1	200	40	2	5

FRIES, MEDIUM

Cheddar	as served	500	35	11	1170	39	4	11
Mexi	as served	390	26	4.5	990	38	4	4

OTHER FAVORITES

Chimichanga, Chicken	1 chimichanga	610	20	11	2620	63	10	37
Chimichanga, Ground Beef	1 chimichanga	650	27	13	2520	63	11	31
Enchilada, Chicken	1 enchilada	230	5	3	610	17	1	23
Enchilada, Ground Beef	1 enchilada	290	12	5	830	21	3	18
Nachos, Grande	1 nacho	930	43	21	3580	96	10	37
Taco Burger	1 burger	460	26	8	1180	31	3	21
Tostada, Bean	1 tostada	230	13	4	1320	21	3	8
Tostada, Ground Beef	1 tostada	380	20	6	1830	25	5	21

SALADS

Taco, Chicken, Regular	1 salad	310	13	4	680	22	2	25

	SERVING SIZE	CALORIES	TOTAL FAT (G)	SAT FAT (G)	SODIUM (MG)	CARBS (G)	FIBER (G)	PROTEIN (G)
Taco, Ground Beef, Regular	1 salad	370	20	6	810	24	4	20
Tostada Delight, Chicken	1 salad	450	19	7	2050	35	4	30
Tostada Delight, Ground Beef	1 salad	490	26	10	1970	36	6	24
TACOS								
Crisp Ground Beef	1 taco	260	17	5	460	12	2	14
Soft, Chicken	1 taco	360	9	4.5	860	40	7	28
Soft, Ground Beef	1 taco	420	16	7	1020	43	9	23
Super Soft, Chicken	1 taco	530	16	8	2180	59	6	34
Super Soft, Ground Beef	1 taco	590	23	10	2410	62	8	30

Target Café
ENTRÉES

	SERVING SIZE	CALORIES	TOTAL FAT (G)	SAT FAT (G)	SODIUM (MG)	CARBS (G)	FIBER (G)	PROTEIN (G)
Beef Hot Dog	1 hot dog	340	20	7	980	27	0	14
Cheese Pizza	1 pizza	400	13	6	960	54	4	19
Chicken Tenders	1 serving	270	10	2.5	870	18	0	27
Pepperoni Pizza	1 pizza	450	17	8	1170	54	4	21
SANDWICHES & FLATBREADS								
Chicken Marinara	1 item	180	8	3.5	510	15	2	11
Chicken Spinach Artichoke	1 item	160	7	3	490	17	2	9
Ham & Swiss	1 sandwich	410	8	4	1940	53	3	31
Turkey & Provolone	1 sandwich	330	12	7	1050	36	1	22
Turkey Club	1 sandwich	420	19	9	1270	34	1	28
SNACKS & TREATS								
Bavarian Pretzel, w/Butter & Salt	1 item	490	6	1.5	2310	93	3	15
Bavarian Pretzel, w/Butter, Cinnamon, & Sugar	1 item	520	6	1.5	780	102	3	15
Cheddar Pretzel	1 item	540	15	8	1530	87	3	18
Cookies, Average of All Flavors	1 cookie	497	24	9	390	66	3	6
French Fries	as served	230	9	1	330	33	4	3
Nachos, w/Cheese & Jalapeños	1 serving	530	25	6	1370	89	4	9
Popcorn	1 bag	300	16	3	500	33	5	5
Smoothies, Average of Strawberry & Mango	12 fl oz	230	0	0	13	57	1	0
Yogurt Parfait	1 item	320	5	1.5	190	59	2	9

TCBY
FROZEN YOGURT, SOFT SERVE

	SERVING SIZE	CALORIES	TOTAL FAT (G)	SAT FAT (G)	SODIUM (MG)	CARBS (G)	FIBER (G)	PROTEIN (G)
Cake Batter	1/2 cup	120	2	1	65	23	3	4
Cheesecake	1/2 cup	110	2	1	65	23	3	4

restaurants

	SERVING SIZE	CALORIES	TOTAL FAT (G)	SAT FAT (G)	SODIUM (MG)	CARBS (G)	FIBER (G)	PROTEIN (G)
Chocolate	1/2 cup	110	2	1	90	23	3	4
Chocolate, No Added Sugar	1/2 cup	70	0	0	70	21	6	4
Coffee	1/2 cup	120	2	1	80	23	3	4
Golden Vanilla	1/2 cup	120	2	1	65	23	3	4
Kiwi Strawberry Sorbet	1/2 cup	100	0	0	15	24	0	0
Mango Sorbet	1/2 cup	110	0	0	10	26	0	0
Mountain Blackberry, No Added Sugar, Fat-Free	1/2 cup	80	0	0	70	22	4	4
Raspberry Sorbet	1/2 cup	100	0	0	10	25	0	0
Vanilla, No Added Sugar	1/2 cup	80	0	0	65	21	4	4
White Chocolate Mousse	1/2 cup	120	2	1	65	23	3	4
Ted Drewes Frozen Custard								
Frozen Custard, No Sugar	1/2 cup	180	8	5	170	26	0	6
Frozen Custard, Vanilla	1/2 cup	200	10	7	70	21	0	6
Thunder Cloud Subs								
CLASSIC SUBS, LARGE								
Avocado	1 sub	421	18	2	585	54	4	8
BLT	1 sub	585	28	9	1320	48	0	24
Capicola	1 sub	673	38	12	2126	48	0	25
Chicken Salad	1 sub	594	26	4	628	48	0	33
Egg Salad	1 sub	599	32	6	883	49	0	19
Genoa Salami	1 sub	398	11	3	1344	49	0	18
Ham & Cheese	1 sub	506	17	8	1906	52	0	24
Roast Beef	1 sub	410	6	1	988	48	0	22
Smoked Chicken	1 sub	375	6	0	1163	48	0	25
Turkey	1 sub	358	5	0	1390	50	0	22
HOT SUBS, LARGE								
NADA Chicken	1 sub	585	15	2	1680	78	6	29
Meatball	1 sub	910	47	17	1916	73	6	38
Pastrami	1 sub	514	15	5	1822	49	0	30
SIGNATURE SUBS, LARGE								
American Classic	1 sub	698	35	15	2485	54	0	32
Austin Club, w/Cheese	1 sub	704	36	11	1800	54	3	32
California Club, w/Cheese	1 sub	692	35	11	1946	55	3	30
Office Favorite	1 sub	1004	46	10	1723	97	0	32
Roast Beef & Avocado	1 sub	641	26	9	1509	54	0	36

	SERVING SIZE	CALORIES	TOTAL FAT (G)	SAT FAT (G)	SODIUM (MG)	CARBS (G)	FIBER (G)	PROTEIN (G)
Texas Tuna	1 sub	819	52	8	1170	54	4	27
The Club, w/Cheese	1 sub	589	23	9	2146	52	0	32
Veggie Delite, w/Hummus	1 sub	471	14	2	948	68	8	16

Tim Hortons
BAGELS
12 Grain	1 bagel	330	9	1	580	52	6	10
Blueberry	1 bagel	270	1	0	470	55	2	10
Cheddar Cheese	1 bagel	220	3	1	410	41	2	9
Cinnamon Raisin	1 bagel	270	1	0	350	55	3	10
Everything	1 bagel	280	2	0	460	53	3	10
Onion	1 bagel	260	2	0	460	53	3	9
Plain	1 bagel	260	2	0	450	52	2	9
Sesame Seed	1 bagel	270	3	0	430	53	3	9
Wheat 'N Honey	1 bagel	300	3	0.4	600	60	4	10

BEVERAGES
Cappuccino	15 fl oz	100	0	0	150	15	0	9
Fruit Smoothies, w/Yogurt, Average of All	16 fl oz	287	2	1	75	66	1	58
Fruit Smoothies, w/o Yogurt, Average of All	16 fl oz	213	0	0	20	55	1	0
Hot Chocolate	15 fl oz	300	7	6	460	57	3	2
Iced Cappuccino, Cream	16 fl oz	410	21	11	115	56	0	1
Iced Cappuccino, Milk	16 fl oz	250	2	1.5	60	54	0	4
Mocha Latte	15 fl oz	230	7	6	200	32	0	9

BREAKFAST
Bagel BELT, w/Cheese	1 sandwich	460	16	6	1020	59	3	21
Breakfast Sausage & Biscuit	1 sandwich	420	27	14	580	32	1	11
Hashbrown	1 serving	100	5	0.5	210	12	1	1
Sandwich, Bacon, Egg & Cheese	1 sandwich	440	25	14	860	35	2	17
Sandwich, Egg & Cheese	1 sandwich	390	21	13	780	35	2	14
Sandwich, Sausage, Egg & Cheese	1 sandwich	560	35	19	1070	36	2	20
Wrap, Bacon & Cheese	1 wrap	270	16	5	630	18	2	13
Wrap, Egg & Cheese	1 wrap	220	12	3.5	550	17	2	10
Wrap, Sausage & Cheese	1 wrap	390	28	9	840	18	2	16

COOKIES
Peanut Butter	1 cookie	280	16	7	260	27	2	6
Average of All Other Flavors	1 cookie	234	10	5.5	233	34	1	3

restaurants

	SERVING SIZE	CALORIES	TOTAL FAT (G)	SAT FAT (G)	SODIUM (MG)	CARBS (G)	FIBER (G)	PROTEIN (G)
DONUTS								
Cruller, Honey	1 donut	320	19	9	220	37	0	1
Dip, Average of All Flavors	1 donut	210	8	3.5	190	31	1	4
Filled, Blueberry	1 donut	230	8	3.5	210	36	1	4
Filled, Boston Cream	1 donut	250	9	4	260	37	1	4
Filled, Canadian Maple	1 donut	260	9	4	260	41	1	4
Filled, Strawberry	1 donut	230	8	3.5	220	36	1	4
Fritter, Apple	1 donut	300	11	5	350	49	2	4
Fritter, Blueberry	1 donut	330	10	4.5	340	55	2	6
Glazed, Chocolate	1 donut	260	10	4.5	300	39	2	4
Old Fashion, Dip	1 donut	300	20	10	230	27	1	3
Old Fashion, Glazed	1 donut	320	19	9	230	35	1	3
Old Fashion, Plain	1 donut	260	19	9	230	20	1	3
Sour Cream Plain	1 donut	270	17	8	230	27	1	3
Walnut Crunch	1 donut	360	23	10	320	35	1	4
MUFFINS								
Banana Nut	1 muffin	390	16	2.5	490	52	2	6
Blueberry	1 muffin	340	11	2	570	55	2	5
Chocolate Chip	1 muffin	440	16	5	440	69	2	5
Double Berry, Low-Fat	1 muffin	290	3	0.5	500	59	2	4
Raisin Bran	1 muffin	360	10	1.5	790	65	6	6
Whole Grain, Average of All	1 muffin	377	14	2.8	507	59	4	5
SOUPS & CHILI, REGULAR								
Chili	1 bowl	420	22	8	1690	25	7	29
Creamy Sundried Tomato & Roasted Garlic	1 bowl	290	18	10	1050	26	2	7
Hearty Potato Bacon	1 bowl	320	18	8	1080	31	2	8
TIMBITS								
Filled, Average of All	1 each	60	2	1	55	10	0	1
Fritter, Apple	1 each	50	2	1	55	9	0	1
Glazed, Chocolate	1 each	70	3	1	75	10	0	1
Glazed, Sour Cream	1 each	90	5	2	65	12	0	1
Honey Dip	1 each	60	2	1	50	9	0	1
Old Fashion, Plain	1 each	70	5	2.5	60	5	0	1
TIM HORTONS WRAP SNACKERS								
Chicken Caesar	1 wrap	210	10	3	570	17	2	13
Chicken Ranch	1 wrap	190	8	2.5	620	17	2	13
Tuna Salad	1 wrap	170	7	0.5	420	18	2	9

	SERVING SIZE	CALORIES	TOTAL FAT (G)	SAT FAT (G)	SODIUM (MG)	CARBS (G)	FIBER (G)	PROTEIN (G)
TIM'S OWN SANDWICHES, REGULAR, WHITE BUN								
BLT	1 sandwich	420	18	5	830	47	3	17
Chicken Salad	1 sandwich	350	9	1	880	48	4	20
Egg Salad	1 sandwich	360	13	3	760	45	3	16
Ham & Swiss	1 sandwich	400	12	5	1310	48	3	24
Toasted Chicken Club	1 sandwich	390	7	2	1000	52	3	29
Turkey Bacon Club	1 sandwich	380	7	2	1340	55	3	20
Turkey Caesar	1 sandwich	370	11	2	1320	48	3	18

Togo's Sandwiches

	SERVING SIZE	CALORIES	TOTAL FAT (G)	SAT FAT (G)	SODIUM (MG)	CARBS (G)	FIBER (G)	PROTEIN (G)
SALAD DRESSINGS								
Asian	2.5 oz	380	33	4.5	830	10	0	0
Spicy Pepitas	2.5 oz	340	35	6	450	3	0	3
SALAD WRAPS								
Asian Chicken Salad	1 wrap	670	32	4.5	1140	74	8	28
BBQ Chicken Ranch	1 wrap	640	30	5	1390	72	8	25
Chicken Caesar	1 wrap	550	20	4.5	1310	67	8	31
Farmer's Market	1 wrap	440	14	3	980	72	9	12
Santa Fe Chicken Salad	1 wrap	800	44	9	1260	75	13	34
SALADS, FULL								
Asian Chicken	1 salad	200	9	0	400	17	3	21
BBQ Chicken Ranch	1 salad	390	20	3.5	1240	32	5	22
Chicken Caesar	1 salad	210	6	2.5	650	17	3	24
Farmer's Market	1 salad	160	6	2.5	550	20	5	7
Santa Fe Chicken	1 salad	370	16	4.5	950	33	10	27
SANDWICHES, HALF, ON CLASSIC WHITE BREAD								
Avocado & Cheese, Cold	1/2 sandwich	350	13	5	930	46	5	13
Capicola, Dry Salami & Provolone, Cold	1/2 sandwich	460	17	7	2520	44	2	36
Chicken, Hot	1/2 sandwich	290	2	0.5	1115	46	2	24
Chicken Salad, Cold	1/2 sandwich	330	9	1.5	1090	47	3	14
Meatball, Hot	1/2 sandwich	370	13	5	1150	49	3	17
Mortadella, Salami & Provolone, Cold	1/2 sandwich	430	15	6	2170	46	2	30
Pacific Cobb	1/2 sandwich	450	21	5	1290	46	5	17
Roast Beef	1/2 sandwich	340	2	1.5	1355	43	2	31
Roast Beef & Avocado, Cold	1/2 sandwich	330	7	1.5	1085	45	4	22
Turkey & Cranberry, Cold	1/2 sandwich	310	2	0.5	1005	57	3	19

	SERVING SIZE	CALORIES	TOTAL FAT (G)	SAT FAT (G)	SODIUM (MG)	CARBS (G)	FIBER (G)	PROTEIN (G)
Turkey, Ham, Salami & Cheese, Cold	1/2 sandwich	420	12	5	2385	45	2	36
Turkey, Roast Beef & Cheese, Cold	1/2 sandwich	340	6	2.5	1285	44	2	30
Turkey, Salami & Cheese, Cold	1/2 sandwich	410	11	4	2145	45	2	35
SOUPS, 8 OZ								
Broccoli Cheddar	1 bowl	270	16	6	1060	22	2	8
Chili	1 bowl	200	4	1.5	730	30	7	11
Fresh Mushroom & Brie	1 bowl	200	14	8	700	16	2	5
Garden Vegetable	1 bowl	80	1	0	600	16	3	3
Moroccan Lentil	1 bowl	130	1	0	940	23	8	7
New England Clam Chowder	1 bowl	280	18	6	1010	24	< 1	7
Roasted Yukon Baked Potato	1 bowl	300	20	12	880	19	1	10
Southwestern Chicken & Green Chile	1 bowl	260	18	11	1000	14	1	12
TOASTED SUBS, REGULAR								
Chili Cheese 'N' Beef	1 sub	1010	53	12	1760	85	6	44
Clubhouse	1 sub	660	23	9	2130	80	7	35
Pepper Jack Pastrami	1 sub	980	57	20	2270	68	1	45
Uncle Tony's Italian	1 sub	880	47	18	3550	73	5	46

Tropical Smoothie Café

	SERVING SIZE	CALORIES	TOTAL FAT (G)	SAT FAT (G)	SODIUM (MG)	CARBS (G)	FIBER (G)	PROTEIN (G)
BREAKFAST								
All American Wrap	1 wrap	620	26	8.9	1823	53	2	36
Buffalo Kick Start Ciabatta	1 sandwich	585	25	10	2198	49	2	41
Early Bird Wrap	1 wrap	848	51	13.7	1609	54	2	40
Salsa Sunrise Wrap	1 wrap	683	32	11.7	2156	54	3	41
The Classic Ciabatta	1 sandwich	809	49	21.4	1489	50	2	39
The Classic Ciabatta, Bacon	1 sandwich	654	33	16	1344	49	2	37
SALADS								
Chicken Caesar	1 salad	324	21	4.3	757	10	4	24
Southwest Chicken	1 salad	542	29	3.7	1740	44	11	26
SMOOTHIES, LOW-FAT								
Blimey Limey	24 fl oz	476	0	0	65	124	4	2
Blue Lagoon	24 fl oz	305	1	0.1	6	79	6	1
Hawaiian Breeze	24 fl oz	370	0	0.2	171	93	1	2
Jetty Punch	24 fl oz	333	1	0	7	87	6	2
Kiwi Quencher	24 fl oz	423	0	0.2	57	109	4	3
Mango Magic	24 fl oz	390	0	0.2	169	100	4	2
Paradise Point	24 fl oz	384	1	0.1	118	100	6	2

	SERVING SIZE	CALORIES	TOTAL FAT (G)	SAT FAT (G)	SODIUM (MG)	CARBS (G)	FIBER (G)	PROTEIN (G)
Peaches 'N' Silk	24 fl oz	324	0	0.1	8	86	5	1
Pineapple Delight	24 fl oz	405	0	0.1	118	104	3	2
Rockin' Raspberry	24 fl oz	379	1	0.1	5	99	7	2
Strawberry Beach	24 fl oz	439	1	0.3	59	113	6	3
Sunny Day	24 fl oz	497	1	0.2	6	128	5	4
Sunrise Sunset	24 fl oz	423	0	0	64	109	5	3
SMOOTHIES, SIMPLY INDULGENT								
Bahama Mama	24 fl oz	460	4	3	155	123	5	2
Beach Bum	24 fl oz	512	5	3.7	96	123	8	5
Chocolate Chiller	24 fl oz	529	7	5.9	178	118	2	5
Mocha Madness	24 fl oz	639	14	12.8	272	129	2	7
Tropi-Colada	24 fl oz	458	1	1.1	121	129	4	1
SMOOTHIES, SUPERCHARGED								
Acai Berry Boost	24 fl oz	445	1	0.1	8	115	7	1
Get Up & Goji	24 fl oz	417	0	0.2	38	108	4	2
Health Nut	24 fl oz	311	6	0.3	37	97	7	25
Lean Machine	24 fl oz	423	1	0.1	7	111	6	2
Muscle Blaster	24 fl oz	433	3	0.1	34	89	6	24
Peanut Paradise	24 fl oz	648	19	3.8	233	99	5	33
Pomegranate Plunge	24 fl oz	381	0	0.1	5	83	3	1
TOASTED WRAPS & SANDWICHES								
Baja Chicken	1 sandwich	454	17	4.8	1152	47	3	29
Chicken Pesto	1 sandwich	452	18	5.2	1097	44	3	30
Jamaican Jerk Chicken	1 wrap	670	18	5.8	1834	85	4	38
King Caesar	1 wrap	626	29	6.3	1627	56	3	32
Thai Chicken	1 wrap	605	17	1.8	1738	81	4	27
Turkey Guacamole	1 sandwich	499	10	1.2	1654	66	8	40
Wasabi Caesar Roast Beef	1 sandwich	470	13	4.9	1509	49	3	37

Tubby's Grilled Submarines
BURGER SUBS, REGULAR

	SERVING SIZE	CALORIES	TOTAL FAT (G)	SAT FAT (G)	SODIUM (MG)	CARBS (G)	FIBER (G)	PROTEIN (G)
All-American Cheeseburger	1 sub	810	48	24	n/a	56	4	39
Big Tub	1 sub	671	56	21	n/a	55	4	34
Burger Special	1 sub	898	59	21	n/a	59	6	39
Cheeseburger	1 sub	911	60	21	n/a	59	9	42
Mushroom Burger	1 sub	868	59	21	n/a	53	5	38
Pizza Burger	1 sub	929	60	21	n/a	62	10	43

restaurants

	SERVING SIZE	CALORIES	TOTAL FAT (G)	SAT FAT (G)	SODIUM (MG)	CARBS (G)	FIBER (G)	PROTEIN (G)
Taco	1 sub	827	47	20	n/a	67	5	39
CHICKEN SUBS, REGULAR								
Chicken & Broccoli	1 sub	552	23	6	n/a	56	5	35
Chicken & Cheddar	1 sub	543	23	6	n/a	54	4	34
Chicken Club	1 sub	705	41	10	n/a	53	4	37
Chicken Parmesan	1 sub	426	14	5	n/a	51	4	32
Chicken Fajita	1 sub	445	12	5	n/a	57	4	33
Grilled Chicken	1 sub	346	5	0.7	n/a	52	4	28
DELI SUBS, REGULAR								
Club	1 sub	705	41	10	n/a	53	4	37
Famous	1 sub	664	39	10	n/a	55	4	26
Ham & Cheese	1 sub	568	30	6	n/a	54	4	27
Turkey & Cheese	1 sub	626	32	7	n/a	51	4	34
Turkey Club	1 sub	850	39	9	n/a	83	6	45
SPECIALTY SUBS, REGULAR								
BLT	1 sub	636	42	8	n/a	50	4	21
Cold Veggie	1 sub	462	14	8	n/a	66	8	23
Hot Veggie Stir-Fry	1 sub	652	27	6	n/a	89	8	21
Italian Sausage	1 sub	729	45	14	n/a	56	4	32
Tuna	1 sub	417	18	4	n/a	47	4	38
STEAK SUBS, REGULAR								
Mushroom Steak	1 sub	833	26	6	n/a	52	4	13
Pepper Steak	1 sub	709	46	15	n/a	52	4	29
Philly Cheese Steak	1 sub	685	40	19	n/a	49	4	37
Pizza Steak	1 sub	986	57	20	n/a	85	7	42
Portabella Mushroom	1 sub	801	48	22	n/a	54	5	43
Steak & Cheese	1 sub	823	56	20	n/a	51	4	36

Uno Chicago Grill
APPETIZER & SIDES

Buffalo Boneless Bites	1/3 item	360	19	2.5	1370	24	0	28
Buffalo Chicken Quesadillas	1/3 item	330	14	7	790	36	2	17
Calamari	1/3 item	350	31	3.5	690	28	1	13
Crispy Cheese Dippers	1/3 item	280	16	6	830	27	1	12
Pizza Skins	1/5 item	410	28	9	600	29	1	12
Uno Breadstick	1 item	210	13	4	460	18	1	6
BURGER								
Bring Home the Bacon	1/2 entrée	520	38	15	1100	15	1	30

	SERVING SIZE	CALORIES	TOTAL FAT (G)	SAT FAT (G)	SODIUM (MG)	CARBS (G)	FIBER (G)	PROTEIN (G)
Cabot Aged Cheddar & Mushroom	1/2 entrée	450	31	12	780	15	1	26
Firecracker	1/2 entrée	470	33	12	850	16	2	22
Uno	1/2 entrée	390	27	10	690	14	1	22
DEEP DISH PIZZA, INDIVIDUAL								
Cheese & Tomato	1/3 entrée	580	40	12	830	39	2	21
Chicago Classic	1/3 entrée	770	55	18	1550	40	2	33
Farmer's Market	1/3 entrée	540	35	9	750	42	3	15
Numero Uno	1/3 entrée	640	44	12	1170	41	2	21
Prima Pepperoni	1/3 entrée	610	42	12	970	39	2	20
Spinicolli	1/3 entrée	620	45	11	780	40	3	16
ENTRÉES								
Chicken Broccoli Alfredo	1/2 entrée	620	35	11	820	53	3	28
Chicken Spinoccoli	1/2 entrée	590	29	13	1150	54	3	31
Fish & Chips	1/2 entrée	460	35	4.5	860	36	5	21
Lobster & Shrimp Scampi	1/2 entrée	590	32	12	1030	53	3	25
Macaroni & Cheese	1/2 entrée	1000	67	32	1550	62	2	41
Rattlesnake Pasta	1/2 entrée	640	37	12	910	52	3	29
Romano Crusted Chicken Parmesan	1/2 entrée	560	19	4.5	1270	69	5	37
Sirloin Steak Tips	1/2 entrée	290	14	4	1030	4	1	31
SALAD								
Chicken Caesar	1/2 salad	290	19	5	770	13	3	20
Chicken Milanese	1/2 salad	430	29	5	1120	21	3	28
Classic Cobb	1/2 salad	440	33	10	970	13	5	25
SANDWICHES								
Crunchy Chicken Wrap	1/2 wrap	520	29	8	1070	40	6	31
Lobster Melt	1/2 wrap	370	17	4.5	750	30	1	23
Turkey Bacon Swiss	1/2 entrée	420	14	5	670	41	2	31
SOUPS, W/O CRACKERS								
Broccoli & Cheddar	2/3 bowl	200	14	6	1060	12	2	7
Chili	2/3 bowl	270	8	3.5	830	36	7	14
French Onion	2/3 bowl	220	15	6	1080	14	2	8
New England Clam Chowder	2/3 bowl	280	18	10	780	21	1	9
Vocelli Pizza								
APPETIZERS								
BBQ Wings, Bone-In	1/2 dish	760	53	13	720	14	0	53
Buffalo Wings, Bone-In	1/2 dish	720	54	13	1010	2	0	53
Cheesesticks	1/4 dish	340	16	7	330	36	1	13

restaurants

	SERVING SIZE	CALORIES	TOTAL FAT (G)	SAT FAT (G)	SODIUM (MG)	CARBS (G)	FIBER (G)	PROTEIN (G)
Garlic Bread	1/4 dish	230	11	2	350	27	1	5
Pepperoni Roll	1/4 dish	380	22	9	570	33	1	13
GOURMET PIZZAS, LARGE								
Buffalo Chicken	1/8 entrée	310	12	5	480	34	1	16
Deluxe	1/8 entrée	350	14	7	630	38	2	15
Hawaiian	1/8 entrée	370	14	8	710	40	1	19
Meat Magnifico	1/8 entrée	370	16	8	850	37	1	19
Philly Steak	1/8 entrée	370	17	8	340	36	1	18
Spring Veggie	1/8 entrée	290	9	4.5	420	38	2	13
HOT SUBS, ON CIABATTA BREAD								
Chicken Parm	1/2 sub	440	18	8	1130	45	4	24
Chicken Pesto	1/2 sub	410	17	9	1310	34	3	29
Italiano	1/2 sub	380	20	9	1390	27	2	22
Meatball	1/2 sub	460	23	11	1120	36	3	27
PASTA								
Chicken Alfredo	1 entrée	1080	55	16	1910	100	5	43
Chicken Parmesan	1 entrée	1030	35	9	2150	132	11	43
Chicken Pesto	1 entrée	1110	59	15	1980	99	6	44
Meatball Marinara	1 entrée	950	34	9	1720	121	10	34
SALAD, REGULAR								
Antipasta	1 salad	270	16	8	2600	17	6	18
Caesar	1 salad	130	3	1	570	5	2	21
Mediterranean	1 salad	270	18	12	2740	17	5	14
Tuscan Chicken	1 salad	290	13	7	910	12	3	32
STROMBOLI								
Italian Sausage	1/2 entrée	650	26	12	940	76	2	28
Pepperoni	1/2 entrée	610	24	12	800	72	2	25

Wahoo's Fish
BANZAI BURRITO, W/WHITE RICE & BLACK BEANS

	SERVING SIZE	CALORIES	TOTAL FAT (G)	SAT FAT (G)	SODIUM (MG)	CARBS (G)	FIBER (G)	PROTEIN (G)
Blackened Chicken	1 entrée	609	16	4	2006	83	9	37
Blackened Fish	1 entrée	654	21	6	1408	83	9	36
Vegetarian	1 entrée	519	14	4	1331	88	11	16
QUESADILLA								
Carne Asada	as served	243	13	6	583	17	0	15
Chicken	as served	246	13	6	595	16	0	15
Fish	as served	260	14	6	431	16	0	15

	SERVING SIZE	CALORIES	TOTAL FAT (G)	SAT FAT (G)	SODIUM (MG)	CARBS (G)	FIBER (G)	PROTEIN (G)
Shrimp	as served	218	12	6	409	16	0	9
STARTERS								
Baja Rolls	as served	168	8	3	483	17	1	9
Jumbo French Fries	as served	130	4	1	23	20	2	2
Maui Onion Rings	as served	128	5	1	255	18	2	1
TAQUITOS, THREE PER ORDER								
Carne Asada	as served	326	10	2	943	42	5	21
Carnitas	as served	417	15	4	795	42	5	27
Chicken	as served	334	9	1	973	41	5	21
Fish	as served	384	15	3	790	41	5	18
WAHOO BOWLS, W/WHITE RICE & BLACK BEANS								
Blackened Chicken Bowl	1 entrée	858	15	4	2531	127	17	56
Blackened Fish Bowl	1 entrée	926	22	7	1634	126	17	55
Vegetarian	1 entrée	761	11	4	1575	141	22	26
WET BANZAI BURRITOS, GREEN SAUCE, W/WHITE RICE & BEANS								
Blackened Chicken	1 entrée	901	34	13	3029	98	10	51
Charbroiled Fish	1 entrée	948	38	15	2454	98	10	50
Vegetarian	1 entrée	810	31	13	2354	103	11	30
WET BANZAI BURRITOS, RED SAUCE, W/WHITE RICE & BLACK BEANS								
Blackened Chicken	1 entrée	875	34	13	2920	92	11	52
Blackened Fish	1 entrée	920	39	15	2322	92	11	51
Vegetarian	1 entrée	784	32	13	2245	97	12	31
Wawa								
BAGEL MELTS								
Ham & Cheese	1 bagel	490	12	7	2080	62	3	29
Italian	1 bagel	550	19	9	1740	63	3	31
Pepperoni & Cheese	1 bagel	750	40	19	2040	62	3	35
Pork Roll	1 bagel	690	35	15	1790	62	3	32
BREAKFAST								
Bacon, Egg & Cheese Bagel Sizzli	1 bagel	370	15	6	1050	42	2	18
Bacon, Egg & Cheese Burrito	1 burrito	390	21	8.5	1230	35	1	20
Sausage, Egg & Cheese Burrito	1 burrito	590	39	15	1600	35	1	26
CHICKEN STRIPS								
Breaded Chicken Strips	5 pieces	400	22	4.5	1510	27	0	24

restaurants

	SERVING SIZE	CALORIES	TOTAL FAT (G)	SAT FAT (G)	SODIUM (MG)	CARBS (G)	FIBER (G)	PROTEIN (G)
HOT HOAGIES, CLASSIC ROLL, W/O ADDITIONAL TOPPINGS								
Beef Cheesesteak	1 sandwich	700	25	11	1950	71	3	48
Chicken Cheesesteak	1 sandwich	700	22	11	1980	71	3	51
Meatball	1 sandwich	880	43	14	3420	98	12	36
HOT TO GO BOWLS								
Mac & Cheese w/Beef Stew	1 bowl	560	24	10	1540	42	0	20
Mac & Cheese w/Chili	1 bowl	500	23	9	1740	48	2	22
SANDWICHES, CLASSIC ROLL, W/O ADDITIONAL TOPPINGS								
BLT	1 sandwich	490	14	5	1650	71	3	27
Chicken Salad	1 sandwich	850	46	6.5	1800	77	3	36
Egg Salad	1 sandwich	850	49	9.5	1305	77	3	27
Genoa Salami	1 sandwich	440	14	4.5	1340	68	3	16
Ham	1 sandwich	520	10	2.5	2380	72	3	40
Italian	1 sandwich	660	24	8.5	2780	72	3	40
Premium Turkey	1 sandwich	500	6	0.5	2260	72	3	44
Roast Beef	1 sandwich	580	8	0.5	1660	72	3	56
Tuna	1 sandwich	970	58	9.5	1950	80	6	33
Wendy's **BURGERS & SANDWICHES**								
1/4 lb Single	1 burger	580	33	14	1240	42	3	31
3/4 lb Triple	1 burger	1060	67	30	2020	42	3	72
Bacon Deluxe Double	1 burger	890	56	24	1830	42	3	55
Baconator Single	1 burger	660	40	17	1440	40	2	36
Crispy Chicken Caesar Wrap	1 wrap	430	25	7	950	35	2	17
Crispy Chicken Sandwich	1 sandwich	380	20	4	720	37	2	15
Double Stack	1 burger	400	21	9	1080	26	1	27
Grilled Chicken Go Wrap	1 wrap	260	10	3.5	730	25	1	19
Jr. Bacon Cheeseburger	1 burger	400	24	9	930	25	2	21
Jr. Cheeseburger Deluxe	1 burger	350	19	7	850	27	2	17
Jr. Hamburger	1 burger	250	10	4	620	25	1	15
Spicy Chicken Fillet Sandwich	1 sandwich	530	22	6	1140	55	3	31
Spicy Chicken Go Wrap	1 wrap	340	16	4.5	770	31	1	17
Ultimate Chicken Grill Sandwich	1 sandwich	390	10	3.5	1080	42	3	33
CRISPY CHICKEN NUGGETS								
Chicken Nuggets	5 pieces	220	14	3	460	13	1	10

	SERVING SIZE	CALORIES	TOTAL FAT (G)	SAT FAT (G)	SODIUM (MG)	CARBS (G)	FIBER (G)	PROTEIN (G)
FROSTY TREATS								
Caramel Frosty Shake, Large	1 shake	1000	19	11	500	195	0	14
Chocolate Frosty, Small	1 frosty	300	8	5	140	49	0	7
Chocolate Frosty Shake, Large	1 shake	880	17	11	370	165	4	15
Strawberry Frosty Shake, Large	1 shake	810	16	10	230	153	1	13
Vanilla Frosty, Small	1 frosty	280	7	4.5	135	47	0	7
Vanilla Bean Frosty Shake, Large	1 shake	870	16	10	700	169	0	13
Wild Berry Frosty Shake, Large	1 shake	740	16	10	240	134	2	13
GARDEN SALADS								
Apple Pecan Chicken	1 salad	340	11	7	1150	28	5	35
Baja	1 salad	540	32	14	1600	34	12	32
BLT Cobb	1 salad	450	25	11	1610	9	3	46
Spicy Chicken Caesar	1 salad	470	25	12	1240	26	5	37
SIDES								
Baked Potato, Sour Cream & Chives	1 item	320	4	2	50	63	7	8
Chili, Small	1 item	210	6	2.5	880	21	6	17
Natural-Cut Fries, Medium	as served	420	21	4	460	55	6	5

Whataburger

	SERVING SIZE	CALORIES	TOTAL FAT (G)	SAT FAT (G)	SODIUM (MG)	CARBS (G)	FIBER (G)	PROTEIN (G)
BREAKFAST								
Hash Brown Sticks	4 pieces	200	12	0.5	280	60	0	2
Honey Butter Chicken Biscuit	1 biscuit	560	34	13	1008	50	2	14
Taquito, w/Bacon, Egg & Cheese	1 taquito	420	24	9	1157	27	3	19
Taquito, w/Potato, Egg & Cheese	1 taquito	470	27	8	1094	57	3	17
Taquito, w/Sausage, Egg & Cheese	1 taquito	450	28	11	1134	27	3	19
BURGERS & SANDWICHES								
A.1. Thick & Hearty Burger	1 burger	1040	62	24	2037	63	2	50
Justaburger	1 burger	290	15	4.5	727	26	1	13
Whataburger	1 burger	620	30	10	1262	58	2	26
Whataburger w/Bacon & Cheese	1 burger	780	43	16	1997	59	2	36
Whataburger, Double Meat	1 burger	870	49	18	1510	58	2	43
Whataburger, Triple Meat	1 burger	1120	68	26	1759	58	2	61
Whatacatch Sandwich	1 sandwich	450	24	4	881	44	3	16
Whatachick'n Sandwich	1 sandwich	560	27	6	978	65	8	21
CHICKEN								
Chicken Strips, w/Gravy	3 pieces	530	27	11	1368	42	2	26
SALADS, W/O DRESSING								
Chicken Strips	1 salad	350	16	6	606	33	5	19

	SERVING SIZE	CALORIES	TOTAL FAT (G)	SAT FAT (G)	SODIUM (MG)	CARBS (G)	FIBER (G)	PROTEIN (G)
Grilled Chicken	1 salad	250	8	1	753	30	4	26
SHAKES & MALTS, MEDIUM								
Malt, Average of Chocolate & Strawberry	1 malt	670	15	10.5	274	123	1	13
Malt, Vanilla	1 malt	600	17	12	259	98	0	13
Shake, Average of Chocolate & Strawberry	1 shake	630	16	11	258	111	1	14
Shake, Vanilla	1 shake	560	17	12	243	87	0	14
SIDES, MEDIUM								
French Fries	as served	480	27	4.5	347	55	7	5
Onion Rings	as served	400	25	8	787	37	3	5

White Castle
BREAKFAST

	SERVING SIZE	CALORIES	TOTAL FAT (G)	SAT FAT (G)	SODIUM (MG)	CARBS (G)	FIBER (G)	PROTEIN (G)
Awrey Cheese Danish	as served	450	24	6	390	52	1	6
Bacon, Egg & Cheese	1 slider	210	12	5	510	13	1	12
French Toast Sticks	4 pieces	460	31	5	410	39	2	5
Hamburger, Egg & Cheese	1 slider	220	13	5.5	340	13	1	13
Sausage, Egg & Cheese	1 slider	310	22	8	630	13	1	15
SIDES								
Angus Steak Chili, Small	1 cup	160	5	1.5	450	16	5	14
Average of Chicken Rings	9 rings	803	71	14	1200	20	1	26
Cheese Fries, Medium	as served	400	27	5	350	35	3	4
Chili Cheese Fries, Medium	as served	350	22	4.5	480	31	4	8
Clam Strips, Medium	as served	210	17	2.5	620	5	0	8
Fish Nibblers, Medium	as served	320	16	3	700	28	1	16
French Fries, Medium	as served	350	23	4.5	50	33	3	3
Fully Loaded Fries, Medium	as served	460	38	8	900	20	2	4
Mozzarella Cheese Sticks	5 sticks	740	55	15	1420	36	2	21
Onion Chips, Medium	as served	670	50	9	970	46	8	5
Sweet Potato Fries, Medium	as served	480	30	4	380	47	6	4
SLIDERS								
Bacon Cheeseburger	1 slider	220	14	6	640	13	1	11
Cheeseburger	1 slider	170	9	4	550	15	1	8
Chicken Ring	1 slider	350	28	5	320	16	1	8
Chicken Ring, w/Cheese	1 slider	380	30	7	460	16	1	10
Chicken Breast	1 slider	360	26	4.5	510	20	1	11
Chicken Breast, w/Cheese	1 slider	390	28	6	650	20	1	13
Double Bacon Cheeseburger	1 slider	400	27	12	1220	21	1	21

	SERVING SIZE	CALORIES	TOTAL FAT (G)	SAT FAT (G)	SODIUM (MG)	CARBS (G)	FIBER (G)	PROTEIN (G)
Double Bacon Jalapeño Cheeseburger	1 slider	390	27	12	1230	21	1	21
Double Cheeseburger	1 slider	300	17	8	940	20	1	15
Double Fish	1 slider	550	43	7	420	24	23	17
Double Fish, w/Cheese	1 slider	610	48	10	700	25	23	19
Double Jalapeño Cheeseburger	1 slider	280	17	8	860	21	1	15
Double Original	1 slider	240	12	5	660	21	1	12
Fish Slider	1 slider	310	22	3.5	270	18	12	9
Fish Slider, w/Cheese	1 slider	340	24	5	410	18	12	11
Jalapeño Cheeseburger	1 slider	160	9	4	460	14	1	8
Original	1 slider	140	6	2.5	360	13	1	7
Surf & Turf, w/Cheese	1 slider	540	38	11	990	27	13	22
Traditional Bun, w/Cheese	1 slider	90	3	1.5	260	12	1	4

Wienerschnitzel
BURGERS & SPECIALTIES

	SERVING SIZE	CALORIES	TOTAL FAT (G)	SAT FAT (G)	SODIUM (MG)	CARBS (G)	FIBER (G)	PROTEIN (G)
Chili Burger	1 burger	280	n/a	3	750	29	n/a	n/a
Chili Cheeseburger	1 burger	330	n/a	6	1000	30	n/a	n/a
Corn Dog	1 corn dog	250	n/a	6	490	15	n/a	n/a
Double Classic Burger	1 burger	390	n/a	6	700	30	n/a	n/a
Double Classic Cheeseburger	1 burger	490	n/a	11	1210	31	n/a	n/a
Ultimate Chili Cheeseburger	1 burger	520	n/a	11	2080	35	n/a	n/a

FRIES & SIDES

	SERVING SIZE	CALORIES	TOTAL FAT (G)	SAT FAT (G)	SODIUM (MG)	CARBS (G)	FIBER (G)	PROTEIN (G)
Bacon Ranch Chili Cheese Fries	as served	700	n/a	22	1610	40	n/a	n/a
Chili Cheese Fries	as served	540	n/a	19	1380	39	n/a	n/a
Jalapeño Poppers	3 poppers	210	n/a	6	670	21	n/a	n/a
Regular Fries	as served	300	n/a	11	400	25	n/a	n/a
Ultimate Chili Cheese Fries	as served	600	n/a	22	1390	41	n/a	n/a

HOT DOGS

	SERVING SIZE	CALORIES	TOTAL FAT (G)	SAT FAT (G)	SODIUM (MG)	CARBS (G)	FIBER (G)	PROTEIN (G)
Angus All Beef Chicago Dog, Pretzel Bun	1 hot dog	600	n/a	9	2760	69	n/a	n/a
Angus All Beef Chicago Dog, Seeded Bun	1 hot dog	520	n/a	9	2780	50	n/a	n/a
Angus All Beef Chili Cheese Dog, Pretzel Bun	1 hot dog	620	n/a	5	2040	59	n/a	n/a
Angus All Beef Chili Cheese Dog, Seeded Bun	1 hot dog	540	n/a	12	1960	40	n/a	n/a
Angus All Beef Chili Dog, Pretzel Bun	1 hot dog	570	n/a	9	1860	58	n/a	n/a
Angus All Beef Chili Dog, Seeded Bun	1 hot dog	490	n/a	9	1870	39	n/a	n/a
Angus All Beef Kraut Dog, Pretzel Bun	1 hot dog	530	n/a	9	1740	56	n/a	n/a
Angus All Beef Kraut Dog, Seeded Bun	1 hot dog	450	n/a	9	1760	37	n/a	n/a

restaurants

	SERVING SIZE	CALORIES	TOTAL FAT (G)	SAT FAT (G)	SODIUM (MG)	CARBS (G)	FIBER (G)	PROTEIN (G)
Angus All Beef Plain Dog, Pretzel Bun	1 hot dog	530	n/a	9	1470	55	n/a	n/a
Angus All Beef Plain Dog, Seeded Bun	1 hot dog	450	n/a	9	1480	36	n/a	n/a
Bacon Wrapped Hot Dog, Standard Bun	1 hot dog	370	n/a	8	860	27	n/a	n/a
Bacon Wrapped Street Dog, Standard Bun	1 hot dog	400	n/a	9	950	29	n/a	n/a
Original Chicago Dog, Pretzel Bun	1 hot dog	460	n/a	5	2100	67	n/a	n/a
Original Chicago Dog, Standard Bun	1 hot dog	330	n/a	4	2040	41	n/a	n/a
Original Chili Cheese Dog, Pretzel Bun	1 hot dog	480	n/a	7	1450	57	n/a	n/a
Original Chili Cheese Dog, Standard Bun	1 hot dog	350	n/a	6	1390	31	n/a	n/a
Original Chili Dog, Pretzel Bun	1 hot dog	430	n/a	5	1200	57	n/a	n/a
Original Chili Dog, Standard Bun	1 hot dog	300	n/a	4	1130	31	n/a	n/a
Original Kraut Dog, Pretzel Bun	1 hot dog	400	n/a	5	1080	54	n/a	n/a
Original Kraut Dog, Standard Bun	1 hot dog	270	n/a	4	1020	28	n/a	n/a
Original Plain Dog, Pretzel Bun	1 hot dog	400	n/a	5	810	53	n/a	n/a
Original Plain Dog, Standard Bun	1 hot dog	270	n/a	4	740	27	n/a	n/a
Turkey Chicago Dog, Pretzel Bun	1 hot dog	450	n/a	4	1970	68	n/a	n/a
Turkey Chicago Dog, Standard Bun	1 hot dog	320	n/a	3	1910	42	n/a	n/a
Turkey Chili Cheese Dog, Pretzel Bun	1 hot dog	470	n/a	6	1320	58	n/a	n/a
Turkey Chili Cheese Dog, Standard Bun	1 hot dog	340	n/a	5	1260	32	n/a	n/a
Turkey Chili Dog, Standard Bun	1 hot dog	290	n/a	3	1000	32	n/a	n/a
Turkey Chili Dog, Pretzel Bun	1 hot dog	420	n/a	4	1070	58	n/a	n/a
Turkey Kraut Dog, Pretzel Bun	1 hot dog	390	n/a	4	950	55	n/a	n/a
Turkey Kraut Dog, Standard Bun	1 hot dog	260	n/a	3	890	29	n/a	n/a
Turkey Plain Dog, Standard Bun	1 hot dog	260	n/a	3	610	28	n/a	n/a
Turkey Plain Dog, Pretzel Bun	1 hot dog	390	n/a	4	680	54	n/a	n/a

Winchell's Donut House
DONUTS

	SERVING SIZE	CALORIES	TOTAL FAT (G)	SAT FAT (G)	SODIUM (MG)	CARBS (G)	FIBER (G)	PROTEIN (G)
Bar, Buttermilk, Glazed	1 donut	420	18	8	330	61	3	3
Bar, Chocolate, Iced	1 donut	380	19	8	490	44	2	6
Bar, Maple, Iced	1 donut	380	19	8	480	44	2	6
Bar, Vanilla, Iced	1 donut	370	19	8	480	44	2	6
Cake, Chocolate, Chocolate Iced	1 donut	210	9	3	300	33	3	3
Cake, White, Vanilla Iced	1 donut	270	12	5	310	40	2	3
Filled, Apple Jelly, w/Cinnamon Crumb	1 donut	370	15	6	600	53	3	7
Filled, Raspberry Jelly, w/Glaze	1 donut	390	13	5	500	61	2	6
Filled, Vanilla Crème, w/Chocolate Icing	1 donut	350	13	6	580	51	2	6

	SERVING SIZE	CALORIES	TOTAL FAT (G)	SAT FAT (G)	SODIUM (MG)	CARBS (G)	FIBER (G)	PROTEIN (G)
French, Glazed	1 donut	270	14	6	330	32	1	3
Mini Cake, White, Plain	1 donut	100	6	2	150	12	1	2
Mini Fancy, Fritter, Apple	1 donut	350	13	6	410	55	3	5
Mini Fancy, Fritter, Blueberry	1 donut	310	13	6	290	43	1	3
Old Fashioned, Glazed	1 donut	410	17	7	360	60	2	4
Raised Ring, Cinnamon Crumb	1 donut	220	9	4	310	31	1	4
Raised Ring, Glazed	1 donut	220	9	4	290	31	1	4
Twist, Glazed	1 donut	390	19	8	540	48	2	7
Wheat & Spice, Glazed	1 donut	270	13	5	260	36	3	4
OTHER								
Donut Hole, Glazed	1 donut hole	90	5	2	80	12	1	1
Fancy, Cinnamon Roll	1 roll	630	31	13	710	80	5	9
Mini Fancy, Cinnamon Roll	1 roll	310	15	6	340	39	2	4
Puffies, w/Vanilla Creme Filling	3 puffies	150	8	4	250	16	1	2

Woody's Bar-B-Q
DINNERS, W/O SIDES

	SERVING SIZE	CALORIES	TOTAL FAT (G)	SAT FAT (G)	SODIUM (MG)	CARBS (G)	FIBER (G)	PROTEIN (G)
Baby Back Combo	1 entrée	680	48	16	624	1	0	6
Baby Backs	1 entrée	520	40	18	720	2	0	38
Beef Brisket	1 entrée	520	38	14	1160	0	0	42
Beef Prime Rib	1 entrée	760	62	26	1400	1	0	46
Carolina Pulled Pork	1 entrée	375	29	11	855	6	0	24
Loaded Chicken Breast	1 entrée	740	35	16	2460	6	0	85
Pork Sampler	1 entrée	1010	62	25	745	4	0	105
Southern Trio	1 entrée	860	55	18	1277	2	0	78
Taste of Woody's	1 entrée	1220	65	21	740	2	0	120

SANDWICHES, W/O SIDES

	SERVING SIZE	CALORIES	TOTAL FAT (G)	SAT FAT (G)	SODIUM (MG)	CARBS (G)	FIBER (G)	PROTEIN (G)
Bacon Cheddar Burger	1 sandwich	1002	62	30	1006	49	2	59
Beef Brisket	1 sandwich	674	36	13	1436	44	2	44
Pork BBQ Wrap	1 wrap	440	21	10	820	31	12	40
Pulled Chicken	1 sandwich	480	10	3	1460	61	2	37
Pulled Pork	1 sandwich	540	23	7	1190	48	2	33
Sloppy Woody	1 sandwich	560	22	7	1310	59	2	31

STARTERS

	SERVING SIZE	CALORIES	TOTAL FAT (G)	SAT FAT (G)	SODIUM (MG)	CARBS (G)	FIBER (G)	PROTEIN (G)
Awesome Onion Rings	as served	366	1	0	2200	83	10	10
Bar-B-Q Cheese Fries	as served	607	31	14	502	63	6	16
Beef Chili Cheese Fries	as served	807	38	17	572	63	6	50

restaurants

	SERVING SIZE	CALORIES	TOTAL FAT (G)	SAT FAT (G)	SODIUM (MG)	CARBS (G)	FIBER (G)	PROTEIN (G)
Chili	as served	405	20	8	530	10	2	10
Corn Nuggets	as served	220	12	1.5	480	27	1	2
WOODY'S FAMOUS BAR-B-Q SALADS, W/O DRESSING								
3 Meat	1 salad	330	16	6	520	9	3	41
Beef	1 salad	280	11	3.5	160	8	3	39
Pork	1 salad	380	23	10	200	9	3	38
Smoked Turkey Breast	1 salad	190	6	0	940	9	3	25
Zaxby's								
MEALZ DEALZ, W/O DRINK								
Boneless Wings Meal, w/o Sauce	1 entrée	840	50	7	1495	71	4	26
Buffalo Wings Meal, w/o Sauce	1 entrée	900	56	10	1025	51	5	47
Chicken Finger Nibbler Meal	1 entrée	1330	71	13	2470	137	8	46
Chicken Finger Sandwich Meal	1 entrée	1100	56	9	2140	106	7	41
Chicken Parmesan Sandwich Meal	1 entrée	1110	58	9.5	2350	105	7	42
Chicken Salad Sandwich Meal	1 entrée	1020	63	10	1430	77	6	29
Grilled Chicken Sandwich Meal	1 entrée	1130	57	10	2180	104	7	50
Kickin' Chicken Sandwich Meal	1 entrée	1065	55	9	2550	104	7	41
Sweet and Smoky Sandwich Meal	1 entrée	1160	49	8	2100	139	7	41
SANDWICHES								
Cajun Club Sandwich Basket	1 entrée	1140	58	12.5	2545	98	6	53
Club Sandwich Basket	1 entrée	1250	73	15	2415	99	7	43
WINGS & FINGERZ								
Boneless Wings, 10 Pieces, w/o Sauce	1 entrée	760	47	7	1660	43	1	38
Buffalo Fingers, 10 Pieces, w/o Sauce	1 entrée	1050	65	9	2830	27	2	92
Buffalo Wings, 10 Pieces, w/o Sauce	1 entrée	880	60	12	700	4	1	81
Chicken Fingerz, 10 Pieces	1 entrée	1230	80	11	3780	36	3	92
ZALADS, W/O DRESSING								
The Blue, Blackened Chicken	1 salad	605	29	12.5	1690	34	3	48
The Blue, Buffalo Chicken	1 salad	780	42	13	2370	50	4	49
The Caesar, w/Fried Chicken	1 salad	730	39	10	1855	39	5	49
The House, w/Fried Chicken	1 salad	765	42	13	1720	44	4	48
ZAPPETIZERS								
Onion Rings	1 serving	560	36	4	1320	52	3	7
Fried White Cheddar Bites w/ Marinara Sauce	1 serving	820	52	20	960	38	1	16
Spicy Fried Mushrooms	1 serving	620	46	6.5	1380	43	5	8

ero's Subs
12"

	SERVING SIZE	CALORIES	TOTAL FAT (G)	SAT FAT (G)	SODIUM (MG)	CARBS (G)	FIBER (G)	PROTEIN (G)
	1 sub	822	39	2	1858	96	6	24
mo Vegetarian Deluxe	1 sub	923	45	20	2008	95	9	39
mo Vegetarian, w/o Cheese, Oil & inegar	1 sub	468	7	0	1060	93	9	13
lled Veggie	1 sub	733	24	12	3207	102	11	34
m & Cheese	1 sub	810	33	13	2350	87	6	43
t Italian Sausage	1 sub	1326	74	27	3286	90	6	71
eatball & Cheese	1 sub	1080	56	25	2255	100	7	40
pperoni & Cheese	1 sub	991	54	24	2771	84	4	44
illy Steak & Cheese, w/Mushrooms & Green Peppers	1 sub	821	20	9	3466	99	7	65
oast Beef & Cheese	1 sub	867	34	13	2928	90	6	54
oast Beef, w/o Cheese, Oil & Vinegar	1 sub	611	11	2	2476	89	6	43
e Club	1 sub	938	42	12	2780	87	6	52
na & Cheese	1 sub	986	48	15	1890	93	6	49
rkey & Cheese	1 sub	833	29	10	2508	87	6	51
rkey, w/o Cheese, Oil & Vinegar	1 sub	577	6	0	2056	86	6	40

pizza
ZZA CLASSICS

merican, Small	1 slice	240	13	5	650	19	1	12
heese, Large	1 slice	200	6	3	440	24	1	11
pperoni, Large	1 slice	210	7	3.5	500	24	1	11

IZZA RUSTICAS

urry Chicken & Yam	1 slice	133	4	1	280	17	1	6
lediterranean	1 slice	147	8	2	333	12	1	5
loroccan	1 slice	120	6	2	213	13	1	5
ear & Gorgonzola	1 slice	133	5	3	293	13	1	7

ALADS, SMALL

rugula	1 salad	450	37	6	450	23	4	13
hicken Caesar	1 salad	400	28	6	850	12	3	23
reek	1 salad	260	19	4.5	1140	20	5	7
ear & Gorgonzola	1 salad	529	44	14	923	25	7	16
BQ Salad	1 salad	220	11	1.5	660	17	3	15

ANDWICHES & CALZONES

urry Chicken	1 sandwich	500	8	0.5	1120	82	5	30

restaurants

	SERVING SIZE	CALORIES	TOTAL FAT (G)	SAT FAT (G)	SODIUM (MG)	CARBS (G)	FIBER (G)	PROTEIN (G)
Pollo Latino	1 sandwich	500	7	0	1510	78	5	33
Veggie Calzone	1 calzone	600	22	7	1380	80	7	20
Yuppie Veggie	1 sandwich	760	37	11	1740	85	6	23
ZPIZZA CREATIONS, SMALL								
Berkeley Vegan	1 slice	180	8	1.5	580	19	2	9
California	1 slice	150	6	2.5	380	19	1	7
Casablanca	1 slice	190	9	4	390	18	1	10
Italian	1 slice	180	8	3	540	17	1	10
Mexican	1 slice	180	7	3.5	360	19	2	10
Provence	1 slice	160	7	2.5	400	20	2	8
Santa Fe	1 slice	180	7	3	380	20	2	8
Thai	1 slice	170	6	2.5	350	19	1	10
Tuscan	1 slice	160	7	3.5	340	18	1	8
ZBQ	1 slice	170	5	2.5	410	21	1	10